P9-DEN-101

EVALUATION AND TREATMENT OF SWALLOWING DISORDERS

Evaluation and Treatment of Swallowing Disorders

Second Edition

Jeri A. Logemann

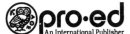
pro·ed
An International Publisher
8700 Shoal Creek Boulevard
Austin, Texas 78757-6897
800/897-3202 Fax 800/397-7633
Order online at http://www.proedinc.com

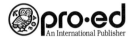

© 1998, 1983 by PRO-ED, Inc.
8700 Shoal Creek Boulevard
Austin, Texas 78757-6897
800/897-3202   Fax 800/397-7633
www.proedinc.com

All rights reserved. No part of the material protected by this
copyright notice may be reproduced or used in any form or by
any means, electronic or mechanical, including photocopying,
recording, or by any information storage and retrieval system,
without the prior written permission of the copyright owner.

NOTICE: PRO-ED grants permission to the user of this material
to copy pages 122–131. Duplication of this material for commercial
use is prohibited.

Library of Congress Cataloging-in-Publication Data

Logemann, Jeri A., 1942–
   Evaluation and treatment of swallowing disorders / Jeri A.
Logemann. — 2nd ed.
      p.   cm.
   Includes bibliographical references and index.
   ISBN-13: 978-089079728-0 (alk. paper)
   ISBN-10: 0-89079-728-5 (alk. paper)
   1. Deglutition disorders. I. Title.
   [DNLM: 1. Deglutition Disorders. 2. Deglutition—physiology.   WI
   250 L832e 1998]
RC815.2.L63 1998
616.3' 1—dc21
DNLM/DLC
for Library of Congress   97-20659
                                                               CIP

This book is designed in Goudy and Eras.

Printed in the United States of America

9   10   07

CONTENTS

PREFACE

When the first edition of this book was released in 1983, one could say that the field was in its infancy relative to our current knowledge about normal and abnormal swallow physiology and methods for the evaluation and treatment of oropharyngeal swallowing disorders. In most of the literature at that time, oropharyngeal swallowing was described as a single behavior with little recognition of its systematic variations with the characteristics of the bolus and the voluntary control exerted in various situations. Methods for assessment of oropharyngeal swallowing largely involved radiographic studies utilizing a relatively simple protocol. Our knowledge regarding the particular oropharyngeal swallowing disorders to be expected as a result of various loci of neurologic or structural damage or various treatments for head and neck cancer was rudimentary. Many of the available studies of dysphagic patients who had suffered neurologic damage, had developed head and neck cancer, or had undergone treatment for the disease included heterogeneous groups of patients at various stages of recovery or degeneration and with various loci of structural or neurologic damage.

Over the past 14 years, the knowledge base regarding normal swallow physiology and the pathophysiology of oropharyngeal swallow has both broadened and deepened. One might say that the field is now in its early adolescence regarding the understanding of normal swallowing, and dysphagia and its sequelae. Although we now realize that normal swallowing physiology varies systematically with the nature of the food to be swallowed and with the volitional control exerted over it, we still do not understand all of the predictable variations that exist, particularly the effects of important variables such as bolus taste and the individual's level of alertness. This limits the ability to treat some dysphagic patients and to understand their complaints.

During these 14 years, the screening techniques, diagnostic technologies, and treatment strategies for oropharyngeal dysphagia have increased; however, our understanding of the optimal application of diagnostic and treatment procedures to various populations requires a great deal more research. Many major questions remain to be answered in all aspects of normal and abnormal physiology of the swallowing mechanism and its relationship to control of respiration and speech production.

Many friends and colleagues encouraged me to write a second edition of this book much earlier. I delayed not only because of time constraints but because of my strong belief that our knowledge base in assessment and treatment of swallowing disorders was rapidly growing. I wanted the second edition of this text to reflect some significant changes and an increased knowledge base, which, I believe, it does. I also believe that enough new information is now available to stop and take stock of where we are and where we need to go.

This second edition is designed as a text and a clinical reference, to provide students with the knowledge base for effective clinical decision making in dysphagia and to stimulate experienced clinicians with new ideas about patient assessment and management. This text is an attempt to review and synthesize the current state of knowledge in dysphagia in relation to both where the profession has been and where it is going and needs to go in the evaluation and treatment of oropharyngeal dysphagic patients. The first edition of this book was based on my experiences with 5,000 dysphagic patients. This second edition utilizes my experience with over 20,000 dysphagic patients.

At least 50% of this text is new, when compared with the 1983 edition. There are additional chapters on swallow assessment procedures and on clinical decision making in treatment of dysphagic patients, as well as information on the influence of voluntary swallowing maneuvers on dysphagic patients, the effects of head injury and dementia on swallowing function, and a number of other topics. In addition to these new chapters and topics, there are entirely rewritten sections on normal swallow physiology, new imaging procedures for assessment of swallow, and new treatment procedures. I have kept all the relevant aspects of the 1983 text, such as the treatment procedures, and have added and expanded on those areas that are relatively new since 1983.

The book is designed for the clinician interested in evaluation and treatment of swallowing disorders within the context of the total neuromotor control of the upper aerodigestive tract. For example, the relationship between respiration and swallowing is a critical one, just being recognized in research and clinical work. I have included suggested procedures for assessing this relationship.

I believe this book also provides clinicians with a set of evaluation and treatment strategies that are workable in a variety of settings, including the schools. As dysphagia has grown in recognition, children and adults with dysphagia are being treated in a variety of settings; this is further encouraged by the changes put in place in the health care system, such as managed care, and the increased inclusion of sick children within school systems.

Throughout the text, I have stressed the critical importance of maintaining safety both for the clinician and for the patient. My baseline philosophy has not changed: There is never an excuse to place a patient at risk, including increased risk for aspiration as well as malnutrition, when evaluating and treating dysphagia.

It is my sincere hope that this text and clinical reference will assist clinicians in further expanding their assessment and treatment portfolios for the good of their dysphagic patients and provide them with the knowledge base for successful and effective clinical problem solving. There are no "cookbooks" in dysphagia, no single set of strategies that will be effective for all patients. The recipe for success involves thorough information gathering regarding each patient, thoughtful assessment, and active intervention. All should be based on a clear understanding of the normal anatomy and physiology of swallowing and the patient's abnormalities in anatomy and physiology of deglutition.

I would like to express my appreciation to a number of individuals who have assisted in the production of this book and in the collection of the research and clinical data incorporated in it. I would like to thank all of my Chicago campus staff, but in particular Cathy Lazarus and Sharon Veis for the support they have given me throughout the production of this book. I owe a large debt of gratitude to my secretaries, Mary Malooly and Mary Smessaert, as well as individuals in my laboratory, in particular, Christina Smith, for not only their hard work, but their consistent support in my ups and downs during the production of this manuscript. Special appreciation goes to my mentor and long-time friend, Hilda Fisher, and to my friends and colleagues, JoAnne Robbins and Peter Kahrilas, for their continuous patience and input of ideas to me as I conceptualize my approach to evaluation and treatment of swallowing disorders. Finally, thanks go to all the patients who have contributed their clinical experiences with swallowing problems, which stimulated my initial and continued interest in this area.

INTRODUCTION: DEFINITIONS AND BASIC PRINCIPLES OF EVALUATION AND TREATMENT OF SWALLOWING DISORDERS

Dysphagia has many definitions. The most frequently used one is difficulty moving food from mouth to stomach. Recently, some clinicians have used another definition that expands the meaning of dysphagia to include all of the behavioral, sensory, and preliminary motor acts in preparation for the swallow, including cognitive awareness of the upcoming eating situation, visual recognition of food, and all of the physiologic responses to the smell and presence of food such as increased salivation (Leopold & Kagel, 1996).

Swallowing disorders occur in all age groups, from newborns to the elderly, and can occur as a result of a variety of congenital abnormalities, structural damage, and/or medical conditions. They may present themselves acutely, for example, as a result of a cerebrovascular accident (CVA) or may worsen slowly over time, as in tumors of the pharynx or progressive neurologic disease (Lazarus & Logemann, 1987; Logemann, 1989; McConnel, Mendelsohn, & Logemann, 1987; Robbins, Logemann, & Kirshner, 1986; Veis & Logemann, 1985). Patients with swallowing disorders may be acutely aware of their problem and able to describe it to the clinician in great detail, or may be entirely oblivious to any difficulty with deglutition. Patients who do report oropharyngeal swallowing disorders and are able to describe them are typically highly accurate in their localization and definition of the problem (Kirchner, 1967; Logemann, 1983). In contrast, patients with esophageal disorders may be highly inaccurate

1

in describing and localizing their dysfunction. They may have symptoms of their problems at the level of the actual physiologic or anatomic disorder or above that level in the gastrointestinal tract. This occurs because the patient may perceive the food collecting above the dysfunctional region. Some patients with esophageal disorders may even exhibit pharyngeal symptoms.

This text presents in-depth discussion of the swallowing problems occurring in the preparatory, oral, and pharyngeal stages of the swallow. Swallowing disorders occurring in the esophageal stage of the swallow are mentioned but not discussed in detail because they are generally not amenable to techniques of swallowing therapy and are usually treated medically or surgically.

Literature on deglutition or swallowing falls into three categories. A number of studies have been devoted to the physiology of normal swallowing, including discussions and measures of the oral stage of the swallow, triggering of the pharyngeal phase of swallow, and the pharyngeal and esophageal stages of deglutition (Ardran & Kemp, 1951, 1956, 1967; Bosma, 1957, 1973; Dellow, 1976; Jacob, Kahrilas, Logemann, Shah, & Ha, 1989; Kahrilas, Dodds, Dent, Logemann, & Shaker, 1988; Kahrilas, Lin, Logemann, Ergun, & Facchini, 1993; Kahrilas, Logemann, Lin, & Ergun, 1992; Logemann, Kahrilas, Cheng, et al., 1992; Miller, 1972; Robbins, Hamilton, Lof, & Kempster, 1992; Tracy et al., 1989).

Another large body of research in the past 10 years has dealt with the changes in physiology of swallowing as a result of a variety of medical conditions (Lazarus & Logemann, 1987; Veis & Logemann, 1985). Some of these studies focus on particular neuromuscular aspects of deglutition, such as tongue movement in the oral stage of the swallow or airway closure during the pharyngeal stage of the swallow (Bisch, Logemann, Rademaker, Kahrilas, & Lazarus, 1994; Fujiu, Logemann, & Pauloski, 1995; Linde & Westover, 1962; Logemann, Rademaker, Pauloski, Kahrilas, et al., 1994; Sloan, 1977). Others examine a small number of patients in each of a variety of disorders and make broad or specific comparisons of swallowing physiology among these subgroups (Conley, 1960; Lazarus, Logemann, Rademaker, et al., 1993; Logemann & Bytell, 1979). Still other research examines in greater detail the swallowing physiology of a specific group of patients, such as those who have undergone hemilaryngectomy or supraglottic laryngectomy or have bulbar polio, myotonic dystrophy, or oculopharyngeal dystrophy (Duranceau, Letendre, Clermont, Levisque, & Barbeau, 1978; Kaplan, 1951; Lazarus & Logemann, 1987; Lazarus et al., 1996; Leopold & Kagel, 1996; Logemann & Kahrilas, 1990; Logemann, 1989; Logemann, Rademaker, Pauloski, et al., 1994; Logemann, Shanahan, et al., 1993; Margulies, Brunt, Donner, & Silbiger, 1968; Pauloski et al., 1993; Rademaker et al., 1993).

Finally, there is a body of information in the literature that presents methodologies for screening, diagnosis, and management of patients with dysphagia (Aguilar, Olson, & Shedd, 1979; Dobie, 1978; Gaffney & Campbell, 1974; Kirchner, 1967; Lazarus, Logemann, & Gibbons, 1993; Lazarus, Logemann, Rademaker, et al., 1993; Linden & Siebens, 1980; Logemann, 1993, 1997;

Logemann, Pauloski, et al., 1995; Pauloski et al., 1993; Pauloski, et al., 1994; Rasley et al., 1993). Articles in this category can be divided into two groups: those that describe procedures to improve the oral stages of the swallow, including both manipulation of food in the preparatory stage prior to swallowing and the transport of food through the oral cavity (Davis, Lazarus, Logemann, & Hurst, 1987; Logemann, 1989; Logemann, Kahrilas, Hurst, Davis, & Krugler, 1989), and those that discuss techniques to improve the triggering of the swallow and the pharyngeal stage of the swallow, in addition to the preparatory stage of oral manipulation and the oral stage (Lazarus & Logemann, 1987; Lazarus, Logemann, & Gibbons, 1993; Lazzara, Lazarus, & Logemann, 1986; Logemann, Kahrilas, Kobara, & Vakil, 1989). Articles in the former group generally describe procedures that can be called *feeding techniques*, whereas those in the latter category describe methodologies for *swallowing therapy*.

Typically, the term *feeding* is limited to the placement of food in the mouth; the manipulation of food in the oral cavity prior to the initiation of the swallow, including mastication if necessary; and the oral stage of the swallow when the bolus is propelled backward by the tongue. Therapy procedures designed to improve feeding generally attempt to improve (1) positioning of food in the mouth; (2) manipulating food in the mouth with the tongue; (3) chewing a bolus of varying consistencies; (4) recollecting the bolus into a cohesive mass prior to initiation of the oral stage of swallow; and (5) organizing lingual action to propel the bolus posteriorly. Thus, feeding techniques deal with the oral preparatory and oral stages of the swallow that terminate when the pharyngeal swallow is triggered.

In contrast, procedures used in *swallowing* therapy include techniques for reducing any delay in triggering the pharyngeal swallow, and improving pharyngeal transit time and the individual neuromotor actions comprising the pharyngeal stage of swallow, as well as all of the techniques used to improve the oral preparatory and oral stage of the swallow. Thus, the term *swallowing* refers to the entire act of deglutition from placement of food in the mouth through the oral, pharyngeal, and esophageal stages of the swallow until the material enters the stomach through the gastroesophageal junction. Throughout this book, the term swallowing rather than feeding is used, as the physiology of deglutition is examined in all stages, and techniques for modification of disorders in each stage of the swallow except the esophageal are discussed.

Signs and Symptoms of Dysphagia

Signs of swallowing difficulty or dysphagia include but are not limited to the inability to recognize food; difficulty in placing food in the mouth; inability to control food or saliva in the mouth; coughing before, during, or after a swallow; frequent coughing toward the end or immediately after a meal; recurring

pneumonia; weight loss when no other reason can be defined; gurgly voice quality or increase in secretions in the pharynx or chest after a swallow or toward the
end of a meal or after a meal; and patient complaints of swallowing difficulties.
The first task of a swallowing therapist is to identify patients who are at high risk
for oropharyngeal dysphagia. This is usually done in a screening process, which
involves a 10- to 15-minute review of the patient's chart and a very brief observation of the patient.

Screening: Identifying the Patient at High Risk for Oropharyngeal Dysphagia

Screening involves looking for signs and symptoms that the patient is at high
risk for oropharyngeal dysphagia. Screening should involve a quick, efficient,
cost-effective, and safe method for identifying patients at highest risk for oropharyngeal dysphagia in order to refer these patients for an in-depth physiologic
assessment of their swallowing mechanism and identify the underlying anatomic
or physiologic abnormalities so that the clinician can proceed to plan and
implement effective treatment.

Screening procedures identify signs and symptoms of oropharyngeal dysphagia. They do not define anatomy or physiology of the oropharynx. To identify
and distinguish a screening procedure from a diagnostic procedure, the clinician
should ask the question, "What information does this procedure provide me?"
The technique is a screening procedure if it provides information on the presence or absence of symptoms of dysphagia, including aspiration, inefficient swallowing, such as residual food left in the mouth or pharynx; or behaviors such as
gurgly voice or coughing while eating. If the technique provides physiologic
data, such as identification and measurement of the duration of a delay in triggering the pharyngeal swallow, poor laryngeal elevation or anterior motion, poor
tongue base posterior motion, and so forth, it is a diagnostic procedure. Most dysphagic patients are initially identified through screening, which is followed by
an in-depth physiologic diagnostic procedure if symptoms of pharyngeal stage
dysphagia are seen. In some cases, the patient's medical diagnosis so frequently
causes pharyngeal dysphagia that it alone indicates the immediate need for
an in-depth diagnostic assessment and initial screening procedures are not
needed. In some situations, the patient's nurse, physician, or dietitian performs
the screening function and refers the patient for a radiographic (X-ray) or other
type of in-depth physiologic assessment. Even if this is the case, the swallowing
therapist usually completes some form of bedside, clinical assessment prior to the
physiologic evaluation to be sure that the patient is ready and appropriate for a
radiographic or other physiologic study.

Recently, various clinicians have attempted to identify new procedures for screening patients for possible oropharyngeal dysphagia. Some of these procedures are considered invasive and may place the patient at high risk; neither of these characteristics should be present in a screening procedure. These and other, more appropriate screening procedures are described in Chapter 5.

The following symptoms of oropharyngeal dysphagia are often observed during a diagnostic assessment procedure:

1. *Aspiration* or the entry of food or liquid into the airway below the true vocal folds

2. *Penetration* or entry of food or liquid into the larynx at some level down to but not below the true vocal cords

3. *Residue* or food that is left behind in the mouth or pharynx after the swallow

4. *Backflow* of food from the esophagus into the pharynx and/or from the pharynx into the nasal cavity

The swallowing therapist's job is to identify the symptom(s) during a diagnostic procedure and, from the symptom(s), identify the underlying abnormality(ies) in anatomy or physiology that cause the symptom(s). In Chapter 4 these symptoms observed during diagnostic assessment are related to anatomic and/or physiologic swallowing disorders.

Complications of Dysphagia

Pneumonia, malnutrition, and dehydration may be symptoms of a swallowing disorder. In fact, they are also complications of dysphagia, which result from either unsafe swallowing, which causes aspiration and the risk of pneumonia, or inefficient swallowing, which results in an insufficient amount of food or liquid reaching the stomach.

Multidisciplinary Approach

The approach to management of swallowing disorders discussed here represents a multidisciplinary model for the safe evaluation and treatment of patients with a swallowing problem that makes oral feeding difficult or impossible. In addition to the swallowing therapist, the dysphagia team typically includes the patient's physician(s), nursing staff, dietitian, occupational therapist, physical therapist, pharmacist, and radiologist. Although the bedside examination is conducted by the swallowing therapist, the radiographic examination is usually conducted by both the radiologist and the swallowing therapist (usually the speech–language pathologist), and resulting chart notes and recommendations are the consensus of the two professionals. Once a management–therapy program has been outlined by the swallowing therapist in conjunction with the patient's attending physician, the swallowing therapist may involve the nursing staff for day-to-day carryover of desired procedures, and interacts closely with the dietitian to ensure adequate nutrition through the program.

The philosophy reiterated throughout this book is that swallowing therapy is superimposed on continuously adequate nutrition and hydration. Nutrition is never jeopardized during the course of management of the patient's swallowing problem. Thus, from the day of the initial evaluation, the swallowing therapist must interact closely with the patient's physicians, nursing staff, and dietitian to outline the best program to maintain nutrition and increasingly improve the patient's swallowing function.

In some settings, the occupational therapist and/or physical therapist may be serving as the swallowing therapist. In other settings, the occupational therapist may be providing therapy to improve arm and hand control for self-feeding or may devise feeding devices to assist the patient's self-feeding. Together with the physical therapist, the occupational therapist may improve sitting balance and design optimal seating for the patient.

Establishing the multidisciplinary team is discussed in Chapter 13 of this text.

Patient Safety

A concern second only to maintenance of adequate nutrition and hydration in the management of a patient with difficulty in swallowing is safety of the patient during oral feedings if oral feeding is appropriate. In general, aspiration (entry of material into the airway below the true vocal cords) should be kept to a minimum. Currently, no clear guidelines exist as to the amount of aspiration that can be tolerated by a patient before such complications as aspiration pneumonia arise. Also, the interaction between such parameters as pulmonary function and tolerance for aspiration is not clearly understood, despite the dramatic increase in research regarding dysphagia. Aspiration is kept to a minimum by giving the patient only a small amount of material during the bedside clinical examination, by *beginning* the radiographic examination with a small amount of material (generally 1 ml) and increasing volume as tolerated, and by carefully monitoring, radiographically, the gross amount of aspiration the patient experiences per bolus. Any patient whose aspiration is larger than approximately 10% per bolus of a particular food consistency despite optimal interventions should be restricted from eating that consistency of food by mouth. This recommendation is based on data collected from 50 surgically treated head and neck cancer patients who aspirated food postoperatively. Each of these patients was aware of the aspiration after it entered the airway below the vocal cords, and was able to expectorate most of the aspirated material. These patients spontaneously stopped eating the food consistencies on which they had aspiration greater than approximately 10% because the continuous coughing quickly made their chests sore and uncomfortable. Patients who could not swallow any food consistency without more than approximately 10% aspiration stopped eating all foods by mouth and required nasogastric feedings (Logemann, Sisson, & Wheeler, 1980). Many physicians consider chronic aspiration of more than small trace amounts (liquid or solid) as a hazard to normal pulmonary function. Others are more tolerant of larger amounts of aspiration for short periods of time. This variance results from each physician's individual experience and the absence of clear guidelines for management beyond those presented above.

It is equally important to ensure that a patient's airway not be blocked by a bolus of material that may be 100% aspirated. Thus, throughout this text, frequent references are made to the use of small amounts of material initially until the patient's swallow is well understood. Small swallows are insufficient to ever completely block or even severely narrow an adult patient's airway.

Patient safety during swallowing therapy can also be assured by completing a radiographic diagnostic examination in addition to any bedside clinical evaluation. A radiographic examination will identify any silent aspirators (i.e., those patients whose sensitivity is reduced and who aspirate food or liquid without coughing or other visible or audible sign). Approximately 50% of patients who aspirate do not cough in response to this aspiration. Research has shown that even the most experienced clinicians fail to identify approximately 40% of the patients who aspirate during a bedside examination (Logemann, Lazarus, & Jenkins, 1982). Also, bedside clinical evaluation is notoriously unable to identify the anatomic and physiologic cause(s) of the aspiration, information that is necessary for effective treatment planning. Therefore, radiographic evaluation of any patient who is suspected of aspiration is absolutely necessary to (a) identify the presence of aspiration; (b) define the etiology of the aspiration; (c) examine immediate effects of selected treatment procedures and design appropriate therapy for the patient; and (d) determine the best method of nutritional intake (i.e., oral, nonoral, or some combination of the two).

Focus of this Book

The vast majority of this book is devoted to evaluation and treatment of oral and pharyngeal swallowing disorders. However, some information on esophageal disorders is provided in order for the swallowing therapist to be able to identify signs and symptoms of esophageal abnormalities. Often, the swallowing therapist is the first health care professional to take a complete history of the dysphagic patient's eating complaints from the patient or caregivers. These complaints can point the clinician to the need for an esophageal assessment by a gastroenterologist in addition to the oropharyngeal evaluation. It is not uncommon for patients with oropharyngeal swallowing disorders to have concurrent esophageal dysfunction. For example, children born with neurologic impairments have a higher than normal incidence of both oropharyngeal swallowing problems and esophageal abnormalities. Similarly, older individuals (over age 60) are at higher risk for both acquired oropharyngeal disorders, because of a stroke, Parkinson's disease, motor neuron disease, and so on, and esophageal dysfunction, because of their age.

This text provides the clinician with the requisite knowledge base regarding the anatomy and physiology of the upper aerodigestive tract as swallow coordinates with respiration and phonation, and the available screening and diagnostic tools for assessment of the mechanism during swallow in order to evaluate the dysphagic patient's swallowing abnormalities accurately and plan an appropriate and effective treatment strategy. The process of evaluation and treatment of swallowing disorders requires a thorough knowledge base in anatomy and physiology of the normal mechanism, as well as effects of aging and disease processes on the mechanism over time. To effectively and efficiently treat oropharyngeal swallowing disorders, the clinician must be able to define the anatomic and/or physiologic abnormalities in the mechanism that are causing the swallowing disorders so that treatment can be directed at these underlying abnormalities. Symptomatic treatment, on the other hand, results in longer, more expensive care and less effective long-term health for the patient when examined over the total course of the patient's management.

This text is not designed to review all of the literature in oropharyngeal dysphagia. Rather, it presents a logical, safe, and efficient physiologically based approach to assessment and treatment of oropharyngeal dysphagia, based on my experience with over 20,000 patients.

References

Aguilar, N. V., Olson, M. L., & Shedd, D. P. (1979). Rehabilitation of deglutition problems in patients with head and neck cancer. *American Journal of Surgery, 138*, 501–507.

Ardran, G., & Kemp, F. (1951). The mechanism of swallowing. *Proceedings of the Royal Society of Medicine, 44*, 1038–1040.

Ardran, G., & Kemp, F. (1956). Closure and opening of the larynx during swallowing. *British Journal of Radiology, 29*, 205–208.

Ardran, G. M., & Kemp, F. (1967). The mechanism of the larynx II: The epiglottis and closure of the larynx. *British Journal of Radiology, 40*, 372–389.

Bisch, E. M., Logemann, J. A., Rademaker, A. W., Kahrilas, P. J., & Lazarus, C. L. (1994). Pharyngeal effects of bolus volume, viscosity and temperature in patients with dysphagia resulting from neurologic impairment and in normal subjects. *Journal of Speech and Hearing Research, 37,* 1041–1049.

Bosma, J. F. (1957). Deglutition: Pharyngeal stage. *Physiological Reviews, 37,* 275–300.

Bosma, J. (1973). Physiology of the mouth, pharynx and esophagus. In M. Paparella & D. Shumrick (Eds.), *Otolaryngology: Volume 1. Basic sciences and related disciplines* (pp. 356–370). Philadelphia: Saunders.

Conley, J. (1960). Swallowing dysfunctions associated with radical surgery of the head and neck. *Archives of Surgery, 80,* 602–612.

Davis, J. W., Lazarus, C., Logemann, J. A., & Hurst, P. (1987). Effect of a maxillary glossectomy prosthesis on articulation and swallowing. *Journal of Prosthetic Dentistry, 57*(6), 715–719.

Dellow, P. (1976). The general physiological background of chewing and swallowing. In B. Sessle & A. Hannan (Eds.), *Mastication and swallowing.* Toronto: University of Toronto Press.

Dobie, R. A. (1978). Rehabilitation of swallowing disorders. *American Family Physician, 17,* 84–95.

Duranceau, C., Letendre, J., Clermont, R., Levisque, H., & Barbeau, A. (1978). Oropharyngeal dysphagia in patients with oculopharyngeal muscular dystrophy. *Canadian Journal of Surgery, 21,* 326–329.

Fujiu, M., Logemann, J. A., & Pauloski, B. R. (1995). Increased postoperative posterior pharyngeal wall movement in patients with anterior oral cancer: Preliminary findings and possible implications for treatment. *American Journal of Speech-Language Pathology, 4,* 24–30.

Gaffney, T., & Campbell, R. (1974). Feeding techniques for dysphagic patients. *American Journal of Nursing, 74,* 2194–2195.

Jacob, P., Kahrilas, P., Logemann, J., Shah, V., & Ha, T. (1989). Upper esophageal sphincter opening and modulation during swallowing. *Gastroenterology, 97,* 1469–1478.

Kahrilas, P., Dodds, W., Dent, J., Logemann, J., & Shaker, R. (1988). Upper esophageal sphincter function during deglutition. *Gastroenterology, 95,* 52–62.

Kahrilas, P. J., Lin, S., Logemann, J. A., Ergun, G. A., & Facchini, F. (1993). Deglutitive tongue action: Volume accommodation and bolus propulsion. *Gastroenterology, 104,* 152–162.

Kahrilas, P. J., Logemann, J. A., Lin, S., & Ergun, G. A. (1992). Pharyngeal clearance during swallow: A combined manometric and videofluoroscopic study. *Gastroenterology, 103,* 128–136.

Kaplan, S. (1951). Paralysis of deglutition. A post poly-poliomyelitis complication treated by sections of the cricopharyngeus muscle. *Annals of Surgery, 133,* 572–924.

Kirchner, J. A. (1967). Pharyngeal and esophageal dysfunction: The diagnosis. *Minnesota Medicine, 50,* 921–924.

Lazarus, C., & Logemann, J. A. (1987). Swallowing disorders in closed head trauma patients. *Archives of Physical Medicine and Rehabilitation, 68,* 79–87.

Lazarus, C., Logemann, J. A., & Gibbons, P. (1993). Effects of maneuvers on swallowing function in a dysphagic oral cancer patient. *Head & Neck, 15,* 419–424.

Lazarus, C. L., Logemann, J. A., Pauloski, B. R., Colangelo., L. A., Kahrilas, P. J., Mittal, B. B., & Pierce, M. (1996). Swallowing disorders in head and neck cancer patients treated with radiotherapy and adjuvant chemotherapy. *Laryngoscope, 106,* 1157–1166.

Lazarus, C. L., Logemann, J. A., Rademaker, A. W., Kahrilas, P. J., Pajak, T., Lazar, R., & Halper, A. (1993). Effects of bolus volume, viscosity and repeated swallows in non-stroke subjects and stroke patients. *Archives of Physical Medicine and Rehabilitation, 74,* 1066–1070.

Lazzara, G., Lazarus, C., & Logemann, J. A. (1986). Impact of thermal stimulation on the triggering of the swallowing reflex. *Dysphagia, 1,* 73–77.

Leopold, N. A., & Kagel, M. A. (1996). Prepharyngeal dysphagia in Parkinson's disease. *Dysphagia, 11*, 14–22.

Linde, L., & Westover, J. (1962). Esophageal and gastric abnormalities in dysautonomia. *Pediatrics, 29*, 303–306.

Linden, P., & Siebens, A. (1980, November). *Videofluoroscopy: Use in evaluation and treatment of dysphagia.* Miniseminar at the American Speech-Language-Hearing Association annual meeting, Detroit.

Logemann, J. A. (1983). *Evaluation and treatment of swallowing disorders.* Austin, TX: PRO-ED.

Logemann, J. (Ed.). (1989). Oral intake disorders after head injury. *Journal of Head Trauma Rehabilitation, 4*(4), 24–33.

Logemann, J. A. (1993). *A manual for videofluoroscopic evaluation of swallowing* (2nd ed.). Austin, TX: PRO-ED.

Logemann, J. A. (1997). Role of the modified barium swallow in management of patients with dysphagia. *Otolaryngology—Head and Neck Surgery, 116*(3), 335.

Logemann, J., & Bytell, E. (1979). Swallowing disorders in three types of head and neck surgical patients. *Cancer, 44*, 1075–1105.

Logemann, J. A., & Kahrilas, P. J. (1990). Relearning to swallow post CVA: Application of maneuvers and indirect biofeedback—A case study. *Neurology, 40*, 1136–1138.

Logemann, J. A., Kahrilas, P. J., Cheng, J., Pauloski, B. R., Gibbons, P. J., Rademaker, A. W., & Lin, S. (1992). Closure mechanisms of the laryngeal vestibule during swallow. *American Journal of Physiology, 262 (Gastrointestinal Physiology, 25)*, G338–G344.

Logemann, J., Kahrilas, P., Hurst, P., Davis, J., & Krugler, C. (1989). Effects of intraoral prosthetics on swallowing in oral cancer patients. *Dysphagia, 4*, 118–120.

Logemann, J., Kahrilas, P., Kobara, M., & Vakil, N. (1989). The benefit of head rotation on pharyngoesophageal dysphagia. *Archives of Physical Medicine and Rehabilitation, 70*, 767–771.

Logemann, J. A., Lazarus, C., & Jenkins, P. (1982, November). *The relationship between clinical judgment and radiographic assessment of aspiration.* Paper presented at the American Speech-Language-Hearing Association annual meeting, Toronto.

Logemann, J. A., Pauloski, B. R., Colangelo, L., Lazarus, C., Fujiu, M., & Kahrilas, P. J. (1995). Effects of a sour bolus on oropharyngeal swallowing measure in patients with neurogenic dysphagia. *Journal of Speech and Hearing Research, 38*, 556–563.

Logemann, J. A., Pauloski, B. R., Rademaker, A. W., McConnel, F. M. S., Heiser, M. A., Cardinale, S., Shedd, D., Stein, D., Beery, Q., Johnson, J., & Baker, T. (1993). Speech and swallow function after tonsil/base of tongue resection with primary closure. *Journal of Speech and Hearing Research, 36*, 918–926.

Logemann, J. A., Rademaker, A. W., Pauloski, B. R., & Kahrilas, P. J. (1994). Effects of postural change on aspiration in head and neck surgical patients. *Otolaryngology—Head and Neck Surgery, 110*, 222–227.

Logemann, J. A., Rademaker, A. W., Pauloski, B. R., Kahrilas, P. J., Bacon, M., Bowman, J., & McCracken, E. (1994). Mechanisms of recovery of swallow after supraglottic laryngectomy. *Journal of Speech and Hearing Research, 37*, 965–974.

Logemann, J. A., Shanahan, T., Rademaker, A. W., Kahrilas, P. J., Lazar, R., & Halper, A. (1993). Oropharyngeal swallowing after stroke in the left basal ganglion/internal capsule. *Dysphagia, 8*, 230–234.

Logemann, J., Sisson, J., & Wheeler, R. (1980). The team approach to rehabilitation of surgically treated oral cancer patients. In *Proceedings of the National Forum on Comprehensive Cancer Rehabilitation and its Vocational Implications* (pp. 222–227).

Margulies, S., Brunt, P., Donner, M., & Silbiger, M. (1968). Familial dysautonomia. A cineradiographic study of the swallowing mechanism. *Radiology, 90*, 107–112.

McConnel, F. M. S., Mendelsohn, M. S., & Logemann, J. A. (1987). Manofluorography of deglutition after supraglottic laryngectomy. *Head & Neck Surgery, 9*, 142–150.

Miller, A. (1972). Characteristics of the swallowing reflex induced by peripheral nerve and brain stem stimulation. *Experimental Neurology, 34*, 210–222.

Pauloski, B. R., Logemann, J. A., Rademaker, A., McConnel, F., Heiser, M. A., Cardinale, S., Shedd, D., Lewin, J., Baker, S., Graner, D., Cook, B., Milianti, F., Collins, S., & Baker, T. (1993). Speech and swallowing function after anterior tongue and floor of mouth resection with distal flap reconstruction. *Journal of Speech and Hearing Research, 36*, 267–276.

Pauloski, B. R., Logemann, J. A., Rademaker, A. W., McConnel, F. M. S., Stein, D., Beery, Q., Johnson, J., Heiser, M. A., Cardinale, S., Shedd, D., Graner, D., Cook, B., Milianti, F., Collins, S., & Baker, T. (1994). Speech and swallowing function after oral and oropharyngeal resections: One-year follow-up. *Head & Neck, 16*(4), 313–322.

Rademaker, A. W., Logemann, J. A., Pauloski, B. R., Bowman, J., Lazarus, C., Sisson, G., Milianti, F., Graner, D., Cook, B., Collins, S., Stein, D., Beery, Q., Johnson, J., & Baker, T. (1993). Recovery of postoperative swallowing in patients undergoing partial laryngectomy. *Head & Neck, 15*, 325–334.

Rasley, A., Logemann, J. A., Kahrilas, P. J., Rademaker, A. W., Pauloski, B. R., & Dodds, W. J. (1993). Prevention of barium aspiration during videofluoroscopic swallowing studies: Value of change in posture. *American Journal of Roentology, 160*, 1005–1009.

Robbins, J., Hamilton, J. W., Lof, G. L., & Kempster, G. B. (1992). Oropharyngeal swallowing in normal adults of different ages. *Gastroenterology, 103*, 823–829.

Robbins, J., Logemann, J., & Kirshner, H. (1986). Swallowing and speech production in Parkinson's disease. *Annals of Neurology, 19*, 283–287.

Sloan, R. (1977). Cinefluorographic study of cerebral palsy deglutition. *Journal of the Osaka Dental University, 11*, 58–73.

Tracy, J., Logemann, J., Kahrilas, P., Jacob, P., Kobara, M., & Krugler, C. (1989). Preliminary observations on the effects of age on oropharyngeal deglutition. *Dysphagia, 4*, 90–94.

Veis, S., & Logemann, J. (1985). The nature of swallowing disorders in CVA patients. *Archives of Physical Medicine and Rehabilitation, 66*, 372–375.

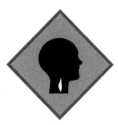

ANATOMY AND PHYSIOLOGY
OF NORMAL DEGLUTITION

Understanding the normal anatomy and physiology of swallowing provides the foundation for evaluation and treatment of swallowing disorders. Diagnosis of dysphagia is designed to identify the abnormal elements of each patient's anatomy and physiology. Treatment is designed to compensate for or improve function in those abnormal elements.

Anatomic Structures

The anatomic areas involved in deglutition include the oral cavity, pharynx, larynx, and esophagus, shown in midsagittal section in Figure 2.1. Structures in the oral cavity are labeled in Figures 2.1 and 2.2, and include the lips anteriorly, the teeth (24 deciduous, 32 permanent), hard palate, soft palate, uvula, mandible or lower jaw, floor of mouth, tongue, and faucial arches. Between the anterior and posterior faucial arches are the palatine tonsils, as seen in Figure 2.2, easily viewed during an oral examination. The pockets or side cavities created by the normal juxtaposition of structures are important in swallowing because in patients with swallowing disorders, these natural cavities or spaces are usually where food or liquid collects and may remain after the swallow. For example, the sulcus is the space formed between the alveolus and cheek or lip musculature both superiorly and inferiorly. There are sulci between the lips and the maxilla

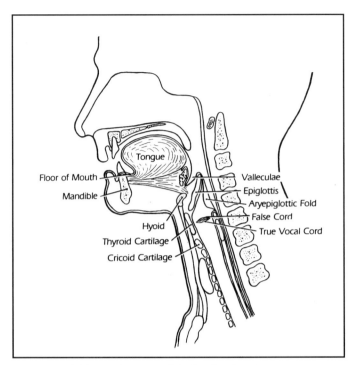

Figure 2.1. Midsagittal section of the head and neck.

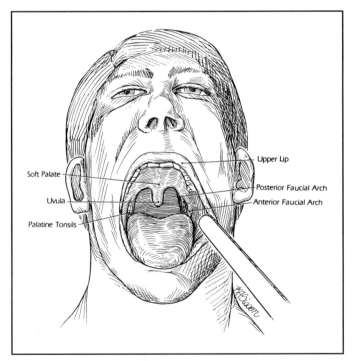

Figure 2.2. Frontal view of the oral cavity, showing anterior and posterior faucial arches.

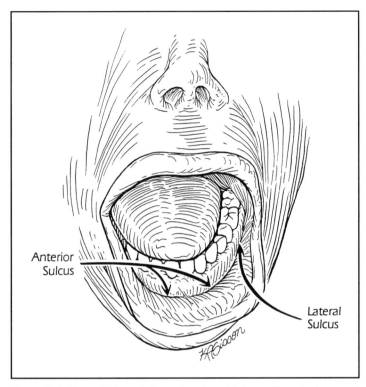

Figure 2.3. Frontal view of the oral cavity with lower lip pulled outward to reveal the anterior and lateral lower sulci.

and mandible and between the cheeks and the maxilla and mandible, both laterally and anteriorly, as shown in Figure 2.3.

Musculature forming the floor of the mouth includes the mylohyoid, geniohyoid, and anterior belly of digastric, all of which attach to the body of the mandible anteriorly and the body of the hyoid bone posteriorly. The hyoid bone forms the foundation for the tongue, the body of which sits on the hyoid. The hyoid bone is embedded in the base of the tongue, articulating with no other bone. The hyoid is suspended in the soft tissue by the floor of mouth muscles and the posterior belly of digastric and the stylohyoid, both attached posterolaterally from the region of the temporal bone, as shown in Figure 2.4. The larynx is suspended from the hyoid bone by the thyrohyoid ligament and thyrohyoid muscle. If the hyoid elevates and moves forward, the larynx will move upward and forward unless it is stabilized by other muscles.

The tongue is composed almost entirely of muscle fibers going in all directions. Functionally, for swallowing, the tongue can be divided into an oral portion and a pharyngeal portion. The oral tongue includes the tip, blade, front, center, and back, as indicated in Figure 2.5. Anatomically, the oral tongue ends

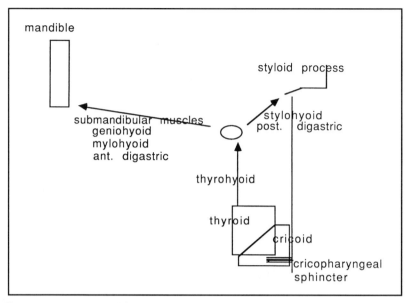

Figure 2.4. Diagram of the suspension of the hyoid bone in the neck from a lateral view. The hyoid (the center oval) is suspended by the submandibular muscles from the mandible anteriorly, and by the stylohyoid and posterior digastric muscle from the styloid process laterally and posteriorly.

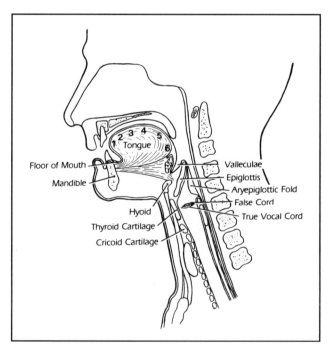

Figure 2.5. Lateral view of the oral cavity with the parts of the oral tongue labeled: tip (1), blade (2), front (3), center (4), and back (5). The tongue base (6) extends from the circumvallate papillae or approximately the tip of the uvula to the hyoid bone.

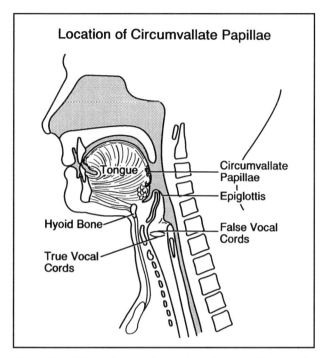

Location of Circumvallate Papillae

Tongue

Circumvallate Papillae

Epiglottis

Hyoid Bone

False Vocal Cords

True Vocal Cords

Figure 2.6. The oral cavity from a lateral view indicating the location of the circumvallate papillae.

at the circumvallate papillae, shown in Figure 2.6. The oral tongue is active during speech and during the oral stages of swallow and is under cortical or voluntary neural control. The pharyngeal portion of the tongue, or tongue base, begins at the circumvallate papillae and extends to the hyoid bone. The tongue base is active during the pharyngeal stage of swallow. The tongue base is under involuntary neural control coordinated in the brainstem (medullary swallow center), but can be placed under some degree of voluntary control.

The roof of the mouth is formed by the maxilla or hard palate, the velum or soft palate, and the uvula. The soft palate may be pulled down and forward against the back of the tongue by the palatoglossus muscle in the anterior faucial arch or may be elevated and retracted to contribute to velopharyngeal closure by a combination of muscle pulls, including the palatopharyngeus located in the posterior faucial arch, the levator palatal muscle, and the fibers of the superior pharyngeal constrictor.

Three large salivary glands are on each side: the parotid glands, the submandibular glands, and the sublingual glands. Many small glands are also in the mucous membrane of the tongue, lips, cheeks, and roof of the mouth. The salivary glands produce two kinds of fluid, a viscid, mucuslike fluid which is thicker, and a serous fluid which is thinner and more watery. The parotid gland produces

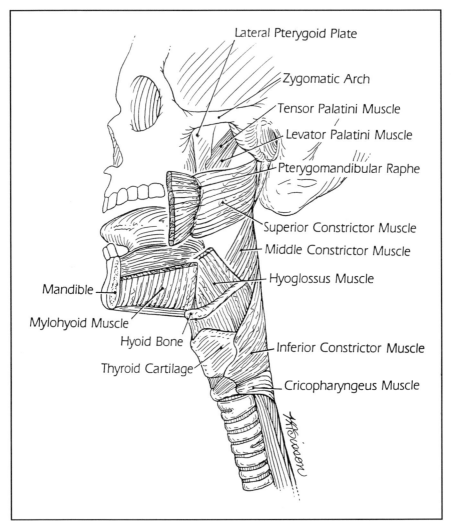

Figure 2.7. Lateral view of the pharyngeal constrictors (superior, medial, and inferior) and their anterior attachments.

the serous fluid, whereas the other glands produce some of both types of fluid, although the submandibular glands tend to produce more serous fluid and the sublingual glands more mucous. Saliva not only serves to maintain oral moisture and reduce tooth decay, but assists in digestion and is a natural neutralizer of stomach acid that may reflux into the esophagus.

Pharyngeal structures involved in deglutition include the three pharyngeal constrictors, superior, medial, and inferior, which form the posterior and lateral

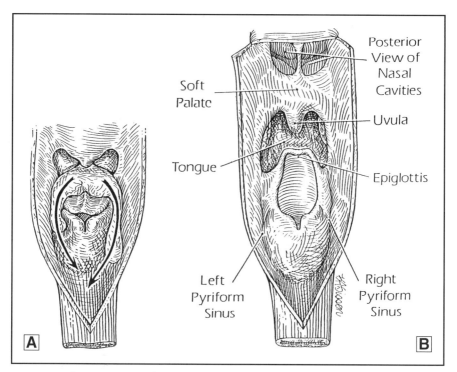

Figure 2.8. Posterior views of the pharynx with the pharyngeal constrictors cut at posterior midline and laid back to reveal the structures anterior to the pharynx. The pyriform sinuses can be seen as spaces created between the sides of the larynx and the pharyngeal constrictors attaching anteriolaterally to the larynx. Arrows on the figure (A) indicate the pathway of food and liquid down the pyriform sinuses on each side during the swallow.

pharyngeal walls. As pictured in Figure 2.7, fibers comprising these muscles arise from the median raphe in the midline of the posterior pharyngeal wall, and run laterally to attach to bony and soft tissue structures located anteriorly. Structures to which these fibers attach anteriorly include the pterygoid plates on the sphenoid bone, the soft palate, the base of the tongue, the mandible, the hyoid bone, and the thyroid and cricoid cartilages. Thus, all of these structures form the anterior wall of the pharynx. Inferior fibers of the superior constrictor that attach to the tongue base are known as the glossopharyngeus muscle. This muscle is probably responsible for tongue base retraction and simultaneous anterior bulging of the posterior pharyngeal wall at the tongue base level.

As the fibers of the inferior constrictor attach to the sides of the thyroid cartilage anteriorly, spaces are formed between these fibers and the thyroid cartilage on each side, as illustrated in Figure 2.8. These spaces are known as the pyriform sinuses. These end inferiorly at the cricopharyngeal muscle, which is the most inferior structure of the pharynx. Cricopharyngeal muscle fibers attach to the posterolateral surface of the cricoid lamina. The cricopharyngeal muscle fibers have been described by some investigators as part of the inferior constrictor. At rest, these fibers are in some degree of tonic contraction in the awake individual to prevent air from entering the esophagus during respiration. During sleep the muscle loses its tonic contraction. Together with the cricoid lamina, the cricopharyngeal muscle fibers form the valve into the esophagus known as the cricopharyngeal (CP) region, the upper esophageal sphincter (UES), or the pharyngoesophageal sphincter (PE segment) (Jacob, Kahrilas, Logemann, Shah, & Ha, 1989). A secondary role for the UES is to reduce the risk of material backflowing from the esophagus and into the pharynx (Kirchner, 1958; Parrish, 1968). The UES is defined as a 2- to 4-cm zone of elevated pressure capable of withstanding pressures of up to 11 cm of water in the esophagus. The cricopharyngeal sphincter has greatest pressure immediately prior to the swallow and during inspiration. Increase in pressure during inhalation ensures that no air is pulled into the esophagus (Parrish, 1968). At the appropriate moment during swallowing, the cricopharyngeal sphincter opens to allow the bolus to pass into the esophagus. The opening of this sphincter is complex.

The esophagus is a collapsed muscular tube approximately 23 to 25 cm long with a sphincter or valve at each end: the upper esophageal sphincter (UES) at the top and the lower esophageal sphincter (LES) at the bottom. This is in contrast to the pharynx, which is a part of the upper airway and is an open cavity except during the moment of the pharyngeal swallow when the larynx closes. The esophagus has two layers of muscle, the inner circular and the outer longitudinal. Each layer is made up of striated muscle in the upper third, a combination of striated and smooth muscle in the middle third, and smooth muscle in the lower third (Hansky, 1973; Ponzoli, 1968). The esophagus passes through the neck, then the chest, through the diaphragm to attach to the stomach. In the neck the esophagus sits behind the trachea, sharing a soft tissue wall so that the posterior wall of the trachea is the anterior wall of the esophagus. The valve at the bottom of the esophagus is the LES, marking the boundary between the esophagus and the stomach. Its primary purpose is to keep food and secretions, including stomach acid, in the stomach.

At the base of the tongue, the pharynx opens into the larynx, which serves primarily as a valve to keep food from entering the airway during swallowing, as shown in Figure 2.1. The topmost structure of the larynx is the epiglottis, the top third to half of which rests against the base of the tongue, attached into the hyoid bone by a ligament, the hyoepiglottic ligament. The base of the epiglottis is attached by ligament to the thyroid notch. The wedge-shaped space formed between the base of the tongue and the epiglottis is the valleculae. The vallecu-lae is subdivided by the hyoepiglottic ligament so that on an anterior–posterior radiographic view, the valleculae appears "scallop shaped," with the hyoepiglot-tic ligament in the middle. Together, the valleculae and the two pyriform sinuses

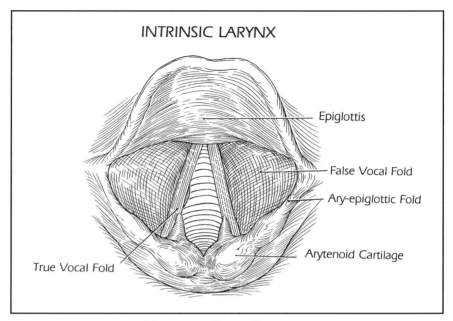

INTRINSIC LARYNX

Epiglottis

False Vocal Fold

Ary-epiglottic Fold

Arytenoid Cartilage

True Vocal Fold

Figure 2.9. Superior view of the instrinsic laryngeal structures.

are known as the pharyngeal recesses or side pockets, into which food may fall and reside before or after the pharyngeal swallow triggers. The lingual tonsils are located against the base of the tongue and take up a small amount of the vallecular space. The opening into the larynx is known as the laryngeal vestibule, or laryngeal additus, and is bounded by the epiglottis, aryepiglottic folds, and arytenoid cartilage, and ends at the superior surface of the false vocal folds.

The intrinsic structures of the larynx are shown in Figures 2.9 and 2.10. The aryepiglottic folds, containing the aryepiglottic muscle, quadrangular membrane, and cuneiform cartilages, are attached to the lateral margins of the epiglottis and run laterally, posteriorly, and inferiorly to surround the arytenoid cartilages. The aryepiglottic folds form the lateral walls of the laryngeal vestibule. The two arytenoids are positioned on the rim of the cricoid cartilage posteriorly. Muscular pull on these arytenoid cartilages controls movement of the true vocal folds. The posterior cricoarytenoid muscle, attaching from the posterior surface of the cricoid lamina to the muscular process of the arytenoid, opens or abducts the arytenoids and the true vocal folds for respiration. The lateral cricoarytenoid (attaching from the top edge of the cricoid cartilage at the side to the muscular process of the arytenoid) and the interarytenoid muscles (attaching between the two arytenoid cartilages) adduct or close the arytenoids and thus close the true vocal folds across the top of the airway (Pressman & Keleman, 1955).

The arytenoids also tilt anteriorly during swallowing. This motion is thought

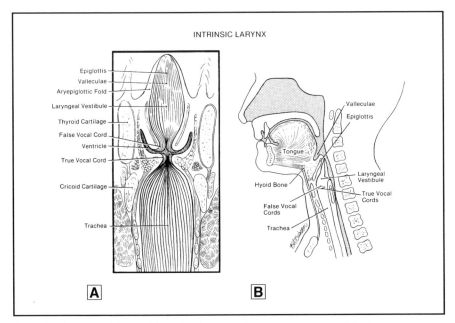

Figure 2.10. Frontal (A) and lateral (B) views of intrinsic structures of the larynx.

to result from the pull of the thyroarytenoid muscle fibers. This anterior tilt-ing contributes to closure of the airway entrance. As shown in Figure 2.10, the aryepiglottic folds end inferiorly in the false vocal folds, two shelves of muscle and connective tissue running anteriorly to posteriorly immediately above the level of the true vocal folds. The false vocal folds are superior to but parallel with the true vocal folds. Like the true folds, the false vocal folds form shelves of soft tissue projecting from the sides of the larynx, anteriorly to posteriorly. The space that is formed between the false and true vocal folds on each side is known as the laryngeal ventricle. The true vocal folds, composed of vocalis and thyro-arytenoid muscle, are attached from the vocal processes of the arytenoids poste-riorly, to the inside surface of the thyroid lamina laterally, and to the thyroid notch anteriorly. These then form two more shelves of soft tissue that, when adducted or closed, project into the airway and effectively close the larynx. The true vocal folds form the last level of airway protection before entering the tra-chea. Together the epiglottis and aryepiglottic folds; the arytenoids, base of epi-glottis, and false vocal folds; and the true vocal folds form three levels of sphinc-ter in the larynx, capable of completely closing the larynx from the pharynx and preventing penetration of food or liquid during swallowing (Lederman, 1977; Pressman & Keleman, 1955).

The larynx and trachea are suspended in the neck between the hyoid bone superiorly and the sternum inferiorly, as shown in Figure 2.11. A number of

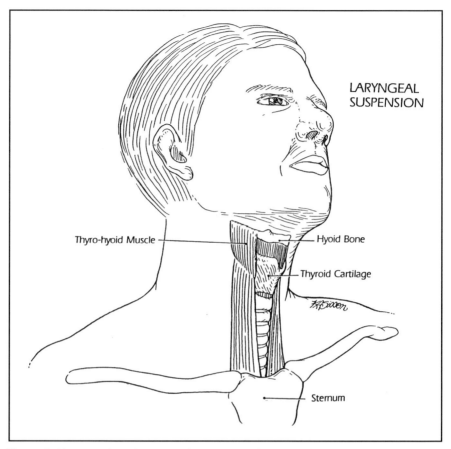

Figure 2.11. Frontolateral view of the strap muscles suspending the larynx in the neck between the hyoid bone and the sternum.

muscles, categorized as the laryngeal strap muscles, contribute to this suspension and, together with the elasticity in the trachea itself, permit the larynx to be elevated, pulled anteriorly, and/or lowered for various activities. The hyoid bone also serves as the foundation for the tongue, which rests on it. Thus, there is a close anatomic relationship between the floor of the mouth, tongue, hyoid bone, and larynx. When one of these structures moves, it often pulls on and moves other structures attached to it.

Physiology

Classically, the act of deglutition is described in four phases: (1) the oral preparatory phase, when food is manipulated in the mouth and masticated if necessary, reducing it to a consistency ready for swallow; (2) the oral phase of the swallow, when the tongue propels food posteriorly until the pharyngeal swallow is triggered; (3) the pharyngeal phase, when the pharyngeal swallow is triggered and the bolus is moved through the pharynx; and (4) the esophageal phase, when esophageal peristalsis carries the bolus through the cervical and thoracic esophagus and into the stomach. The duration and characteristics of each of these phases depend on the type and volume of food being swallowed and the voluntary control exerted over it (Kahrilas, Lin, Chen, & Logemann, 1996; Kahrilas & Logemann, 1993; Kahrilas, Logemann, Krugler, & Flanagan, 1991). Thus, there are many types of normal swallows that occur predictably based on the characteristics of the food swallowed and voluntary control.

The frequency of deglutition varies with activity (Lear, Flanagan, & Moorrees, 1965; Logan, Kavanagh, & Wornall, 1967). Swallowing frequency is greatest during eating and least during sleep, with other activities taking an intermediate place. Mean deglutition frequency is approximately 580 swallows per day. Records during sleep have shown periods of 20 minutes or more when no swallow occurs.

Swallowing and respiration are reciprocal functions; that is, respiration halts during the pharyngeal phase of deglutition in humans of all ages, including infants. Storey (1976) described swallowing as an airway-protective reflex because of this reciprocity. For purposes of this discussion, the neuromuscular functions of the oropharyngeal swallow are discussed first according to these phases even though some types of swallows do not involve all phases. For example, swallows of saliva in the pharynx usually do not include any oral preparation or oral stage of swallow. The normal systematic variations in swallow observed under various conditions are discussed later in this chapter.

Oral Preparatory Phase

Sensory recognition of food approaching the mouth and being placed in the mouth is critical before any oral preparatory movements can be initiated. Movement patterns in the oral preparatory phase of the swallow vary, depending on the viscosity of the material to be swallowed and the amount of oral manipulation the individual uses in savoring a particular food. From the time the material is placed in the mouth, labial seal is maintained to ensure that no food or liquid falls from the mouth. This requires an open nasal airway and nasal breathing. During liquid swallows, the extent of oral manipulation of the bolus varies greatly from individual to individual. When placed into the mouth, a liquid bolus has a certain degree of cohesiveness that may be maintained as the bolus is held between the tongue and the anterior hard palate in preparation for the pharyngeal swallow. In this case, the tongue cups around the liquid bolus with the sides of the tongue sealed against the lateral alveolus. The food may be held between the midline of the tongue and the hard palate with the tongue tip elevated and contacting the anterior alveolar ridge, or it may be held on the floor of the mouth in front of the tongue. Dodds et al. (1989) termed these two normal hold positions "tippers" and "dippers," respectively. Approximately 20% of normal swallowers are dippers. Some individuals may desire to move the liquid around in the mouth prior to swallowing it, and may in the process spread the bolus evenly or unevenly throughout the oral cavity. However, prior to initiating the swallow, the material is generally pulled together into a cohesive ball or bolus by the tongue, and held in either the tipper or the dipper position. Holding the bolus more anteriorly between the tongue and the anterior teeth is an abnormal preswallow position in adults, and often indicates that a tongue thrust swallowing pattern will be used. The tongue thrust pattern, in which the tongue moves anteriorly with the bolus often pushing food from the mouth, is often seen in adults with frontal lobe damage and in children with cerebral palsy.

Oral manipulation of thicker consistency materials again depends somewhat upon the preference of the individual. As with liquids, the material is introduced into the oral cavity as a cohesive bolus. In preparation for the swallow, it may be maintained as such and held in either the tipper or dipper hold position, with the sides and front of the tongue sealed around the maxillary alveolus. Or, the individual may choose to manipulate the bolus in the mouth, lateralize it, and masticate it somewhat by moving the mandible and tongue in a lateral rotary motion before bringing the material into a cohesive bolus and initiating the swallow. The natural cohesiveness of the paste bolus after entry into the oral cavity sometimes makes patients with reduced tongue control prefer this consistency. However, if the consistency of the paste is too thick, it may be more difficult for individuals with reduced tongue control to propel the material posteriorly and to keep it from adhering to the hard palate. During this oral preparatory phase, if there is no active chewing, the soft palate is pulled down and forward (Figure 2.12), sealing off the oral cavity from the pharynx (Fletcher, 1974; Negus, 1949; Robbins, Logemann, & Kirshner, 1982; Shedd, Scatliff, & Kirchner, 1960; Storey, 1976; Wildman, 1976).

The oral preparatory phase of deglutition for materials requiring mastication involves a rotary lateral movement of the mandible and tongue. The tongue positions material on the teeth. When the upper and lower teeth have met and crushed the material, the food falls medially toward the tongue, which moves the material back onto the teeth as the mandible opens. The cycle is repeated numerous times before forming a bolus and initiating the oral phase of the swallow. In addition to this cyclic movement during mastication, the tongue mixes the food with saliva (Lowe, 1981). It has been postulated that the rhythmic movements of mastication are controlled by a central pattern generator. In addition, peripheral feedback is important in positioning the bolus on the teeth and

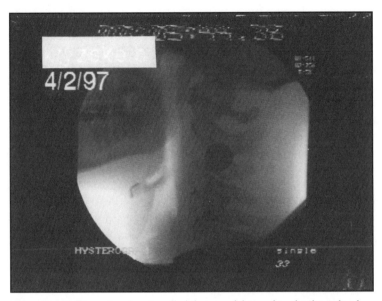

Figure 2.12. The soft palate is pulled down and forward in this lateral video-print while the bolus is being held in the oral cavity prior to initiation of the oral phase of the swallow.

preventing injury to the tongue during chewing (Lowe, 1981). Tension in the buccal musculature closes off the lateral sulcus and prevents food particles from falling laterally into the sulcus between the mandible and the cheek (Bosma, 1973). Rotary tongue and jaw motion is continued until the food has been adequately cleared. After chewing, the tongue pulls the food into a semicohesive bolus or ball before the oral stage of swallow is initiated. During active chewing, the soft palate is not pulled down and forward and premature spillage is common and entirely normal (Palmer, Rudin, Lara, & Crompton, 1992). Such premature spillage is not normal during the hold phase before swallows of liquid and paste or pudding materials.

The volume of bolus swallowed varies with the viscosity of the food. For thin liquids, the volume ranges from 1 ml (saliva bolus) to 17 to 20+ ml (cup drinking). As the bolus viscosity increases, the maximum volume swallowed decreases so that swallows of pudding may be 5 to 7 cc on average, whereas swallows of thicker mashed potatoes may be 3 to 5 cc and meat may average 2 cc. This downsizing with viscosity allows easier passage of the bolus through the pharynx and particularly the upper esophageal sphincter. If larger volumes of these thicker foods are placed in the mouth, the tongue subdivides the food after chewing, forming only part of it into a bolus to be swallowed at one time and sequestering the rest on the side of the mouth for later swallows.

The larynx and pharynx are at rest during the oral preparatory phase of swallowing. The airway is open and nasal breathing continues. Clearly, if an individual loses control of a part of the bolus during this oral preparatory phase and it trickles into the pharynx, the material may continue to drop down and enter the open airway. The pharyngeal swallow rarely triggers in response to this material unless the food starts to enter the larynx, possibly because the oral stage of swallow has not been initiated (Pouderoux, Logemann, & Kahrilas, 1996).

During this oral preparation, a great deal of sensory information is processed from sensory receptors throughout the oral cavity, including the tongue. It is likely that information on bolus volume comes from the shape of the tongue as it surrounds the bolus prior to the swallow. The sequence of the movements of the upper aerodigestive tract during deglutition is illustrated in Figure 2.13.

Oral Phase

The oral stage of the swallow is initiated when the tongue begins posterior movement of the bolus. If the bolus is held in the dipper position, the tongue tip moves forward and lifts the bolus onto the tongue and into the tipper position. This is done in a smooth action, which moves directly into the oral stage of tongue propulsion. Tongue movement during this oral phase has often been described as a stripping action, with the midline of the tongue sequentially squeezing the bolus posteriorly against the hard palate (Ardran & Kemp, 1951; Kahrilas, Lin, Logemann, Ergun, & Facchini, 1993; Lowe, 1981; Negus, 1949; Shawker, Sonies, & Stone, 1984). Another way to describe this tongue movement is as an anterior to posterior rolling action of the midline of the tongue, with tongue elevation progressing sequentially more posteriorly to push the bolus backward. The sides and tip of the tongue remain firmly anchored against the alveolar ridge. During this time, a central groove is formed in the tongue, acting as a ramp or chute for food to pass through as it moves posteriorly (Ramsey, Watson, Gramiak, & Weinberg, 1955; Shedd et al., 1960). As food viscosity thickens, the pressure of the oral tongue against the palate increases, requiring greater muscle activity (Dantas & Dodds, 1990). Thicker foods require more pressure to propel them cleanly and efficiently through the oral cavity and pharynx (Reimers-Neils, Logemann, & Larson, 1994). Several authors also have described the contribution of negative pressure created by slight inward movement and increased tension of the buccal musculature in propelling the bolus posteriorly (Shedd, Kirchner, & Scatliff, 1961). The oral stage of the swallow typically takes less than 1 to 1.5 seconds to complete. It increases slightly as bolus viscosity increases.

In summary, the normal oral stage of the swallow requires intact labial musculature to ensure an adequate seal to prevent material from leaking out of the oral cavity, intact lingual movement to propel the bolus posteriorly, intact buccal musculature to ensure that material does not fall into the lateral sulci,

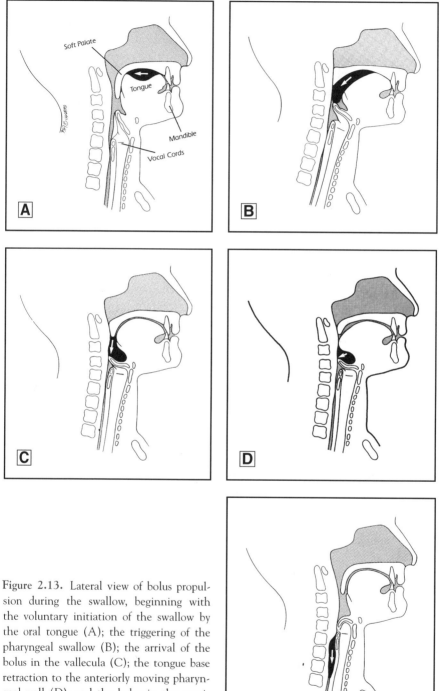

Figure 2.13. Lateral view of bolus propulsion during the swallow, beginning with the voluntary initiation of the swallow by the oral tongue (A); the triggering of the pharyngeal swallow (B); the arrival of the bolus in the vallecula (C); the tongue base retraction to the anteriorly moving pharyngeal wall (D); and the bolus in the cervical esophagus and cricopharyngeal region (E).

normal palatal muscles, and the ability to breathe comfortably through the nose (Campbell, 1981; Cleall, 1965).

Triggering of the Pharyngeal Swallow

As the tongue movement propels the bolus posteriorly, sensory receptors in the oropharynx and tongue itself (particularly deep proprioceptive receptors) are stimulated, sending sensory information to the cortex and brainstem. It is hypothesized that a sensory recognition center in the lower brainstem (medulla) in the nucleus tractus solitarus decodes the incoming sensory information and identifies the swallow stimulus, sending this information to the nucleus ambiguous, which initiates the pharyngeal swallow motor pattern (Doty, Richmond, & Storey, 1967; Miller, 1972). When the leading edge of the bolus, or the "bolus head," passes any point between the anterior faucial arches and the point where the tongue base crosses the lower rim of the mandible (see Figure 2.14), the oral stage of the swallow is terminated and the pharyngeal swallow should be triggered. If the pharyngeal stage is not triggered by that time, the pharyngeal swallow is said to be delayed. In the first edition of this book, the trigger point for the pharyngeal swallow was defined as the anterior faucial arch. This was based on studies of young and middle-aged adults. The point of triggering of the pharyngeal swallow has been lowered in response to more recent observations of older normal swallowers whose pharyngeal swallow triggers when the bolus head has reached the lower level (Robbins, Hamilton, Lof, & Kempster, 1992; Tracy et al., 1989). Individuals of all ages should trigger the pharyngeal swallow by the time the bolus head reaches the point where the mandible crosses the tongue base, as seen radiographically.

In younger, normal individuals, the triggering of the pharyngeal swallow occurs at the anterior faucial arch, and timing is such that posterior movement of the bolus is not interrupted (Jean & Car, 1979; Lederman, 1977; Tracy et al., 1989). There is no pause in bolus movement while the pharyngeal swallow triggers. Pommerenke (1928) and others have established the base of the anterior faucial pillars as the most sensitive place for elicitation of the pharyngeal swallow. Hollshwandner, Brenman, and Friedman (1975) and Storey (1976) postulated receptors in the tongue, epiglottis, and larynx as additional centers for elicitation of the pharyngeal swallow. Older (over age 60) normal individuals are not seen to trigger the pharyngeal swallow until the bolus head reaches approximately the middle of the tongue base (Robbins et al., 1992; Tracy et al., 1989). Observations of neurologically impaired patients corroborate these variations. In some patients, the pharyngeal swallow is not triggered until material has fallen into the pyriform sinuses.

There is much that is not known about the triggering of the pharyngeal swallow. However, it is clear that humans cannot swallow unless there is

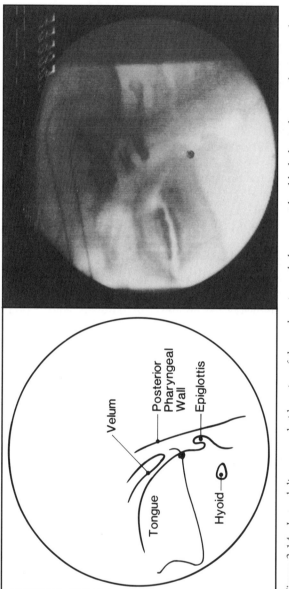

Figure 2.14. Lateral diagram and videoprint of the oral cavity and pharynx with a black dot indicating the point where the mandible crosses the tongue base. When the head of the bolus reaches this point (black dot on the videoprint and diagram), the pharyngeal swallow should be initiated.

something in their mouth, either food, liquid, or saliva. If one attempts to swallow four times in rapid succession, it is difficult to continue past the second or third swallow because these dry swallows have depleted saliva in the mouth.

No doubt, a relationship exists between voluntary attempts to swallow and triggering of the pharyngeal swallow. The exact nature of that relationship, however, is not understood. It is clear that simply placing food or liquid in the mouth will not trigger the pharyngeal swallow unless there is the voluntary initiation of swallowing. Direct stimulation to the areas of the mouth where the pharyngeal swallow is triggered, using a light touch or stronger stimulation, will usually not stimulate the swallow unless saliva or other material is present and the patient is also attempting voluntarily to initiate the swallow. Roueche (1980) probably stated it best: "Both voluntary and reflex components are involved in the normal swallow. Neither mechanism alone is capable of producing swallowing with the regularity and immediacy which is necessary during the normal process of oral feeding."

The pharyngeal stage of the swallow begins as the pharyngeal swallow is triggered. Cumming and Reilly (1972), Dobie (1978), Donner and Silbiger (1966), and others have suggested that the sensory portion of the pharyngeal swallow is carried by cranial nerves IX, X, and XI. The impulses travel to the medullary reticular formation, or swallowing center, located within the brainstem (Doty et al., 1967; Goldberg, 1976; Miller, 1972; Sumi, 1972). This center acts as a neuronal pool to organize the synergy necessary for normal pharyngeal swallowing. The motor portion is carried by nerves IX and X. Nerve VII may additionally contribute to the sensory portion. Nerves V, VII, and XII have been identified as possible contributors to the afferent portion.

The role of the cerebellum in control of swallowing is unclear. The work of Brooks, Kozlovskaya, Atkin, Horvath, and Uno (1973), Kent and Netsell (1975), and Larson and Sutton (1978) indicates cerebellar input into the velocity of movement and, thus, at least into mastication and the preparatory phase of the swallow. Cortical input into the control of swallowing is not well understood, although abnormal swallowing is observed in patients after damage to cortical areas, and swallowing is usually facilitated by voluntary attempts to swallow (Bieger & Hockman, 1976). Cortical recognition of food or liquid approaching the mouth and placed in the mouth is critical to the initiation of the oral phase of swallow or of oral preparation if chewing is needed.

Pharyngeal Swallow

A number of physiological activities occur as a result of pharyngeal triggering, including (1) elevation and retraction of the velum and complete closure of the velopharyngeal port to prevent material from entering the nasal cavity; (2) elevation and anterior movement of the hyoid and larynx; (3) closure of the larynx at all three sphincters—the true vocal folds, the laryngeal entrance (i.e., the false vocal folds, the anteriorly tilting arytenoids, and thickening of the epiglottic base as the larynx elevates), and epiglottis—to prevent material from entering the airway; (4) opening of the cricopharyngeal sphincter to allow material to pass from the pharynx into the esophagus; (5) ramping of the base of the tongue to deliver the bolus to the pharynx followed by tongue base retraction to contact the anteriorly bulging posterior pharyngeal wall; and (6) progressive top to bottom contraction in the pharyngeal constrictors (Bosma, 1957; Cook, Dodds, Dantas, Kern, et al., 1989; Cook, Dodds, Dantas, Massey, et al., 1989; Doty & Bosma, 1956; Jacob et al., 1989; Kahrilas et al., 1991; Kahrilas, Logemann, Lin, & Ergun, 1992; Logemann et al., 1992; Vantrappen & Hellemans, 1967).

Velopharyngeal Closure

Velopharyngeal closure varies somewhat from person to person and may involve some elements of elevation and retraction of the soft palate, inward movement of the posterior and/or lateral pharyngeal walls, and an anteriorly bulging adenoid pad. Velopharyngeal closure enables the buildup of pressure in the pharynx. Functional swallowing is possible without velopharyngeal closure if all other physiologic aspects of the pharyngeal swallow are normal, particularly the tongue base and pharyngeal wall movement and contact.

Elevation and Anterior Movement of the Hyoid and Larynx

During the swallow the larynx and hyoid bone elevate and move anteriorly by the pull of the floor of mouth muscles (i.e., the anterior belly of digastric, mylohyoid, geniohyoid, and the laryngeal elevator, the thyrohyoid). In young men, the hyoid elevates approximately 2 cm (Jacob et al., 1989). The elevation contributes to closure of the airway entrance, and the forward movement contributes to opening of the upper esophageal sphincter.

Closure of the Larynx

Ardran and Kemp (1952, 1956) described the closure of the larynx as beginning at the level of the vocal folds and progressing upward to the laryngeal vestibule. These researchers' cineradiographic studies, as well as more recent studies using videofluoroscopy (Logemann et al., 1992), indicate that closure is effected from below upwards, with the contents of the laryngeal vestibule being expressed into the pharynx. This action clears any penetration (i.e., entry of food, liquid, etc. into the airway to the level of the top surface of the true vocal folds) that may occur. During closure of the airway at the vestibule, there is a downward, forward, and inward rocking movement of the arytenoid cartilages, which narrows the laryngeal opening (Ardran & Kemp, 1967). At the same time, the larynx is elevated and pulled forward. This elevation thickens the base of epiglottis, assisting with closure of the laryngeal vestibule (Ardran & Kemp, 1956; Negus, 1949; Ohmae, Logemann, Kaiser, Hanson, & Kahrilas, 1995). In normal adults the airway entrance is closed for approximately one third to two thirds of a second during single swallows. During sequential cup drinking, the airway may be closed 5 seconds or more (Martin, Logemann, Shaker, & Dodds, 1994). Vocal fold closure occurs when the larynx has elevated to approximately 50% of its maximum elevation (Gilbert et al., 1996).

Cricopharyngeal Opening

Cricopharyngeal opening occurs by a complex series of actions (Cook, Dodds, Dantas, Massey, et al., 1989; Jacob et al., 1989). First, tension in the cricopharyngeal muscular portion of the sphincter is released. Approximately 0.1 second later, laryngeal anterior superior motion is seen to begin to open the sphincter; thus, the sphincter is yanked open by the motion of the larynx resulting from the upward and forward pull of the floor of the mouth muscles. The leading edge of the bolus reaches the sphincter as it opens, and the pressure within the bolus widens the opening (Jacob et al., 1989). As the bolus passes through the sphincter, the larynx lowers and the cricopharyngeus muscle returns to some level of contraction.

Tongue Base and Pharyngeal Wall Action

As the pharyngeal swallow triggers, the tongue base assumes a ramp shape, directing the food into the pharynx. Then, tongue base retraction and pharyngeal wall contraction occur when the bolus tail reaches the tongue base level. The tongue base and pharyngeal walls should make complete contact during the swallow (Kahrilas et al., 1992). As the two structures move toward each other, pharyngeal pressure builds. When the two structures make contact, the pharyngeal wall contraction continues progressively down the pharynx to the upper esophageal sphincter, where esophageal peristalsis takes over bolus propulsion. The pharyngeal contraction wave is no longer called peristalsis because peristalsis is defined as progressive contraction down a muscular tube. The pharynx is not a muscular tube; therefore, the term is inappropriate when describing progressive contractions down the pharyngeal constrictors during swallow. The constrictors comprise only the lateral and posterior pharyngeal walls, and not the anterior pharyngeal wall which is made up of the skull base, palate, tongue base, and larynx. Pressure generated by the tongue base retraction and pharyngeal wall contraction increases as bolus viscosity increases. Pressure is always applied to the tail of the bolus, as shown in Figure 2.15.

Typically, in normal swallowers, velopharyngeal closure and hyolaryngeal

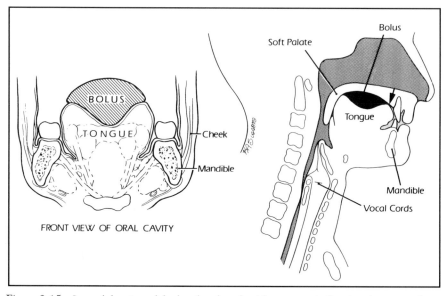

Figure 2.15. Lateral drawing of the head and neck with an arrow indicating the point where pressure is being applied to the bolus tail.

upward and forward movement occur almost simultaneously. Opening of the upper esophageal sphincter and closure of the airway usually begin essentially simultaneously. Pressure on the bolus begins as the oral tongue pushes against the tail of the bolus. When the tail of the bolus reaches the tongue base and pharyngeal walls, these structures move toward each other until they make contact, thus applying pressure to the bolus.

Without the triggering of the pharyngeal swallow, none of these physiologic activities would occur. If the oral tongue propels the bolus posteriorly and no pharyngeal swallow is triggered, the bolus is likely to be propelled by the tongue into the pharynx, where it may come to rest in the valleculae or pyriform sinuses. If the material is liquid, it may splash into the pharynx and into the open airway. No pharyngeal swallow actions will occur until the pharyngeal swallow triggers, so the bolus may rest in the valleculae until the pharyngeal swallow is triggered. Or, depending on consistency, the food may drain from the valleculae, down the aryepiglottic folds and into the pyriform sinuses, or may fall into the airway where it may or may not be expectorated, depending upon the patient's sensitivity in the trachea and larynx. It is important to remember that a swallow comprised of velar, pharyngeal, tongue base, and laryngeal activity occurs only as a result of the triggering of the pharyngeal swallow. Patients can be taught to voluntarily protect their airway or to open the cricopharyngeal sphincter or UES voluntarily, as seen in sword swallowers (Devgan, Bross, McCloy, & Smith, 1978; Kahrilas et al., 1992; Logemann et al., 1992) and some alaryngeal speakers, as described in Chapter 5; however, there is no way to voluntarily initiate or modify pharyngeal wall contraction (Hollis & Castell, 1975). Patients may struggle and exhibit repeated laryngeal and/or tongue base movements, but these are not in the context of a full pharyngeal swallow.

Pharyngeal transit time—the time taken for the bolus to move from the point at which the pharyngeal swallow is triggered through the cricopharyngeal juncture into the esophagus—is normally 1 second or less. During this transit, the bolus does not hesitate for any length of time anywhere in the pharynx, but moves smoothly and quickly over the base of the tongue through the pharynx and into the cervical esophagus. As the bolus moves through the pharynx, it usually divides at the valleculae, with approximately half flowing down each side of the pharynx through the pyriform sinuses. Approximately 20% of normal subjects swallow down only one side (Logemann, Kahrilas, Kobara, & Vakil, 1989). The purpose of the epiglottis appears to be to direct the food around the airway rather than over the top of the airway. The two portions of the bolus join again at about the level of the opening of the esophagus (Ardran & Kemp, 1951). When the pharyngeal phase of the swallow is over, normally very little residual food is left in the pharynx, even in older individuals.

Esophageal Phase

Esophageal transit times can be measured from the point where the bolus enters the esophagus at the cricopharyngeal juncture or UES until it passes into the stomach at the gastroesophageal juncture or LES. Normal esophageal transit time varies from 8 to 20 seconds (Dodds, Hogan, Reid, Stewart, & Arndorfer, 1973; Mandelstam & Lieber, 1970). The peristaltic wave, which begins at the top of the esophagus, pushes the bolus ahead of it and continues in sequential fashion through the esophagus until the lower esophageal sphincter opens to allow the bolus to enter the stomach.

Motility disorders in the esophagus can be defined during a videofluoroscopic study, as described in Chapter 5. However, because the esophageal phase of the swallow is generally not amenable to any kind of therapeutic exercise regimen, the videofluoroscopic study of oropharyngeal deglutition usually does not involve examination of the esophagus. Patients with esophageal disorders should be referred to a gastroenterologist or for a standard barium swallow or upper gastrointestinal series. Unfortunately, the barium swallow does not always define gastroesophageal reflux (i.e., the backflow of food from the stomach into the esophagus). A referral to a gastroenterologist may be more productive in identifying the etiology and optimal treatment for the patient's esophageal disorder.

The Mechanism as a Set of Tubes and Valves

The upper aerodigestive tract can be conceived as a series of tubes and valves. The tubes are the oral cavity, which is a horizontal tube as shown in Figure 2.16, and the pharynx, which is a vertical tube. Within these two tubes, there are a number of valves that serve several functions: (1) directing the food in the appropriate way to keep it from going down the airway or up the nose, for example, and (2) applying pressure to the food to propel it along. The valves consist of (1) the lips anteriorly, which keep food in the mouth; (2) the oral portion of the tongue, which can make complete contact with any point along the hard palate and soft palate or can approximate the palate to any degree; (3) the velopharyngeal region, which closes to keep food from entering the nose; (4) the larynx, whose primary biologic function is to prevent food from entering the trachea; (5) the tongue base and pharyngeal walls, which make complete contact during the pharyngeal swallow to generate pressure and drive the bolus cleanly through the pharynx; and (6) the cricopharyngeal region, which opens at the appropriate time to allow the bolus into the esophagus. A seventh valve is in the digestive tract at the base of the esophagus (i.e., the lower esophageal sphincter). The lower esophageal sphincter (LES) functions quite differently from the UES and is anatomically quite distinct. Whereas the UES or cricopharyngeal

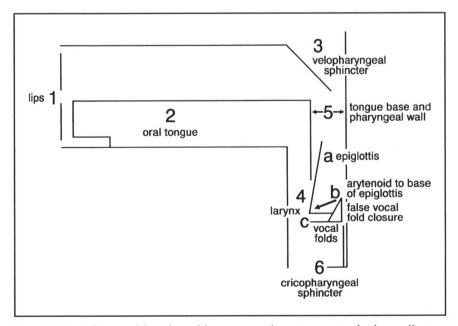

Figure 2.16. A diagram of the valves of the upper aerodigestive tract involved in swallowing

region is a musculoskeletal valve made up of the cricopharyngeus muscle and the cricoid cartilage, the LES is a muscular sphincter that relaxes to open and contracts to close. The LES is designed to keep food and stomach acid in the stomach, that is, to prevent reflux or the backflow of food from the stomach into the esophagus. To produce a normal swallow, all of these valves must function both in appropriate timing and appropriate range of movement. One way to evaluate this mechanism is to systematically examine each of the valve functions to determine whether it is opening and closing at the right times during the swallow and whether its range of movement is normal. Many of these same valves function for speech. However, swallowing generally requires greater muscular contraction, demands greater range of motion, and generates higher pressures than speech (Perlman, Luschei, & DuMond, 1989).

Changes with Age

Variations in Normal Anatomy and Physiology

The normal anatomy of the upper airway in a young infant differs from that of the adult.

Infants and Young Children

In infants and young children, the anatomic relationship between the structures of the oral cavity and the pharynx is different from that in adults. In the infant, the tongue fills the oral cavity, the fat pads in the cheeks narrow the oral cavity laterally, and the hyoid bone and larynx are much higher than in adults (Figure 2.17), affording more natural protection for the airway (Bosma, 1986a, 1986b; Newman, Cleveland, Blickman, & Hillman, 1991). The velum usually hangs lower, with the uvula often resting inside the epiglottis, forming a pocket in the valleculae. As described later, with repeated tongue pumps, the bolus is often collected at the back of the mouth in front of an anteriorly bulging velum or in the vallecular pocket. During the first 21 years of life, the face continues to grow. The jaw grows down and forward, carrying the tongue down and enlarging the space between the tongue and the palate, thereby developing an oral cavity space. The larynx lowers as does the hyoid bone, thereby elongating and enlarging the pharynx. The greatest elongation of the pharynx and downward displacement of the larynx occur during puberty.

According to Dellow (1976), swallowing begins in the fetus, with sucking movements, drinking of amniotic fluid, and occasional presentation of the thumb in the mouth. Swallow physiology in the infant is quite different from that in the adult. When sucking from a nipple, the infant repeatedly pumps the

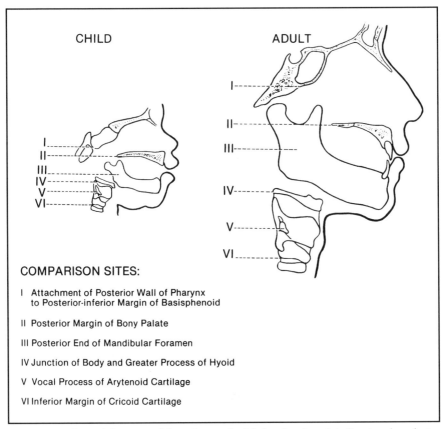

CHILD

ADULT

COMPARISON SITES:

I Attachment of Posterior Wall of Pharynx
 to Posterior-inferior Margin of Basisphenoid

II Posterior Margin of Bony Palate

III Posterior End of Mandibular Foramen

IV Junction of Body and Greater Process of Hyoid

V Vocal Process of Arytenoid Cartilage

VI Inferior Margin of Cricoid Cartilage

Figure 2.17. Lateral drawings of the infant and adult head and neck indicating the relative position of oral and pharyngeal structures.

tongue (initially the tongue and jaw together), expressing milk from the nipple with each pump and collecting this liquid at the faucial arches (in front of the anteriorly bulging soft palate) or in the valleculae. Each infant tends to use a pattern of a particular number of tongue pumps predominantly, with some variability. Normal infants may use anywhere from 2 to 7 tongue pumps (Burke, 1977; Newman et al., 1991). More than that would be considered abnormal. Usually the number of tongue pumps used relates to the amount of liquid expressed from the nipple by a single tongue movement (i.e., fewer tongue pumps if a large amount of liquid is expressed with each tongue movement, more tongue pumps if less liquid is expressed). When a bolus of adequate size has been formed, the pharyngeal swallow triggers. If given a small liquid bolus (1 ml) on a spoon, an infant usually produces an oral and then pharyngeal swallow similar to that of an adult.

The pharyngeal swallow in the infant is similar to that of the adult with two exceptions. Laryngeal elevation is much reduced, since the larynx is anatomically elevated under the tongue base and does not need to move upward. In normal infants, the posterior pharyngeal wall is often seen to move much further anteriorly during swallow than is observed in adults.

According to Bosma (1973), bite is achieved at approximately 7 months, and chewing begins at approximately 10 to 12 months, although there is great variability in the time when the normal adult chewing pattern is achieved, which can be up to 3 to 4 years. Once the infant moves to discrete swallows of pureed or soft foods, the oral and pharyngeal swallow physiology is similar to that of an adult, with the exception of reduced laryngeal elevation.

Older Adults

A number of studies have been done to define the changes in normal swallowing patterns throughout adulthood. Feldman, Kapur, Alman, and Chauncey (1980) studied masticatory function in older adults. High masticatory performance was maintained regardless of age in normal individuals with complete, or almost complete, dentition. These authors did find an increase in the number of chewing strokes used to prepare food for swallowing related to age and dental status. More strokes are needed in patients with poor dentition or dentures.

Several studies have examined the structure and function of swallowing in normal aging adults (Blonsky, Logemann, Boshes, & Fisher, 1975; Mandelstam & Lieber, 1970; Robbins et al., 1992; Tracy et al., 1989). These studies have shown that some minor but statistically significant changes in the physiology of deglutition occur until individuals reach their 80s.

With age, ossification in the thyroid and cricoid cartilages and the hyoid bone increases, so that these structures may appear more prominent during fluoroscopy. Also, as adults reach age 70 and beyond, the larynx may begin to lower in the neck, approaching the 7th cervical vertebra. With age, the incidence of cervical arthritis increases. Arthritic changes in the cervical vertebrae may impinge on the pharyngeal wall, decreasing its flexibility. This may be responsible for some reported reduction in the strength of pharyngeal contraction, resulting in some need to swallow a second time to clear residual material from the pharynx after the swallow.

Some statistically significant changes in oropharyngeal swallow physiology have been noted in normal individuals over age 60 (Robbins et al., 1992; Tracy et al., 1989). Older individuals tend to more frequently hold the bolus on the floor of the mouth and pick it up with the tongue tip as the oral stage of swallowing is initiated—that is, the dipper swallow (Dodds et al., 1989). The oral stage of swallowing is slightly longer in older adults as is the "normal" delay in triggering the pharyngeal swallow (Figure 2.18).

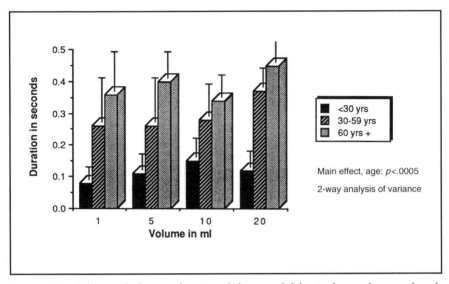

Figure 2.18. A bar graph showing duration of pharyngeal delay in the oropharyngeal swallow in younger and older normal adults. The difference in pharyngeal delay time is significant with age.

A very small increase has been observed in frequency and extent of oral or pharyngeal residue in individuals over 60. Penetration of material into the laryngeal vestibule is reported as increasing in frequency with age, but there is no increase in aspiration in older adults (Robbins et al., 1992; Tracy et al., 1989). Figures 2.19A and 2.19B illustrate the extremes of pharyngeal residue (least and most) observed in older normal subjects in our videofluorographic studies. In contrast to these small changes in oropharyngeal swallow physiology in older adults, esophageal function deteriorates more significantly with age so that esophageal transit and clearance are slower and less efficient (Mandelstam & Lieber, 1970).

My colleagues and I have completed a comparative study of oropharyngeal swallow in young men (21 to 29 years old) and old men (80 to 94 years old) (Logemann, Pauloski, Rademaker, & Kahrilas, 1996). Results revealed reduced maximal laryngeal and hyoid anterior and vertical movement in the old men, indicating reduced neuromuscular reserve. As shown in Figure 2.20, the vertical movement of the hyoid and larynx in the old and young men was identical until each accomplished cricopharyngeal opening. After cricopharyngeal opening was attained, hyoid and laryngeal elevation continued in the young men but remained stable in the old men. The young men had excess laryngeal and hyoid motion. This difference between necessary movement and actual motion is known as "reserve." The old men had no reserve.

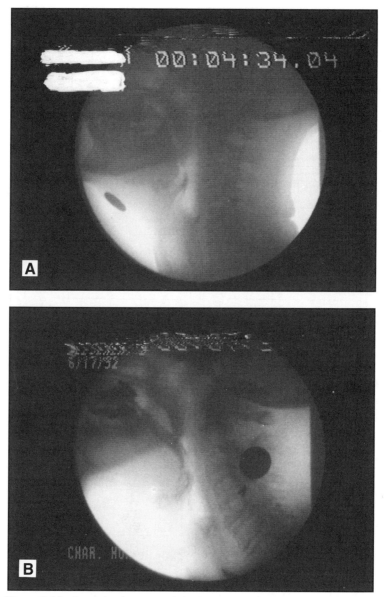

Figure 2.19. Lateral videoprints of the least (A) and most (B) residue in the pharynx in the oldest subjects in our studies, ages 80 to 93.

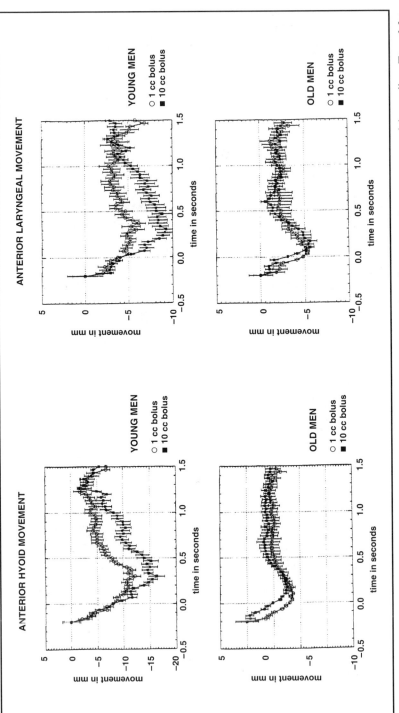

Figure 2.20. The anterior movement of the hyoid and larynx in young and old men from the onset to the termination of the swallow. Time 0.0 is the onset of opening of the upper esophageal sphincter.

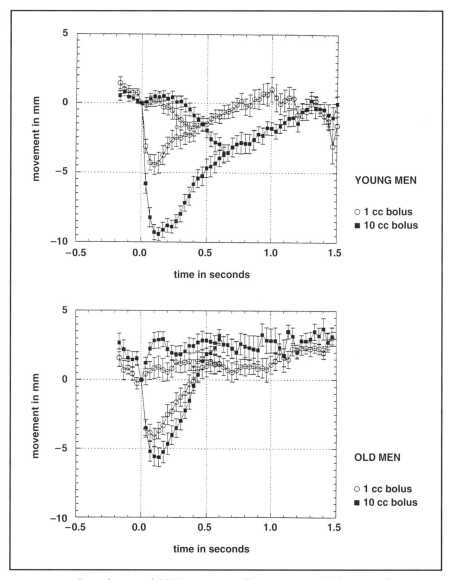

Figure 2.21. Cricopharyngeal (CP) opening profile in young and old men swallowing several volumes of liquid. Time 0.0 is onset of opening of the upper esophageal sphincter.

Examination of changes in cricopharyngeal opening (Figure 2.21) in the two groups revealed reduced flexibility in the old men, that is, less change as volume increased. Reduction in reserve and flexibility in neuromuscular control has been found to characterize normal aging of the motor system. Both of these characteristics in the swallows of the "oldest old" put them at increased risk for developing swallowing problems if they become physically weak as a result of any illness, even if it is not in the region of the head and neck.

Taste

Taste is a chemical sense in the oropharyngeal region and is activated during eating and drinking (Frank, Hettinger, & Mott, 1992). With age, rating of the intensity of taste and smell are reduced (Cowart, 1989), smell perhaps more than taste. Loss of interest in nutritious food may develop in the elderly as taste sensation is affected. Taste supplements may be added to food to increase intake (Schiffman & Warwick, 1989) but must be done carefully as foods can be sweetened or salted to unhealthy levels. Some medications can result in an unpleasant metallic taste in the mouth, including tetracycline (an antibiotic), lithium carbonate (an antipsychotic), penicillamine (an antiarthritic), and captopril (an antihypertensive) (Coulter, 1988; Greenberg et al., 1989; Hochberg, 1986; Magnasco & Magnasco, 1985).

Coordination of Respiration and Swallowing

Several studies have examined the coordination between respiration and swallowing in normal individuals of various ages (Martin et al., 1994; Nishino & Hiraga, 1991; Preiksaitis, Mayrand, Robins, & Diamant, 1992). During swallow, the airway closes for a fraction of a second. The airway closure period, when there is no respiration, is known as the apneic period. The apneic period usually corresponds to the closure of the airway during the pharyngeal stage of swallowing and the cessation of chest wall movement. The duration of the airway closure tends to increase as bolus volume increases (Logemann et al., 1992). The airway is open during the oral preparatory, oral, and esophageal stages of swallow. There is a predominant pattern of swallow–respiratory coordination, with a great deal of variability. The predominant pattern of coordination involves the swallow interrupting the exhalatory phase of the respiratory cycle (Martin et al., 1994; Nishino, Yonezawa, & Honda, 1985; Preiksaitis et al., 1992; Selley, Flack, Ellis, & Brooks, 1989a, 1989b; Smith, Wolkove, Colacone, & Kreisman, 1989). Usually the individual returns to exhalation after the swallow. This coordination is thought to be safer than interrupting inhalation to swallow. By interrupting exhalation and returning to exhalation, the normal individual has a slight airflow through the larynx and pharynx after the swallow, which may help to clear any mild residue from around the airway entrance. At least one study has found that at larger bolus volumes, more swallows were preceded by inspiration (Preiksaitis et al., 1992).

There are indications that dysphagic patients may more often interrupt inhalation to swallow, which may increase their risk of aspiration (Selley et al., 1989b). There are also data indicating that it takes infants approximately 2 to 3 months to stabilize their swallow–respiratory coordination to be more like the adult pattern (i.e., so that swallowing interrupts the exhalatory phase of respiration) (McPherson et al., 1992).

Variations in Normal Swallowing

Normal swallowing consists of a number of different types of swallows. This helps to explain why some patients indicate they can swallow a certain type or volume of food but not another. The characteristics of the food are a major factor in making systematic changes in the oropharyngeal swallow. The other factor is volitional control exerted over the swallow.

Volume Effects

In general, changes in bolus volume create the greatest systematic changes in the oropharyngeal swallow. Whereas a small volume swallow (1 to 3 ml) is characterized by an oral phase followed by pharyngeal swallow triggering, the pharyngeal phase, and then the esophageal phase, a large volume swallow (10 to 20 ml) is usually characterized by simultaneous oral and pharyngeal activity. This is necessary in order to safely clear the large bolus from both the oral cavity and the pharynx (Kahrilas & Logemann, 1993; Shaker et al., 1993). As bolus volume increases, the timing of tongue base retraction to contact the anteriorly and medially moving pharyngeal walls occurs later in the swallow. The commonality across swallows is that the tongue base and pharyngeal walls move toward each other and make contact at the time when the tail of the bolus reaches the tongue base. This ensures that all of the pressure generated by the movement of the tongue base and pharyngeal walls toward each other is directed at the bolus tail.

Increasing Viscosity

As bolus viscosity increases, the pressure generated by the oral tongue, tongue base, and pharyngeal walls increases and muscular (electromyographic) activity increases (Dantas & Dodds, 1990; Dantas et al., 1990; Reimers-Neils et al., 1994). In addition, valve functions, such as velopharyngeal closure and upper esophageal opening and laryngeal closure, all increase slightly in duration as viscosity increases.

Cup Drinking

Cup drinking, if it is sequential, is characterized by early airway closure and some preelevation of the larynx as the cup is approaching the lips with airway closure extending across all of the sequential swallows. The duration of airway closure on cup drinking may last anywhere from 5 to 10 seconds, depending upon the number of consecutive swallows produced (Martin et al., 1994). During these sequential swallows, the velopharyngeal area is closed, the lips maintain seal around the cup or glass, the tongue repeatedly propels the consecutive swallows from the oral cavity, and the tongue base and pharyngeal walls make contact at the tail of each sequential bolus. The upper esophageal sphincter opens repeatedly as each bolus approaches. Patients with respiratory problems may not be able to cup drink because they cannot sustain the duration of airway closure needed.

Straw Drinking

In straw drinking, the bolus is brought into the mouth via suction created in the oral cavity. To create the suction, the soft palate is lowered against the back of the tongue and the muscles of the cheek and face contract and create suction intraorally to bring material into the mouth. When material has reached the mouth, the suction is discontinued, and the soft palate elevates as the oral stage of swallow is initiated by the tongue. Thus, straw drinking is simply a way to modify food placement into the mouth. There is, however, an inappropriate or dangerous way to straw drink which involves sucking via inhalation rather than intraoral suction. This can usually be easily observed at the bedside by watching the patient attempt to straw drink. If the suction is timed with inhalation, it is likely that the patient is straw drinking inappropriately with the airway open. This increases the patient's risk of material entering the airway as he or she is bringing the material into the oral cavity if it spills over and is sucked into the airway.

"Chug-a-Lug"

Some individuals can "chug-a-lug" a can of soda or other beverage without swallowing. To do this, they pull their larynx forward, which opens the upper esophageal sphincter volitionally; hold their breath to close the airway at the larynx; and then literally dump material through the oral cavity and pharynx by gravity into the esophagus and stomach. This is much the way a sword swallower manages to swallow the sword. The sword swallower aligns the oral cavity, pharynx, esophagus, and stomach vertically; opens the upper esophageal sphincter by forward pull of the larynx; holds his or her breath to protect the airway; and allows the sword to pass straight through the mouth, pharynx, and esophagus. Then the person relaxes the lower esophageal sphincter to enable the sword to enter the stomach. This action clearly represents tremendous volitional control over the mechanism, which indicates the potential that patients may have to compensate for their oropharyngeal dysphagia.

Pharyngeal Swallow with No Oral Swallow

If secretions are collecting in the pharynx or if there is chewing with premature spillage, which is building up in the valleculae and the pyriform sinuses, the individual may produce a pharyngeal swallow with little or no oral swallow. Generally, if chewing is taking place, the individual will stop chewing, produce a pharyngeal stage swallow, and then return to chewing. Thus, it is quite possible to have a pharyngeal stage swallow with no oral swallow at all. This again represents volitional control over the mechanism.

Components of All Swallows

All swallows must have certain physiologic components in order to clear food from the oral cavity and pharynx with no residue and with good airway protection. The components that must be present are (1) oral propulsion of the bolus into the pharynx, (2) airway closure, (3) upper esophageal sphincter opening, and (4) tongue base–pharyngeal wall propulsion to carry the bolus through the pharynx and into the esophagus. The variations on normal swallow generally involve changing the relative timing of these elements, but all must be present and normal for the bolus to be cleared safely and efficiently.

The behaviors characterizing normal swallowing are rapid acts, each involving voluntary and involuntary aspects requiring complex neuromotor control. Although all of the aspects of neural control of swallowing are not entirely understood, the physiology of normal deglutition has been moderately well defined and forms a basis for comparison of the abnormalities in swallowing described in Chapter 3.

References

Ardran, G., & Kemp, F. (1951). The mechanism of swallowing. *Proceedings of the Royal Society of Medicine, 44*, 1038–1040.

Ardran, G., & Kemp, F. (1952). The protection of the laryngeal airway during swallowing. *British Journal of Radiology, 25*, 406–416.

Ardran, G., & Kemp, F. (1956). Closure and opening of the larynx during swallowing. *British Journal of Radiology, 29*, 205–208.

Ardran, G. M., & Kemp, F. (1967). The mechanism of the larynx II: The epiglottis and closure of the larynx. *British Journal of Radiology*, 40, 372–389.

Bieger, D., & Hockman, C. (1976). Suprabulbar modulation of reflex swallowing. *Experimental Neurology*, 52, 311–324.

Blonsky, E., Logemann, J., Boshes, B., & Fisher, H. (1975). Comparison of speech and swallowing function in patients with tremor disorders and in normal geriatric patients: A cinefluorographic study. *Journal of Gerontology*, 30, 299–303.

Bosma, J. F. (1957). Deglutition: Pharyngeal stage. *Physiological Reviews*, 37, 275–300.

Bosma, J. (1973). Physiology of the mouth, pharynx and esophagus. In M. Paparella & D. Shumrick (Eds.), *Otolaryngology volume 1: Basic sciences and related disciplines* (pp. 356–370). Philadelphia: Saunders.

Bosma, J. F. (1986a). *Anatomy of the infant head.* Baltimore: Johns Hopkins University Press.

Bosma, J. F. (1986b). Development of feeding. *Clinical Nutrition*, 5, 210–218.

Brooks, V., Kozlovskaya, I., Atkin, A., Horvath, F., & Uno, M. (1973). Effects of cooling dentate nucleus on tracking task-performance in monkeys. *Journal of Neurophysiology*, 36, 974–995.

Burke, P. (1977). Swallowing and the organization of sucking in the human newborn. *Child Development*, 48, 523–531.

Campbell, S. (1981). Neural control of oral somatic motor function. *Physical Therapy*, 61, 16–22.

Cleall, J. (1965). Deglutition: A study of form and function. *American Journal of Orthodontia*, 51, 566–594.

Cook, I. J., Dodds, W. J., Dantas, R. O., Kern, M. K., Massey, B. T., Shaker, R., & Hogan, W. J. (1989). Timing of videofluoroscopic, manometric events, and bolus transit during the oral and pharyngeal phases of swallowing. *Dysphagia*, 4, 8–15.

Cook, I. J., Dodds, W. J., Dantas, R. O., Massey, B., Kern, M. K., Lang, I. M., Brasseur, J. G., & Hogan, W. J. (1989). Opening mechanism of the human upper esophageal sphincter. *American Journal of Physiology*, 257, G748–G759.

Coulter, D. M. (1988). Eye pain with Nifedipine and disturbance of taste with Captopril: A mutually controlled study showing a method of post marketing surveillance. *British Medical Journal*, 296, 1086–1088.

Cowart, B. J. (1989). Relationships between taste and smell across the adult life span. *Annals of New York Academy of Science*, 561, 31–55.

Cumming, W., & Reilly, B. (1972). Fatigue aspiration. *Pediatric Radiology*, 105, 387–390.

Dantas, R. O., & Dodds, W. J. (1990). Effect of bolus volume and consistency on swallow-induced submental and infrahyoid electromyographic activity. *Brazilian Journal of Medical and Biological Research*, 23, 37–44.

Dantas, R. O., Kern, M. K., Massey, B. T., Dodds, W. J., Kahrilas, P. J., Brasseur, J. G., Cook, I. J., & Lang, I. M. (1990). Effect of swallowed bolus variables on oral and pharyngeal phases of swallowing. *American Journal of Physiology*, 258, G675–G681.

Dellow, P. (1976). The general physiological background of chewing and swallowing. In B. Sessle & A. Hannan (Eds.), *Mastication and swallowing* (pp. 6–21). Toronto: University of Toronto Press.

Devgan, B., Bross, G., McCloy, R., & Smith, C. (1978). Anatomic and physiologic aspects of sword swallowing. *Ear, Nose and Throat*, 57, 445–450.

Dobie, R. A. (1978). Rehabilitation of swallowing disorders. *American Family Physician*, 17, 84–95.

Dodds, W. J., Hogan, W., Reid, D., Stewart, E., & Arndorfer, R. (1973). A comparison between primary esophageal peristalsis following wet and dry swallows. *Journal of Applied Physiology, 35,* 851–857.

Dodds, W. J., Taylor, A. J., Stewart, E. T., Kern, M. K., Logemann, J. A., & Cook, I. J. (1989). Tipper and dipper types of oral swallows. *American Journal of Roentgenology, 153,* 1197–1199.

Donner, M., & Silbiger, M. (1966). Cinefluorographic analyses of pharyngeal swallowing in neuromuscular disorders. *The American Journal of Medical Sciences, 251,* 600–616.

Doty, R., & Bosma, J. (1956). An electromyographic analysis of reflex deglutition. *Journal of Neurophysiology, 19,* 44–60.

Doty, R., Richmond, W., & Storey, A. (1967). Effect of medullary lesions on coordination of deglutition. *Experimental Neurology, 17,* 91–106.

Feldman, R., Kapur, K., Alman, J., & Chauncey, H. H. (1980). Aging and mastication: Changes in performance and in the swallowing threshold with natural dentition. *American Geriatrics Society, 28,* 97–103.

Fletcher, S. (1974). The swallow pattern. In *Tongue thrust in swallowing and speaking.* Austin, TX: Learning Concepts.

Frank, M. E., Hettinger, T. P., & Mott, A. E. (1992). The sense of taste: Neurobiology, aging, and medication effects. *Critical Reviews in Oral Biology and Medicine, 3,* 371–393.

Gilbert, R. J., Daftary, S., Woo, P., Seltzer, S., Shapshay, S. M., & Weisskoff, R. M. (1996). Echoplanar magnetic resonance imaging of deglutitive vocal fold closure: Normal and pathologic patterns of displacement. *Laryngoscope, 106,* 568–572.

Goldberg, L. (1976). Mononeurone mechanisms: Reflex controls. In B. Sessle & A. Hannan (Eds.), *Mastication and swallowing* (pp. 47–59). Toronto: University of Toronto Press.

Greenberg, A. J., Kane, M. L., Keller, M. B., Lavori, P., Rosenbaum, J. F., Cole, K., & Lavelle, J. (1989). Comparison of standard and low serum levels of Lithium for maintenance treatment of bipolar disorder. *New England Journal of Medicine, 321,* 1489–1493.

Hansky, J. (1973). The use of oesophageal motility studies in the diagnosis of dysphagia. *Australian New Zealand Journal of Surgery, 42,* 360–361.

Hochberg, M. C. (1986). Auranofin or D-Penicillamine in treatment of rheumatoid arthritis. *Annals of Internal Medicine, 105,* 528–535.

Hollis, J., & Castell, D. (1975). Effect of dry and wet swallows of different volumes on esophageal peristalsis. *Journal of Applied Physiology, 383,* 1161–1164.

Hollshwandner, C., Brenman, H., & Friedman, M. (1975). Role of afferent sensors in the initiation of swallowing in man. *Journal of Dental Research, 54,* 83–88.

Jacob, P., Kahrilas, P., Logemann, J., Shah, V., & Ha, T. (1989). Upper esophageal sphincter opening and modulation during swallowing. *Gastroenterology, 97,* 1469–1478.

Jean, A., & Car, A. (1979). Inputs to the swallowing medullary neurons from peripheral afferent fibers and the swallowing cortical area. *Brain Research, 178,* 567–572.

Kahrilas, P. J., Lin, S., Chen, J., & Logemann, J. A. (1996). Oropharyngeal accommodation to swallow volume. *Gastroenterology, 111,* 297–306.

Kahrilas, P. J., Lin, S., Logemann, J. A., Ergun, G. A., & Facchini, F. (1993). Deglutitive tongue action: Volume accommodation and bolus propulsion. *Gastroenterology, 104,* 152–162.

Kahrilas, P. J., & Logemann, J. A. (1993). Volume accommodations during swallowing. *Dysphagia, 8,* 259–265.

Kahrilas, P. J., Logemann, J. A., Krugler, C., & Flanagan, E. (1991). Volitional augmentation of upper esophageal sphincter opening during swallowing. *American Journal of Physiology, 260 (Gastrointestinal Physiology, 23)*, G450–G456.

Kahrilas, P. J., Logemann, J. A., Lin, S., & Ergun G. A. (1992). Pharyngeal clearance during swallow: A combined manometric and videofluoroscopic study. *Gastroenterology, 103*, 128–136.

Kent, R., & Netsell, R. (1975). A case study of an ataxic dysarthric: Cineradiographic and spectrographic observations. *Journal of Speech and Hearing Research, 40*, 115–134.

Kirchner, J. (1958). The motor activity of the cricopharyngeus muscle. *Laryngoscope, 68*, 1119–1159.

Larson, C., & Sutton, D. (1978). Effects of cerebellar lesions on monkey jaw-force control: Implications for understanding ataxic dysarthria. *Journal of Speech and Hearing Research, 21*, 295–308.

Lear, C., Flanagan, J., & Moorrees, C. (1965). *Archives of Oral Biology, 10*, 83–89.

Lederman, M. (1977). The oncology of breathing and swallowing. *Clinical Radiology, 28*, 1–14.

Logan, W., Kavanagh, J., & Wornall, A. (1967). Sonic correlates of human deglutition. *Journal of Applied Physiology, 23*, 279–284.

Logemann, J. A., Kahrilas, P. J., Cheng, J., Pauloski, B. R., Gibbons, P. J., Rademaker, A. W., & Lin, S. (1992). Closure mechanisms of the laryngeal vestibule during swallow. *American Journal of Physiology, 262 (Gastrointestinal Physiology, 25)*, G338–G344.

Logemann, J. A., Kahrilas, P. J., Kobara, M., & Vakil, N. (1989). The benefit of head rotation on pharyngo-esophageal dysphagia. *Archives of Physical Medicine and Rehabilitation, 70*, 767–771.

Logemann, J., Pauloski, B., Rademaker, A., & Kahrilas, P. (1996). [Oropharyngeal swallow in young men and old men]. Unpublished data.

Lowe, A. (1981). The neural regulation of tongue movement. *Progress in Neurobiology, 15*, 295–344.

Magnasco, L. D., & Magnasco, A. J. (1985). Metallic taste associated with tetracycline therapy. *Clinical Pharmacology, 4*, 455–456.

Mandelstam, P., & Lieber, A. (1970). Cineradiographic evaluation of the esophagus in normal adults. *Gastroenterology, 58*, 32–38.

Martin, B. J. W., Logemann, J. A., Shaker, R., & Dodds, W. J. (1994). Coordination between respiration and swallowing: Respiratory phase relationships and temporal integration. *Journal of Applied Physiology, 76(2)*, 714–723.

McPherson, K. A., Kenny, D. J., Koheil, R., Bablich, K., Sochaniwskyj, A., & Milner, M. (1992). Ventilation and swallowing interactions of normal children and children with cerebral palsy. *Developmental Medicine and Child Neurology, 34*, 577–588.

Miller, A. (1972). Characteristics of the swallowing reflex induced by peripheral nerve and brain stem stimulation. *Experimental Neurology, 34*, 210–222.

Negus, V. (1949). The second stage of swallowing. *Acta Otolaryngologica* (Suppl.), pp. 75–82.

Newman, L., Cleveland, R., Blickman, J., & Hillman, R. (1991). Videofluoroscopic analyses of the infant swallow. *Investigative Radiology, 26*, 870–873.

Nishino, T., & Hiraga, K. (1991). Coordination of swallowing and respiration in unconscious subjects. *Journal of Applied Physiology, 70*, 988–993.

Nishino, T., Yonezawa, T., & Honda, Y. (1985). Effects of swallowing on the pattern of continuous respiration in human adults. *American Review of Respiratory Disease, 132*, 1219–1222.

Ohmae, Y., Logemann, J. A., Kaiser, P., Hanson, D. G., & Kahrilas, P. J. (1995). Timing of glottic closure during normal swallow. *Head & Neck, 17*, 394–402.

Palmer, J. B., Rudin, N. J., Lara, G., & Crompton, A. W. (1992). Coordination of mastication and swallowing. *Dysphagia, 7*, 187–200.

Parrish, R. (1968). Cricopharyngeus dysfunction and acute dysphagia. *Canadian Medical Association Journal, 99*, 1167–1171.

Perlman, A. L., Luschei, E. S., & DuMond, C. E. (1989). Electrical activity from the superior pharyngeal constrictor during reflexive and non-reflexive tasks. *Journal of Speech and Hearing Research, 32*(4), 749–754.

Pommerenke, W. (1928). A study of the sensory areas eliciting the swallowing reflex. *American Journal of Physiology, 84*, 36–41.

Ponzoli, V. (1968). Zenker's diverticulum. *Southern Medical Journal, 61*, 817–821.

Pouderoux, P., Logemann, J. A., & Kahrilas, P. J. (1996). Pharyngeal swallowing elicited by fluid infusion: Role of volition and vallecular containment. *American Journal of Physiology, 270*, G347–G354.

Preiksaitis, H. G., Mayrand, S., Robins, K., & Diamant, N. E. (1992). Coordination of respiration and swallowing: Effect of bolus volume in normal adults. *American Journal of Physiology, 263*, R624–R630.

Pressman, J., & Keleman, G. (1955). Physiology of the larynx. *Physiological Reviews, 35*, 506–554.

Ramsey, G., Watson, J., Gramiak, R., & Weinberg, S. (1955). Cinefluorographic analysis of the mechanism of swallowing. *Radiology, 64*, 498–518.

Reimers-Neils, L., Logemann, J. A., & Larson, C. (1994). Viscosity effects on EMG activity in normal swallow. *Dysphagia, 9*, 101–106.

Robbins, J., Hamilton, J. W., Lof, G. L., & Kempster, G. B. (1992). Oropharyngeal swallowing in normal adults of different ages. *Gastroenterology, 103*, 823–829.

Robbins, J., Logemann, J., & Kirshner, H. (1982). *Velopharyngeal activity during speech and swallowing in neurologic disease.* Paper presented at the American Speech-Language-Hearing Association annual meeting, Toronto.

Roueche, J. (1980). *Dysphagia: An assessment and management program for the adult.* Minneapolis: Sister Kenny Institute.

Schiffman, S. S., & Warwick, Z. S. (1989). Use of flavor-amplified foods to improve nutritional status in elderly persons: Nutrition and the chemical senses in aging. *Annals of New York Academy of Science, 561*, 267–276.

Selley, W. G., Flack, F. C., Ellis, R. E., & Brooks, W. A. (1989a). Respiratory patterns associated with swallowing: 1. The normal adult pattern and changes with age. *Age and Ageing, 18*, 168–172.

Selley, W. G., Flack, F. C., Ellis, R. E., & Brooks, W. A. (1989b). Respiratory patterns associated with swallowing: 2. Neurologically impaired dysphagic patients. *Age and Ageing, 18*, 173–176.

Shaker, R., Ren, J., Podvrsan, B., Dodds, W. J., Hogan, J. W., Kern, M., Hoffman, R., & Hintz, J. (1993). Effect of aging and bolus variables on pharyngeal and upper esophageal sphincter motor function. *American Journal of Physiology, 264*, G427–G432.

Shawker, T. H., Sonies, B. C., & Stone, M. (1984). Sonography of speech and swallowing. In R. C. Sanders & M. C. Hill (Eds.), *Ultrasound annual* (pp. 237–260). New York: Raven.

Shedd, D., Kirchner, J., & Scatliff, J. (1961). Oral and pharyngeal components of deglutition. *Archives of Surgery, 82*, 371–380.

Shedd, D., Scatliff, J., & Kirchner, J. (1960). The buccopharyngeal propulsive mechanism in human deglutition. *Surgery, 48*, 846–853.

Smith, J., Wolkove, N., Colacone, A., & Kreisman, H. (1989). Coordination of eating, drinking and breathing in adults. *Chest, 96,* 578–582.

Storey, A. (1976). Interactions of alimentary and upper respiratory tract reflexes. In B. J. Sessle & A. G. Hannan (Eds.), *Mastication and swallowing.* Toronto: University of Toronto Press.

Sumi, T. (1972). Role of the pontine reticular formation in the neural organization of deglutition. *Japanese Journal of Physiology, 22,* 295–314.

Tracy, J., Logemann, J., Kahrilas, P., Jacob, P., Kobara, M., & Krugler, C. (1989). Preliminary observations on the effects of age on oropharyngeal deglutition. *Dysphagia, 4,* 90–94.

Vantrappen, G., & Hellemans, J. (1967). Studies on the normal deglutition complex. *American Journal of Digestive Diseases, 12,* 255–266.

Wildman, A. (1976). The motor system: A clinical approach. *Dental Clinics of North America, 20,* 691–705.

C H A P T E R   3

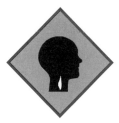

INSTRUMENTAL TECHNIQUES FOR THE STUDY OF SWALLOWING

A number of imaging and nonimaging instrumentation procedures have been used to study various aspects of normal and/or abnormal swallow physiology. Each procedure provides some pieces of information on oropharyngeal anatomy or swallowing physiology or the food as it is being swallowed. It is important that clinicians be familiar with the types of information each procedure provides about swallowing and the basic methodology for each procedure (Langmore & Logemann, 1991). If a physician, other health care provider, patient, or patient's significant other asks about various assessment procedures, the swallowing therapist should be able to explain why each procedure would or would not be appropriate for the patient's particular swallowing problem in the context of his or her age, language, cognition, and medical diagnosis. Some instrumental procedures for the study of swallowing have been used in research more frequently than in clinical care of patients, such as electromyography (Doty & Bosma, 1956; Palmer, 1988; Perlman, 1993; Perlman, Luschei, & DuMond, 1989). Some procedures have been used concurrently, such as videofluorography and electromyography or videofluoroscopy and manometry (Jacob, Kahrilas, Logemann, Shah, & Ha, 1989; Kahrilas, Logemann, Krugler, & Flanagan, 1991; McConnel, Hester, Mendelsohn, & Logemann, 1988; McConnel, Mendelsohn, & Logemann, 1987).

Imaging Studies

Several technologies can be used to image the oropharyngeal region (Bastian, 1991, 1993; Dodds, Logemann, & Stewart, 1990; Dodds, Stewart, & Logemann, 1990; Donner, 1988; Langmore & Logemann, 1991; Langmore, Schatz, & Olson, 1988, 1991; Linden, 1989; Logemann, 1993a, 1993b; Muz, Mathog, Miller, Rosen, & Borrero, 1987). These include ultrasound, videoendoscopy, and video-fluoroscopy. A fourth technique, scintigraphy, enables visualization of food being swallowed, but not of the anatomy and physiology of the oropharyngeal region during deglutition.

Ultrasound

Ultrasound studies of the oral cavity have been used to observe tongue function and to measure oral transit times, as well as motion of the hyoid bone (Shawker, Sonies, Hall, & Baum, 1984; Shawker, Sonies, & Stone, 1984; Shawker, Sonies, Stone, & Baum, 1983). Unfortunately, ultrasound cannot at this time visualize the pharynx because of the mix of tissue types (cartilage, bone, muscle) in the pharynx. The inability to image the pharynx has limited the application of ultrasound to the study of the oral stages of swallow, especially oral tongue function during deglutition and biofeedback for various oral tongue exercises.

Videoendoscopy

Videoendoscopy has been used increasingly in recent years to examine the anatomy of the oral cavity and pharynx from above and to examine the pharynx and larynx before and after swallowing (Bastian, 1991, 1993; Kidder, Langmore, & Martin, 1994; Langmore & Logemann, 1991; Langmore et al., 1991). This procedure has sometimes been called FEES or flexible fiberoptic examination of swallowing. Endoscopy can be performed with a flexible scope inserted into the nose, down to the level of the soft palate, or below, as shown in Figure 3.1. This transnasal position often requires light topical anesthetic in the nose to permit comfortable placement. Endoscopy does not visualize the oral stage of swallowing. If the tube is positioned above the level of the soft palate, the dynamics of velopharyngeal closure can be observed, including the inward movement of the lateral and/or posterior pharyngeal walls and the elevation and retraction of the soft palate. With the endoscopic tube placed so that the tip is behind the tip of the uvula (Figure 3.2), the pharynx is imaged before the pharyngeal swallow triggers and again when the pharynx relaxes after the swallow. The moment when the pharyngeal swallow triggers causes the pharynx to close around the

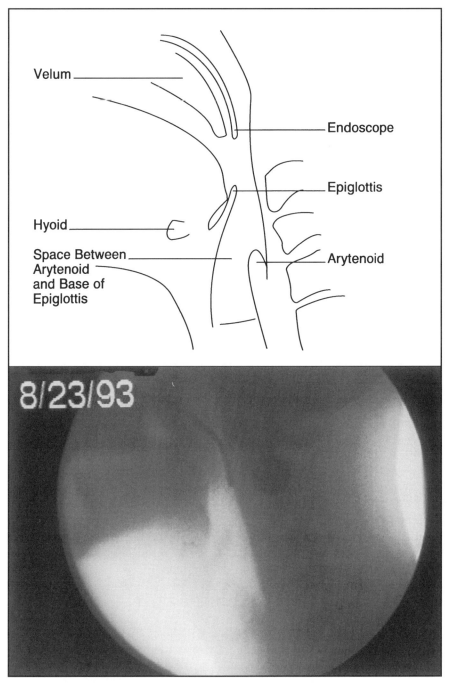

Figure 3.1. Lateral views of the flexible endoscopic tube placement behind the soft palate to view the pharynx before and after swallowing.

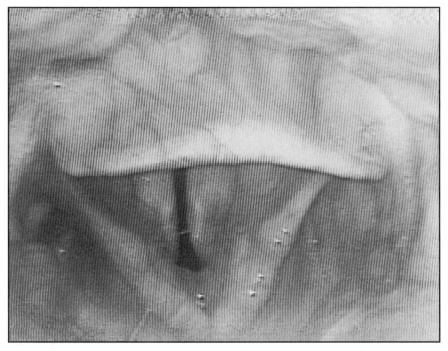

Figure 3.2. Endoscopic view of the pharynx and larynx showing the epiglottis, arytenoids, pyriform sinuses, and vocal folds with the endoscopic tube positioned behind the soft palate.

endoscopic tube, blocking the image during the swallow. Many important events occur during this closed period, as identified from simultaneous videofluoroscopy and videoendoscopy in Figure 3.3.

Because treatment for oropharyngeal swallowing disorders is directed largely at the motor activity during the swallow, videoendoscopy makes it difficult to define the exact nature of the patient's physiologic disorder and the effectiveness of treatment strategies. A clinician can try to infer the nature of the patient's swallow physiology from the location of residual food when the endoscopic image returns to view, but this is an indirect process based on symptoms rather than actual observation of the swallow itself.

Endoscopy can also be performed with a rigid scope placed into the mouth, as shown in Figure 3.4, which often provides a better image of the same pharyngeal and laryngeal structures; however, the patient cannot swallow with the rigid scope in place.

Although flexible, fiberoptic endoscopy of swallow has been reported as possible in children (Willging, 1995), my experience is that children under 6 to 8 years old do not cooperate well with the procedure. Similarly, adults

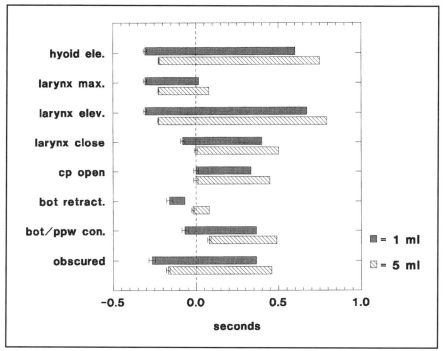

seconds

Figure 3.3. Graph showing the relative timing of various pharyngeal swallow events observed on videofluoroscopy in relation to the obscured period during videoendoscopy. Time 0.0 represents the onset of cricopharyngeal opening. All events are referenced to that time point. The graph shows the onset and termination of hyoid elevation (hyoid ele.), maximal laryngeal elevation (larynx max.), total duration of laryngeal elevation (larynx elev.), closure of the airway entrance (larynx close), cricopharyngeal opening (cp open), base of tongue retraction until contact with the posterior pharyngeal wall (bot retract.), duration of base of tongue contact to the posterior pharyngeal wall (bot/ppw con.), and the duration of obscured period when the image disappears during this swallow (obscured) for 1- and 5-ml swallows of thin liquid.

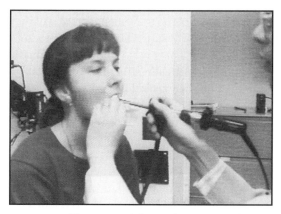

Figure 3.4. Placement of the rigid scope into the oral cavity.

with cognitive disorders or those who are agitated are poor candidates for the procedure.

Videoendoscopy or fiberoptic endoscopic evaluation recorded on videotape can provide an excellent superior view of the pharyngeal anatomy, including the relationship between the epiglottis, airway entrance, valleculae, aryepiglottic folds, and pyriform sinuses. The advantage of videoendoscopy is that there is no radiation exposure. The tube can be used to test sensory awareness by touching pharyngeal and laryngeal structures. However, a tube is placed transnasally, which may interfere with swallowing in some patients and may be uncomfortable and not tolerated well by others. Videoendoscopy is an excellent way to observe the vocal folds if the tube is placed lower (at or below the tip of the epiglottis) (Figure 3.5), and to assess oropharyngeal anatomy. Videoendoscopy can also be used to assess the patient's ability to use airway closure maneuvers, such as the supraglottic swallow (easy breath hold) and the super-supraglottic swallow (effortful breath hold). With endoscopy, these procedures can be viewed prior to the actual swallow but not during the swallow.

Endoscopy can also be used to provide biofeedback to the patient who is having difficulty learning the airway closure maneuvers. The patient can observe his or her laryngeal movement while producing the easy and effortful breath hold.

Videofluoroscopy

The most frequently used technique in the assessment of oropharyngeal swallow is videofluoroscopy (Dodds, Logemann, & Stewart, 1990; Dodds, Stewart, & Logemann, 1990; Donner, 1988; Linden, 1989; Logemann, 1993a, 1993b; Palmer, DuChane, & Donner, 1991). Radiographic procedures have been used to study swallowing since the early 1900s. In the 1930s the development of fluoroscopy permitted examination of the movement patterns of the oral cavity, pharynx, and esophagus during swallowing. The fluoroscopic image, first recorded on movie film and called *cinefluorography*, allowed examination of movement patterns of the bolus and of particular structures in slow motion and frame by frame. The movie film could be exposed at various speeds up to 60 frames per second (Ardran & Kemp, 1951, 1952, 1956; Sloan, Ricketts, Brummett, Bench, & Westover, 1965; Sokol, Heitmann, Wolf, & Cohen, 1966; Wictorin, Hedegard, & Lundberg, 1971).

More recently, fluoroscopic studies have been recorded on videotape (*videofluorography*), which also permits frame-by-frame analysis employing a video recorder–player with frame-by-frame analysis capability (Yotsuya, Nonaka, & Yoshinobu, 1981; Yotsuya, Saito, & Yoshinobu, 1981). Cinefluorography had the disadvantage of requiring more radiation exposure than videofluoroscopy and requiring film development, so immediate review of the study was not possible. Thus, videofluoroscopy quickly became more popular than cinefluorography. By

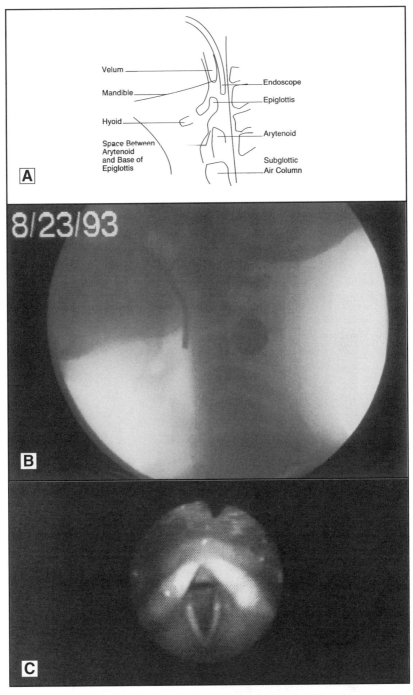

Figure 3.5. (A) A diagram of the placement of the flexible fiberoptic endoscope transnasally to the level of the top of the epiglottis. (B) The tube placement as viewed radiographically. (C) The image of the larynx as viewed with the tube in the position behind the tip of the epiglottis.

recording numbers on each frame of the videotape using a video counter timer, the swallowing studies can be repeatedly examined in slow motion or frame by frame, and the specific frame numbers of greatest interest can be easily located and examined. Because swallowing occurs very rapidly, with normal oral and pharyngeal transit times together taking approximately 1 to 2 seconds, slow motion analysis is most helpful in defining movement disorders. Almost any videotape recorder can be attached to the fluoroscopic equipment so that the fluoroscopic image can be easily recorded on videotape. Thus, no special equipment is generally necessary.

Videofluoroscopic studies provide information on bolus transit times, motility problems, and amount and, most important, etiology of aspiration. Although videofluoroscopy does use radiation, the patient receives a relatively low dose, while the oropharyngeal region is fully viewed in the lateral or posterior–anterior plane (Figure 3.6). Videofluoroscopy enables visualization of (1) oral activity during chewing and the oral stage of swallowing, (2) the triggering of

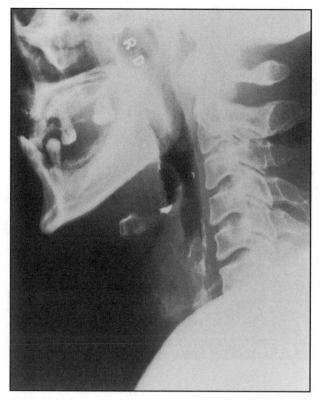

Figure 3.6. Lateral radiographic view of the oral cavity and pharynx.

the pharyngeal swallow in relation to position of the bolus, and (3) the motor aspects of the pharyngeal swallow, including movements of the larynx, hyoid, tongue base, pharyngeal walls, and cricopharyngeal region. Videofluoroscopy does not enable measurement of pressures generated during swallowing, but does enable an indirect observation of pressure through the speed of movement of the bolus in relation to structural motion. The videofluorographic assessment of oropharyngeal swallow generally uses a variety of food types and visualizes the patient initially in the lateral plane. The patient is given measured amounts of liquid, usually from 1 to 10 ml; then liquid to drink from a cup; then some type of soft pureed food such as a pudding; and, finally, a masticated bolus such as a piece of a cookie. However, the patient can be given whatever food types are of interest for observation by the clinician. If patients complain of a food-specific dysphagia, those particular foods should be given with barium applied to or mixed with them.

The lateral radiographic view is used initially to assess the transit times or speed and efficiency of bolus movement and also for better observation of aspiration. In the posterior–anterior view, the airway overlies the esophagus, and the identification of the presence and etiology for aspiration is difficult. The radiographic study, usually called a modified barium swallow, is not designed to determine whether someone aspirates, but rather to understand why they aspirate. Further, the study is designed to define optimal eating strategies to enable the patient to continue at least partial intake.

Once the abnormalities in the patient's anatomy and/or swallow physiology have been identified, the clinician should introduce treatment strategies during the radiographic study in order to facilitate safe and more efficient oral intake. Such strategies usually include changes in head or body posture, heightening sensory input prior to the swallow, and, when possible, the swallowing therapy techniques designed to change specific aspects of swallow physiology, such as swallow maneuvers. Effects of changing bolus viscosity can also be examined. These strategies to improve the patient's swallow are introduced during the radiographic study so the clinician can obtain direct evidence of the efficacy of these interventions.

Scintigraphy

Scintigraphy is a nuclear medicine test in which the patient swallows measured amounts of a radioactive substance (Muz, Hamlet, Mathog, & Farris, 1994; Muz et al., 1987; Silver & Van Nostrand, 1992; Silver, Van Nostrand, Kuhlemeier, & Siebens, 1991). During swallows, the bolus is imaged and recorded by a gamma camera. With this technique the amount of aspiration and residue can be measured, but the physiology of the mouth and pharynx is not visualized so that the dysfunctions causing the residue and aspiration are not identified.

Scintigraphy can be diagnostic for esophageal aspects of swallowing dysfunction, particularly gastroesophageal reflux disease (Hamlet, Choi, Kumpuris, Holliday, & Stachler, 1994; Hamlet et al., 1996; Hamlet, Muz, Farris, Kumpuris, & Jones, 1992). The amount aspirated and the amount of oral and pharyngeal residue left after a swallow are measured. If there is no aspiration and reflux is suspected, the patient is rescanned every 15 to 30 minutes for several hours. If the patient showed no evidence of aspiration on early scans but after several minutes or hours reveals material in the airway and lungs, reflux disease has clearly been the etiology for the aspiration. Scintigraphy has largely been used for research purposes in the oropharynx, rather than as a standard clinical tool.

Nonimaging Procedures

Nonimaging procedures provide a variety of types of information about swallowing but do not result in pictures of the swallowing process or the food being swallowed. Instead, most result in amplitude over time displays of the swallow parameters being examined, such as pressure generated at specific locations in the pharynx (manometry) or amount of electrical energy generated by muscle contractions (electromyography).

Electromyography

Electromyography (EMG) of muscles involved in swallowing can provide information on the timing and relative amplitude of selected muscle contraction during swallowing (Doty & Bosma, 1956; Palmer, 1988; Perlman et al., 1989). Doty and Bosma (1956) studied reflexive deglutition in dogs, cats, and monkeys by placing two electrodes in each muscle to be analyzed. Overall, 22 muscles were examined. Pharyngeal swallowing was activated by stimulating the pharynx with a cotton swab or rapidly injected water, or by stimulating the superior laryngeal nerve. These investigators found no difference in temporal pattern, duration, or amplitude of contraction of participating muscles in swallows elicited by these varying methods. One group of muscles (superior constrictor, palatopharyngeus, palatoglossus, posterior intrinsic muscles of the tongue, styloglossus, stylohyoid, geniohyoid, and mylohyoid) fired concurrently with initiation of the swallow. The activity of four muscles in the oral stage of the swallow was examined in humans by Hrycyshyn and Basmajian (1972). They found no universal firing pattern within the four muscles, the geniohyoid, anterior belly of digastric, mylohyoid, and genioglossus. The type of bolus appeared to affect the duration of muscle activity.

Studies of swallowing with electromyography have utilized surface EMG and hooked-wire EMG, as well as suction cup electrodes (Palmer, Tanaka, & Siebens,

1989; Perlman, 1993; Reimers-Neils, Logemann, & Larson, 1994). Surface electromyography involves the application of electrodes to the skin surface above muscles of interest and has been used in some studies as a marker of the swallow. Most often, in studies of swallowing, surface electromyography records information from muscles of the floor of the mouth by placing one or two electrodes on the soft tissue under the chin or from muscles involved in laryngeal elevation by placing an electrode above the thyroid cartilage on one or both sides (Bryant, 1991; Reimers-Neils et al., 1994). Electrical activity in all of these muscles has been found to occur early in the swallow (Doty & Bosma, 1956). Therefore, surface EMG of these muscles has been used as a marker of the onset of swallow. Both suction cup electrodes and hooked-wire electrodes have been used to study pharyngeal wall activity during swallowing (Palmer et al., 1989; Perlman et al., 1989).

A few investigators have used hooked-wire electromyography to assess muscle function during the swallow. Perlman et al. (1989) utilized hooked-wire electromyography to study superior pharyngeal constrictor activity during a variety of functions, including swallowing, in order to examine the relative level of contraction in this muscle during swallowing versus other voluntary actions, such as producing selected speech sounds, falsetto voice, and gagging. Findings of this study indicated that the electrical activity in the superior pharyngeal constrictor was greatest for swallowing as compared to gagging, Valsalva (effortful bearing down with a breath hold), effortful articulation, falsetto, and other speech and voice productions. The authors compared the relative amplitude of the electromyographic signal within each subject across the various physiologic activities and then compared these relative levels across individuals. The absolute amount of electrical activity produced in muscles across individuals cannot be compared.

Electrical activity in muscles measured by electromyography has also been used as a biofeedback technique during therapy for patients with dysphagia (Bryant, 1991). Most frequently, biofeedback involves surface electromyography of the laryngeal elevators to illustrate the duration of laryngeal elevation during the Mendelsohn maneuver. This maneuver is designed to improve the extent and duration of laryngeal elevation during the swallow and thus to improve the duration and width of cricopharyngeal opening during deglutition. Surface electromyography recording from the laryngeal elevators has been presented on an oscilloscope screen to provide visual feedback regarding the onset and duration of laryngeal elevation to the patient learning the Mendelsohn maneuver.

Surface electromyography can also be used to provide biofeedback for the effortful swallow. The patient can observe the amount of electrical activity in the submandibular muscles when producing a normal swallow and then a very effortful, hard swallow, squeezing hard with all of the muscles. The patient can monitor the muscle activity and try to increase it within the session.

Electroglottography

Electroglottography (EGG) is designed to track vocal fold movement by record-ing the impedance changes as the vocal folds move toward and away from each other during phonation (Perlman & Grayhack, 1991; Perlman & Liang, 1991). The equipment can be modified to track laryngeal elevation (Perlman & Liang, 1991), which can be useful in determining the onset and termination of a pha-ryngeal swallow, and in providing biofeedback on extent and duration of laryn-geal elevation during the swallows in which the patient is attempting to improve these swallow parameters.

Cervical Auscultation: Listening to and Recording the Sounds of Swallowing

Several authors have examined various parameters of deglutition using acoustic procedures (Logan, Kavanagh, & Wornall, 1967; Mackowiak, Brenman, & Friedman, 1967). Hollshwandner, Brenman, and Friedman (1975) studied some temporal measures of swallowing, such as the time elapsing from the final chew of the swallowing cycle to the first sound of deglutition, by attaching a contact microphone to the skin surface paralaryngeally. Using this same technique, Lear, Flanagan, and Moorrees (1965) assessed the frequency of adult deglutition over 24-hour periods. Unfortunately, acoustic techniques are limited by the few parameters of swallowing that can be studied, as many aspects of deglutition appear to be silent.

Recording the sounds produced during the swallow by placing a small micro-phone or accelerometer on the surface of the patient's neck at various locations has identified some repeatable sounds produced across normal subjects (Hamlet, Nelson, & Patterson, 1990; Hamlet, Patterson, Fleming, & Jones, 1992). The "click" associated with the opening of the eustachian tube and the "clunk" asso-ciated with the opening of the upper esophageal sphincter appear to be the most reliable sounds produced during swallowing. Though a number of other sounds have been recorded, the source of their generation has not been clearly iden-tified. Even the source of the clunk sound associated with cricopharyngeal open-ing has not been defined. Further, there have been no studies to determine whether the few sounds of swallowing that have been identified are different in normal swallowers and in patients with specific swallowing abnormalities. The ability of clinicians to identify or distinguish normal from abnormal sounds or to define the meaning of the sounds produced during swallow by patients with swallowing disorders has not been determined. The application of any under-standing of the sounds generated during swallowing needs further research before reliable and broad clinical application is appropriate. Another method for listening to the sounds of swallowing is to apply a stethoscope to the patient's neck. The clinician can then listen to the sounds of swallowing and/or to the sounds of respiration, as described in the next section.

Cervical Auscultation—Sounds of Respiration

The clinician can use the stethoscope to listen to respiration and define the inhalatory and exhalatory phases of the respiratory cycle, as well as the moment when the pharyngeal swallow occurs and in which part (inhalation or exhalation) of the respiratory cycle the swallow occurs. If secretions are in the airway before or after the swallow, these will also be heard, as will any change(s) in secretion levels before and after the swallow. Information on secretion levels and changes in these levels before and after the swallow may be indicators of aspiration so that cervical auscultation could be used as a screening procedure to help identify high-risk patients needing in-depth physiologic assessment.

Pharyngeal Manometry

Pharyngeal manometry requires solid-state pressure sensors (strain gauges) that have a fast enough frequency response to react to the rapid pressure changes during the pharyngeal swallow. Unlike the esophagus, in which normal transit times range from 8 to 20+ seconds, pharyngeal transport of the bolus takes less than 1 second and is often completed in 0.5 seconds. The pressure sensors are encased in a flexible 3-mm tube (see Figure 3.7), which is placed transnasally so that, in most cases, a sensor is located at the tongue base, another at the upper esophageal (cricopharyngeal) sphincter, and a third in the cervical esophagus. Pharyngeal manometry generally requires concurrent videofluoroscopy in order to define the etiology of pressure changes—that is, whether they are the result of the bolus passage, the pharyngeal contractile wave, or other structures touching the manometric sensors (Ergun, Kahrilas, & Logemann, 1993). Accurate interpretation of pharyngeal manometry generally requires visualization of the bolus position in relation to the manometric sensors, as well as the location of various structures in the pharynx in relation to the pressure sensors throughout the swallow (Ergun et al., 1993; Robbins, Hamilton, Lof, & Kempster, 1992).

Pharyngeal manometry allows measurement of intrabolus pressures and the timing of the pharyngeal contractile wave. Pharyngeal manometry also enables indirect examination of the relaxation of the cricopharyngeal muscle by identification of the drop in pressure at the upper sphincter (as measured by a sensor in the sphincter) in relation to the opening of the upper sphincter as seen on videofluorography. In general, the pressure drop to zero at the upper sphincter occurs approximately 0.1 second before the opening of the upper sphincter, as visualized videofluorographically (Cook, Dodds, Dantas, et al., 1989; Jacob et al., 1989; Kahrilas, Logemann, Lin, & Ergun, 1992).

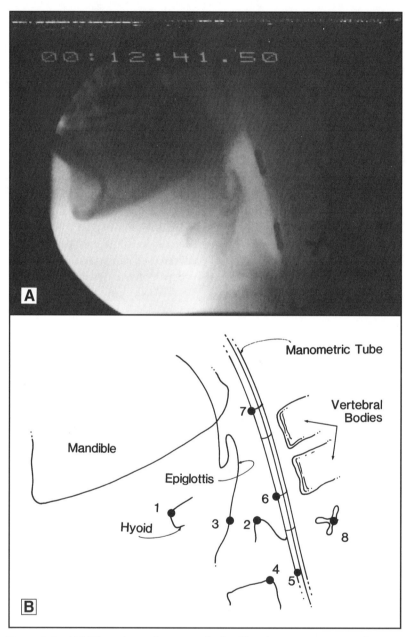

Figure 3.7. (A) The radiographic view of a flexible tube containing several manometric sensors positioned in the pharynx. (B) A diagram of the same radiographic
image with structures labeled and manometric sensors identified: the tip of the arytenoid cartilage (2), the epiglottic base opposite the arytenoid (3), the posterior
superior corner of the undersurface of the vocal folds (4), the cricopharyngeal region
(5), the top edge of the manometric sensors (6 and 7), and an external landmark
placed on the neck to enable measurement of structural movement from the fluoroscopic image (8).

Pharyngeal manometry in concert with videofluoroscopy has been used in a number of studies of normal swallow physiology, but in relatively few studies of the abnormal pharynx (Jacob et al., 1989; Kahrilas et al., 1991; McConnell et al., 1988; McConnel et al., 1987; Robbins et al., 1992). At this time, solid-state manometry is not used as a general diagnostic tool, partially because of its reduced availability as compared with water manometry, which is used in the esophagus, and because it is a relatively invasive technique and technically needs to be combined with videofluoroscopy, which requires significant person-nel and equipment coordination.

Selecting an Instrumental Procedure

The swallowing therapist should select an instrumental procedure for use in swal-lowing assessment and treatment based on the particular information needed. If understanding the patient's pharyngeal anatomy is the question, such as in a postsurgical oropharyngeal cancer patient, then rigid videoendoscopy is prob-ably the procedure of choice. If defining the presence (but not necessarily the cause) of aspiration of saliva is the desired goal, then flexible fiberoptic video-endoscopy (FEES) is the procedure of choice. If understanding pharyngeal phys-iology in relation to symptoms such as aspiration is the issue of interest, then videofluoroscopy should be used. If the pressure generated during swallowing is the information needed, then pharyngeal manometry may be used in combina-tion with videofluoroscopy. In summary, the clinician must define the informa-tion needed for each patient and select the instrumental procedure accordingly.

References

Ardran, G. M., & Kemp, F. (1951). The mechanism of swallowing. *Proceedings of the Royal Society of Medicine, 44*, 1038–1040.

Ardran, G. M., & Kemp, F. (1952). The protection of the laryngeal airway during swallowing. *British Journal of Radiology, 25*, 406–416.

Ardran, G., & Kemp, F. (1956). Closure and opening of the larynx during swallowing. *British Jour-nal of Radiology, 29*, 205–208.

Bastian, R. W. (1991). Videoendoscopic evaluation of patients with dysphagia: An adjunct to the modified barium swallow. *Otolaryngology—Head and Neck Surgery, 104*, 339–350.

Bastian, R. W. (1993). The videoendoscopic swallowing study: An alternative and partner to the videofluoroscopic swallowing study. *Dysphagia, 8*, 359–367.

Bryant, M. (1991). Biofeedback in the treatment of a selected dysphagic patient. *Dysphagia, 6*, 140–144.

Cook, I. J., Dodds, W. J., Dantas, R. O., Massey, B., Kern, M. K., Lang, I. M., Brasseur, S. G., & Hogan, W. J. (1989). Opening mechanism of the human upper esophageal sphincter. *Ameri-can Journal of Physiology, 257*, G748–G759.

Dodds, W. J., Logemann, J. A., & Stewart, E. T. (1990). Radiological assessment of abnormal oral and pharyngeal phases of swallow. *American Journal of Roentology, 154*, 965–974.

Dodds, W. J., Stewart, E. T., & Logemann, J. (1990). Physiology and radiology of the normal oral and pharyngeal phases of swallowing. *American Journal of Roentology, 154*, 953–963.

Donner, M. (1988). The evaluation of dysphagia by radiography and other methods of imaging. *Dysphagia, 1*, 49–50.

Doty, R., & Bosma, J. (1956). An electromyographic analysis of reflex deglutition. *Journal of Neurophysiology, 19*, 44–60.

Ergun, G. A., Kahrilas, P. J., & Logemann, J. A. (1993). Interpretation of pharyngeal manometric recordings: Limitations and variability. *Diseases of the Esophagus, 6*, 11–16.

Hamlet, S., Choi, J., Kumpuris, T., Holliday, J., & Stachler, R. (1994). Quantifying aspiration in scintigraphic deglutition testing: Tissue attenuation effects. *Journal of Nuclear Medicine, 35*, 1007–1013.

Hamlet, S., Choi, J., Zormeier, M., Shamsa, F., Stachler, R., Muz, J., & Jones, L. (1996). Normal adult swallowing of liquid and viscous material: Scintigraphic data on bolus transit and oropharyngeal residues. *Dysphagia, 11*, 41–47.

Hamlet, S., Muz, J., Farris, R., Kumpuris, T., & Jones, L. (1992). Scintigraphic quantification of pharyngeal retention following deglutition. *Dysphagia, 7*, 12–16.

Hamlet, S. L., Nelson, R. J., & Patterson, R. L. (1990). Interpreting the sounds of swallowing: Fluid flow through the cricopharyngeus. *Annals of Otology, Rhinology, and Laryngology, 99*, 749–752.

Hamlet, S. L., Patterson, R. L., Fleming, S. M., & Jones, L. A. (1992). Sounds of swallowing following total laryngectomy. *Dysphagia, 7*, 160–165.

Hollshwandner, G., Brenman, J., & Friedman, M. (1975). Role of afferent sensors in the initiation of swallowing in man. *Journal of Dental Research, 54*, 83–88.

Hrycyshyn, A., & Basmajian, J. (1972). Electromyography of the oral stage of swallowing in man. *American Journal of Anatomy, 133*, 333–340.

Jacob, P., Kahrilas, P., Logemann, J., Shah, V., & Ha, T. (1989). Upper esophageal sphincter opening and modulation during swallowing. *Gastroenterology, 97*, 1469–1478.

Kahrilas, P. J., Logemann, J. A., Krugler, C., & Flanagan, E. (1991). Volitional augmentation of upper esophageal sphincter opening during swallowing. *American Journal of Physiology, 260 (Gastrointestinal Physiology, 23)*, G450–G456.

Kahrilas, P. J., Logemann, J. A., Lin, S., & Ergun, G. A. (1992). Pharyngeal clearance during swallow: A combined manometric and videofluoroscopic study. *Gastroenterology, 103*, 128–136.

Kidder, T. M., Langmore, S. E., & Martin, B. J. W. (1994). Indications and techniques of endoscopy in evaluation of cervical dysphagia: Comparison with radiographic techniques. *Dysphagia, 9*, 256–261.

Langmore, S. E., & Logemann, J. A. (1991). After the clinical bedside swallowing examination: What next? *American Journal of Speech-Language Pathology, 1*, 13–20.

Langmore, S. E., Schatz, K., & Olson, M. (1988). Fiberoptic endoscopic examination of swallowing safety: A new procedure. *Dysphagia, 2*, 216–219.

Langmore, S. E., Schatz, K., & Olson, M. (1991). Endoscopic and videofluoroscopic evaluations of swallowing and aspiration. *Annals of Otology, Rhinology, and Laryngology, 100*, 678–681.

Lear, C., Flanagan, J., & Moorrees, C. (1965). The frequency of deglutition in man. *Archives of Oral Biology, 10*, 83–99.

Linden, P. (1989). Videofluoroscopy in the rehabilitation of swallowing dysfunction. *Dysphagia, 3*, 189–191.

Logan, W., Kavanagh, J., & Wornall, A. (1967). Sonic correlates of human deglutition. *Journal of Applied Physiology, 23*, 279–284.

Logemann, J. A. (1993a). Imaging the oropharyngeal swallow. *Administrators in Radiology, 3*, 20–24, 43.

Logemann, J. (1993b). *Manual for the videofluoroscopic study of swallowing* (2nd ed.). Austin, TX: PRO-ED.

Mackowiak, R., Brenman, H., & Friedman, M. (1967). Acoustic profile of deglutition. *Proceedings of the Society for Experimental Biology, 125*, 1149–1152.

McConnel, F. M. S., Hester, T. R., Mendelsohn, M. S., & Logemann, J. A. (1988). Manofluorography of deglutition after total laryngopharyngectomy. *Plastic and Reconstructive Surgery, 81*, 346–351.

McConnel, F. M. S., Mendelsohn, M. S., & Logemann, J. A. (1987). Manofluorography of deglutition after supraglottic laryngectomy. *Head & Neck Surgery, 9*, 142–150.

Muz, J., Hamlet, S., Mathog, R., & Farris, R. (1994). Scintigraphic assessment of aspiration in head and neck cancer patients with tracheostomy. *Head and Neck, 16*, 17–20.

Muz, J., Mathog, R., Miller, P., Rosen, R., & Borrero, J. (1987). Detection and quantification of laryngotracheopulmonary aspiration with scintigraphy. *Laryngoscope, 97*, 1180–1185.

Palmer, J. B. (1988). Electromyography of the muscles of oropharyngeal swallowing: Basic concepts. *Dysphagia, 3*, 192–198.

Palmer, J. B., DuChane, A. S., & Donner, M. W. (1991). The role of radiology in the rehabilitation of swallowing. In B. Jones & M. W. Donner (Eds.), *Normal and abnormal swallowing: Imaging in diagnosis and therapy* (pp. 214–225). New York: Springer.

Palmer, J. B., Tanaka, E., & Siebens, A. A. (1989). Electromyography of the pharyngeal musculature: Technical considerations. *Archives of Physical Medicine and Rehabilitation, 70*(4), 283–287.

Perlman, A. L. (1993). Electromyography and the study of oropharyngeal swallowing. *Dysphagia, 8*, 351–355.

Perlman, A. L., & Grayhack, J. P. (1991). Use of the electroglottograph for measurement of temporal aspects of the swallow: Preliminary observations. *Dysphagia, 6*, 88–93.

Perlman, A. L., & Liang, X. (1991). Frequency response of the Fourcin electroglottograph and measurement of temporal aspects of laryngeal movement during swallowing. *Journal of Speech and Hearing Research, 34*, 791–795.

Perlman, A. L., Luschei, E. S., & DuMond, C. E. (1989). Electrical activity from the superior pharyngeal constrictor during reflexive and non-reflexive tasks. *Journal of Speech and Hearing Research, 32*, 749–754.

Reimers-Neils, L., Logemann, J. A., & Larson, C. (1994). Viscosity effects on EMG activity in normal swallow. *Dysphagia, 9*, 101–106.

Robbins, J., Hamilton, J. W., Lof, G. L., & Kempster, G. B. (1992). Oropharyngeal swallowing in normal adults of different ages. *Gastroenterology, 103*, 823–829.

Shawker, T., Sonies, B., Hall, T., & Baum, G. (1984). Ultrasound analysis of tongue hyoid and larynx activity during swallowing. *Investigative Radiology, 19*, 82–86.

Shawker, T. H., Sonies, B. C., & Stone, M. (1984). Sonography of speech and swallowing. In R. C. Sander & M. C. Hill (Eds.), *Ultrasound annual* (pp. 237–260). New York: Raven Press.

Shawker, T. H., Sonies, B. C., Stone, M., & Baum, B. (1983). Real-time ultrasound visualization of tongue movement during swallowing. *Journal of Clinical Ultrasound, 11*, 485–494.

Silver, K. H., & Van Nostrand, D. (1992). Scintigraphic detection of salivary aspiration: Description of a new diagnostic technique and case reports. *Dysphagia, 7*, 45–49.

Silver, K. H., Van Nostrand, D., Kuhlemeier, K. V., & Siebens, A. A. (1991). Scintigraphy for the detection and quantification of subglottic aspiration: Preliminary observations. *Archives of Physical Medicine and Rehabilitation, 72*, 902–910.

Sloan, R., Ricketts, R., Brummett, S., Bench, R., & Westover, J. L. (1965). Quantified cinefluorographic techniques used in oral roetgenology. *Oral Surgery, 20*, 456–462.

Sokol, E., Heitmann, P., Wolf, B., & Cohen, B. (1966). Simultaneous cineradiographic and manometric study of the pharynx, hypopharynx, and cervical esophagus. *Gastroenterology, 51*, 960–974.

Wictorin, W., Hedegard, B., & Lundberg, M. (1971). Cineradiographic studies of bolus position during chewing. *Journal of Prosthetic Dentistry, 26*, 236–246

Willging, J. P. (1995). Endoscopic evaluation of swallowing in children. *International Journal of Pediatric Oto-Rhino-Laryngology, 32*, S107–S108.

Yotsuya, H., Nonaka, K., & Yoshinobu, I. (1981). Studies on positional relationships of the movements of the pharyngeal organs during deglutition in relation to the cervical vertebrae by X-ray TV cinematography. *Bulletin of the Tokyo Dental College, 22*, 159–170.

Yotsuya, H., Saito, Y., & Yoshinobu, I. (1981). Studies on temporal correlations of the movements of the pharyngeal organs during deglutition by X-ray TV cinematography. *Bulletin of the Tokyo Dental College, 22*, 171–181.

C H A P T E R 4

DISORDERS OF DEGLUTITION

Disorders of deglutition may be described according to their clinical or radiographic symptomatology and according to the specific abnormalities in anatomy or neuromuscular functioning that result in the disturbed motility seen on X-ray or at the bedside (Logemann, 1993). It is important to differentiate symptoms from anatomic or neuromuscular dysfunctions, as information on the symptoms and the dysfunctions is used differently. Symptoms determined clinically and radiographically alert the clinician that the patient's swallowing is disordered, and point toward the nature of the dysfunction. The anatomic and/or neuromuscular dysfunctions are the actual disorders leading to the symptom for which treatment is designed. Swallowing therapists must educate physicians and others in this distinction to prevent symptomatic management that does not move the patient ahead in rehabilitation. Aspiration and residue are symptoms of a variety of disorders, not disorders themselves. In this chapter, symptoms are related to the swallowing disorders that can cause them.

Usually, the clinician begins to examine a patient with disordered deglutition by identifying clinical symptoms of dysphagia from careful history taking, chart review, patient descriptions, and a thorough bedside examination. The radiographic study (videofluoroscopy) should then be completed on any patient whose disordered deglutition is not clearly limited to the oral cavity (i.e., who has a suspected pharyngeal dysphagia) or who may be aspirating (Logemann, 1997).

The clinician then uses the information from the videofluoroscopic study to

(1) define anatomic and/or neuromuscular dysfunctions present in the patient's swallow; (2) determine the recommendation as to whether or not the patient should eat by mouth and, if so, the best conditions under which to eat and the best consistency(ies) of foods to be given; and (3) plan direct or indirect treatment appropriate for the specific swallowing disorders.

This chapter defines the anatomic and neuromuscular disorders, as well as the symptoms of each disorder, as might be (1) described by a patient, (2) observed in a bedside clinical evaluation, and/or (3) observed radiographically. Table 4.1 summarizes symptomology in relation to the anatomic and neuromuscular dysfunctions affecting mastication and other oral preparatory aspects of the swallow, the oral phase of the swallow, the triggering of the pharyngeal swallow, the pharyngeal phase of the swallow, and the cervical esophageal phase. Following this organizational format, a clinician may use any or all of the three types of information to identify swallowing dysfunctions. A patient's description alone can be erroneous. The swallowing therapist should note the patient's symptoms and use them in the overall analysis of the patient's problem(s) but should not use them as the sole evidence for diagnosis and management.

The Videofluorographic Examination of Swallowing Worksheet in Appendix 4A at the end of this chapter is organized to parallel the sequence of swallowing disorders seen during the modified barium swallow procedure. Thus, the radiographic symptoms of swallowing disorders that may be observed in the oral preparatory, oral, pharyngeal, and cervical esophageal stages of the swallow in the *lateral* view are described first and listed first on the worksheet. The last part of the chapter and the worksheet present those symptoms of swallowing disorders that may be observed in the oral preparatory and pharyngeal stages of the swallow when viewed in the *posterior–anterior* (P–A) plane. The oral stage is not easily viewed in the P–A plane.

On the worksheet, the far right-hand column identifies swallowing disorders, and the far left-hand column presents symptoms. That is, the symptoms or observations noted on the left are indicative of particular swallowing disorders, which are noted in the far right-hand column. For example, the symptom of residue in the pharynx, particularly on the pharyngeal walls and in the pyriform sinus on only one side (as listed in the left-hand column), would be an indication of unilateral dysfunction of the pharyngeal wall (the corresponding disorder listed in the right-hand column). Food residue in the lateral sulcus in the oral cavity (a symptom noted in the left column) is an indication of reduced tension in the buccal musculature (the corresponding disorder noted in the right column). Thus, residue in the lateral sulcus is a radiographic or bedside symptom listed in the left-hand column under the oral stage of swallow, whereas reduced buccal tension is the swallowing disorder causing the symptom and listed in the far right-hand column. The swallowing disorders listed in the right-hand column that relate to the radiographic symptoms in the left-hand column

Table 4.1
Clinical and Radiographic Symptoms Corresponding
to Some of the Neuromuscular and Anatomic Disorders of Swallowing

Patient Description[a]	Clinical (Bedside) Symptom	Radiographic Symptom[b]	Possible Motility (Neuromuscular) Anatomic Disorder
Cannot chew—avoids foods requiring mastication.	Material remains midline on tongue or falls into sulcus. Material falls into sulci.	Material remains midline on tongue or falls into sulcus. Material falls into sulci.	Inability to lateralize material with tongue. Reduced buccal tension.
Cannot "line up" teeth.	Cannot align mandible.	Cannot align mandible and maxilla (posterior–anterior [P–A] view).	Inability to align dentition.
Material goes all over mouth. Food catches in mouth.	Material spreads throughout oral cavity.	Loss of bolus control: Material spreads around oral cavity.	Reduced tongue coordination to form bolus (after mastication). Reduced oral sensation.
Coughing, choking *before* the swallow. Food catches in mouth.	Coughing, choking *before* the swallow.	Material falls over base of tongue into the valleculae or the airway (aspiration *before* the swallow).	Reduced tongue coordination to hold bolus (for liquids and paste materials).
Food catches in mouth. Slow eating, worse with solids.	Slowed oral transit times.	Slowed oral transit times. Reduced tongue elevation. Collection of material on the hard palate.	Reduced tongue elevation.
Slow eating, worse with solids.[a]	Slowed oral transit times.	Slowed oral transit times.	Reduced anterior to posterior tongue movement.

(continues)

Table 4.1. Continued

Patient Description[a]	Clinical (Bedside) Symptom	Radiographic Symptom[b]	Possible Motility (Neuromuscular) Anatomic Disorder
Slow eating.	Slowed oral transit times.	Slowed oral transit times. Repeated pumping tongue motion.	Swallow apraxia. Disorganized anterior to posterior tongue movement. Repeated tongue pumping.
	Slowed oral transit times	Slowed oral transit times.	Scarred tongue contour.
	Slowed oral transit times.	Collection of material in tongue depression from scarring, worsened with tongue movement.	
Food catches at base of tongue, high in the throat.[a]	Delayed elevation of the hyoid bone and thyroid cartilage.	Hesitation of material in the valleculae *prior* to initiation of the pharyngeal swallow.	Delayed pharyngeal swallow.
Food does not go down.	No hyoid/thyroid elevation. Slowed oral transit times.	Hesitation of material in the valleculae, with potential spill over into pyriform sinus and/or airway.	Absent pharyngeal swallow.
Food coughed up. Coughing/choking.	Coughing, choking. Expectoration of material *before* the pharyngeal swallow.	Aspiration *before* swallow. Expectoration of material.	Delayed pharyngeal swallow.
	Coughing, choking *after* the pharyngeal swallow. Expectoration of material after the pharyngeal swallow.	Residue of material in the valleculae after the swallow. Residue of material in the pyriform sinus after the swallow.	Reduced pharyngeal contraction. Reduced tongue base movement. Reduced laryngeal elevation.

Some food "sticks" high in the throat.	Residue of material on one or both sides of valleculae or pyriform sinus. Aspiration *after* swallow.	Unilateral or bilateral pharyngeal paralysis. Reduced tongue base movement.
Coughing, choking. Material catching at bottom of throat. Regurgitation of food.	Aspiration (spillover from pyriform sinuses) *after* the swallow. Collection of material in pyriform sinuses. Prominent pharyngoesophageal segment. Spillover from valleculae	Cricopharyngeal dysfunction. Reduced laryngeal elevation.
Coughing, choking.	Aspiration *after* the swallow. Reduced thyroid elevation. Residue in valleculae, pyriform sinus(es).	Unilateral or bilateral pharyngeal paresis. Reduced tongue base movement. Reduced laryngeal elevation.
Coughing, choking *during* swallow.	Aspiration *during* the swallow. Reduced airway closure (P–A view).	Reduced laryngeal closure.
Hoarseness.[a]	Normal swallow or reduced airway closure.	
Material caught lower in the throat at base of neck.[a]	Collection of material in the cervical esophagus after the swallow.	Reduced esophageal peristalsis or other esophageal disorder.
Regurgitation of food. Coughing, choking *after* the swallow.[a]	Collection of material in a side pocket in the pharynx or esophagus. Backflow.	Esophageal diverticulum.

(continues)

Table 4.1. Continued

Patient Description[a]	Clinical (Bedside) Symptom	Radiographic Symptom[b]	Possible Motility (Neuromuscular) Anatomic Disorder
Regurgitation of food. Coughing, choking *after* the swallow.	Regurgitation of food. Coughing, choking after the swallow.	Aspiration after the swallow from esophageal "overflow."	Partial or total obstruction in esophagus. Reflux.
Coughing, choking *after* the swallow.	Coughing, choking after the swallow.	Material passes from esophagus into trachea.	Tracheoesophageal fistula.
Material leaks out hole.	Material leaks out hole onto skin.	Material leaks through skin.	Pharyngocutaneous fistula.

[a]Some patients are unaware of having a swallowing disorder and may not, therefore, describe any particular problem with eating or drinking.
[b]As viewed laterally unless otherwise noted.

are meant to act as reminders to the clinician of the possible meaning of the symptoms seen radiographically. This list of radiographic symptoms and disorders includes the most common symptoms and disorders; it is not meant to be exhaustive, but rather to serve as a guide to clinicians in interpreting the videofluorographic studies. Disorders other than those listed on the worksheet may occasionally be seen. If so, there is space (marked Other) at the end of each swallowing stage on the worksheet to note other disorders as they occur on the swallows of various volumes and consistencies.

The Lateral View

The lateral view of the oral cavity and pharynx permits examination and measurement of oral and pharyngeal transit times; pharyngeal delay time; movement patterns of the bolus and oropharyngeal structures in the oral preparatory, oral, pharyngeal, and cervical esophageal phases of deglutition; and the approximate amount and cause (etiology) of any aspiration that occurs. Oral transit time (OTT) is defined as the time taken from the initiation of the tongue movement to begin the voluntary oral stage of the swallow until the bolus head reaches the point where the lower edge of the mandible crosses the tongue base (Miller, 1972; Pommerenke, 1928). Normally, this time is approximately 1 to 1.50 seconds (Mandelstam & Lieber, 1970; Tracy et al., 1989). Pharyngeal delay time (PDT) begins when the bolus head reaches the point where the lower edge of the mandible crosses the tongue base and ends when laryngeal elevation begins in the context of the rest of the swallow. Pharyngeal transit time (PTT) is defined as the time elapsed from the triggering of the pharyngeal swallow—that is, the onset of laryngeal elevation as a part of the swallow—until the bolus tail passes through the cricopharyngeal region or the pharyngoesophageal (PE) segment. This time is normally a maximum of 1 second, usually far less (0.35 to 0.48 seconds) (Blonsky, Logemann, Boshes, & Fisher, 1975; Mandelstam & Lieber, 1970; Rademaker, Pauloski, Logemann, & Shanahan, 1994; Tracy et al., 1989).

The lateral view of the oral cavity, pharynx, and larynx also facilitates the observation of whether aspiration occurs, the estimation of the percentage of the bolus aspirated, and the determination of the cause of the aspiration. In the posterior–anterior view, the trachea and the esophagus overlap each other, and it is difficult to assess the occurrence and approximate amount of aspiration and the cause of the aspiration. It is critical to note whether aspiration occurs *before*, *during*, or *after* the pharyngeal swallow and to identify the physiologic or anatomic cause(s) for the aspiration and to include this information in the patient's report. Treatment strategies are introduced into the X-ray study in an attempt to eliminate the aspiration. Therapy is then designed to eradicate the aspiration by eliminating its etiology.

Neuromuscular and Anatomic Swallowing Disturbances

The most important step in evaluation and treatment of disorders of deglutition is relating the symptoms observed clinically or radiographically to the actual anatomic or neuromuscular disorder creating the swallowing disturbance. Disorders are described in this chapter in the order in which they might occur in the mastication and deglutition sequence. Normal mastication, as described in Chapter 2, requires an intact mandible and maxilla and intact buccal and lingual musculature.

Disorders in Oral Preparation for the Swallow

The oral preparatory stage of the swallow is designed to break down food into an appropriate consistency for the swallow, mix it with saliva, and bring part or all of the food together into a cohesive ball or bolus ready for the swallow.

Cannot Hold Food in the Mouth Anteriorly—Reduced Lip Closure

Normally, as food is placed in the mouth, the lips close and remain closed during all phases of the swallow to keep food in the mouth anteriorly. This requires nasal breathing. If the patient is a mouth breather and keeps the lips open during mastication and oral manipulation, the clinician should check the patency of the nasal airway. When food falls from the mouth anteriorly, it is an indication of reduced lip closure, as shown in Figure 4.1.

Cannot Hold a Bolus—Reduced Tongue Shaping/Coordination

Liquid and paste materials are placed into the oral cavity as a cohesive or semi-cohesive bolus. Normally, unless an individual wants to taste material or otherwise manipulate it in the mouth, the liquid or paste is kept in a cohesive bolus, or ball, awaiting the initiation of the oral phase of the swallow. If a patient has reduced ability to shape the tongue around the liquid or paste, he or she will be unable to hold the liquid or paste in a cohesive bolus, and material will immediately spread throughout the oral cavity. During this period the soft palate is pulled down and forward (Figure 4.2) against the back of the tongue, preventing the material from entering the pharynx until the swallow is initiated. If the soft palate cannot or does not bulge anteriorly to contact the back of the tongue, food can be lost into the pharynx prematurely. Premature loss of a bolus over the tongue base and into the pharynx is normal during mastication but not while holding a liquid or pudding bolus. Premature loss of the bolus can result in aspiration before the swallow if the liquid or food falls over the base of the tongue into the pharynx and the open airway.

Whether or not aspiration will occur depends on the amount of food given, its consistency, and the exact posture of the patient. Inability to hold a bolus is

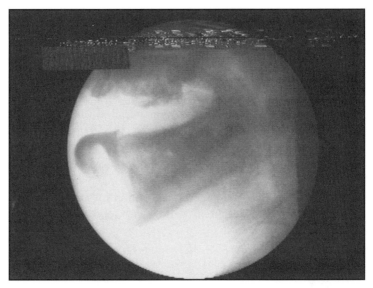

Figure 4.1. Lateral radiographic view of the oral cavity and pharynx in a patient with reduced lip closure. Food is falling from the mouth anteriorly.

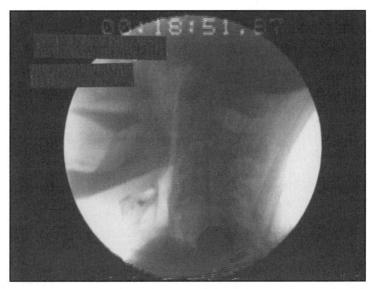

Figure 4.2. Lateral radiographic view of the oral cavity showing the soft palate pulled actively down and forward against the back of the tongue, holding liquid in the oral cavity.

an indication of reduced tongue coordination. Premature loss of liquid or paste into the valleculae is an indication of reduced anterior soft palate positioning and/or poor tongue control.

Cannot Form a Bolus—Reduced Range of Tongue Motion or Coordination

During mastication, or while merely tasting material in the mouth prior to the swallow, food is normally manipulated and moved throughout the oral cavity. When the individual is finished with mastication or oral manipulation, food is pulled together by the tongue into a single ball or bolus to initiate the swallow. If a patient has reduced range or coordination of tongue movement, he or she will have difficulty in pulling this food back together into a cohesive bolus, and thus will often be forced to initiate a swallow with food spread throughout the oral cavity.

Material Falls into Anterior Sulcus—Reduced Labial Tension/Tone

Food falling into the anterior sulcus, after it has been placed in the oral cavity or as the patient is chewing, is an indication of reduced labial and facial muscle tone. Muscle tone in the labial and facial musculature is responsible for closing the anterior sulcus and preventing food from lodging there.

Material Falls into Lateral Sulcus—Reduced Buccal Tension/Tone

Material falling into the lateral sulcus as the patient chews is an indication of reduced muscle tension or tone in the buccal musculature, as shown in Figure 4.3. Normally, tension or tone in the buccal musculature closes the lateral sulcus and prevents material from lodging there by directing it medially toward the tongue.

Abnormal Hold Position—Reduced Tongue Control; Tongue Thrust

Normally, the bolus is held between the tongue and the hard palate in preparation for the initiation of the oral phase of the swallow, or on the floor of the mouth in front of the retracted tongue tip. If held on the floor of the mouth, the tongue moves forward and picks up the bolus and brings it onto the surface of the tongue as the swallow begins. Approximately 20% of normal subjects hold the bolus on the floor of the mouth. This increases oral transit time. This pattern is often seen in older adults (Dodds et al., 1989). To hold and pick up the bolus, the tongue must be able to shape itself around the bolus and seal the sides of the tongue to the lateral alveolar ridge. If tongue shaping is not possible, the patient may hold the bolus in an abnormal position. If the bolus is held against the front teeth, as seen in Figure 4.4, it is likely that the swallow will be accomplished with a tongue thrusting behavior (i.e., a forward movement of the tongue

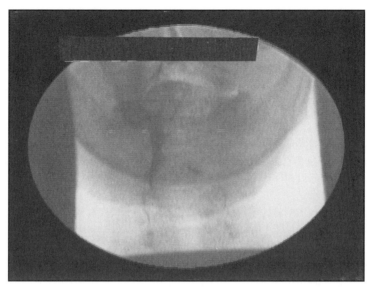

Figure 4.3. Anterior view of the oral cavity showing residual food in the lateral sulcus between the lateral mandible and the facial musculature.

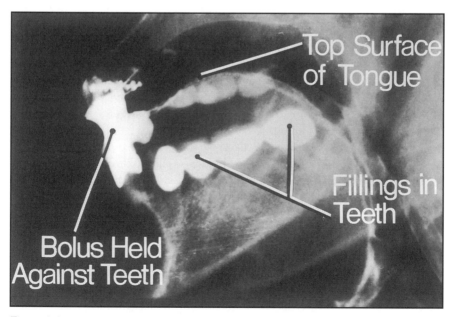

Figure 4.4. Lateral view of the oral cavity illustrating the abnormal hold position against the central incisors prior to initiating the swallow.

toward the lips and central incisors, thereby pushing the bolus forward). Often this tongue thrust is so strong that it actually pushes the food out of the oral cavity. As described here, this tongue thrust relates to neurologic impairment and is seen in some patients with cerebral palsy and in some individuals after stroke or head trauma.

Other

This space is provided for the clinician to note any other abnormal movement patterns that may be observed during the oral preparatory phase of the swallow in the lateral view.

Posture/Treatment Introduced

Space is provided on the worksheet to note any treatment procedures introduced and evaluated during the radiographic study.

Disorders in the Oral Phase of Deglutition

The oral phase of deglutition consists of lingual propulsion of the bolus through the oral cavity. This phase of the swallow is considered under voluntary cortical control, but plays a role in the initiation (triggering) of the pharyngeal swallow. The oral phase of the swallow begins with the lateral and anterior margins of the tongue sealed against the alveolar ridge. The anterior midline of the tongue initiates backward movement of the bolus with an upward, backward motion. Oral transit terminates when the pharyngeal swallow is triggered (Kahrilas, Lin, Logemann, Ergun, & Facchini, 1993; Shawker, Sonies, Stone, & Baum, 1983). The pharyngeal swallow is normally triggered when the head of the bolus reaches any point from the anterior faucial arch to the point where the lower edge of the mandible crosses the base of the tongue from sensory input to (predominantly) cranial nerve IX (i.e., the glossopharyngeal nerve). The total time for oral transit in normal individuals is approximately 1 to 1.25 seconds for all consistencies of material swallowed (Mandelstam & Lieber, 1970; Tracy et al., 1989).

Delayed Oral Onset of Swallow—Apraxia of Swallow; Reduced Oral Sensation

Some patients with severe neurological impairments exhibit significant delay in initiating the oral swallow when given a swallow command. Often the bolus is held in the mouth with no lingual movement. This symptom may indicate a severe swallow apraxia, reduced oral sensation, or lack of recognition of the bolus as something to be swallowed (oral tactile agnosia for food). The clinician can increase sensory stimulation for these patients by increasing the pressure of the spoon on the tongue as the bolus is presented, using a cold bolus, a larger bolus, a stronger tasting bolus, or a textured bolus, which may cause the oral swallow to begin (see Chapter 6). Also, some of these patients will not react to liquid or pureed material placed in the mouth, but will begin chewing in response to a small piece of cookie and, after the chewing, will begin the oral swallow.

Searching Tongue Movements—Apraxia of Swallow

Apraxia of swallow often accompanies severe oral apraxia. Symptoms of swallow apraxia include searching movements with the tongue, exhibiting good range of motion but inability to organize the front-to-back lingual and bolus movement normally characteristic of a swallow, or, in some cases, simply holding the bolus without initiating any oral activity, as discussed previously. Increasing sensory stimulation as the bolus is presented or giving a bolus that has a distinct temperature, flavor, or texture may facilitate more organized tongue movement during the oral swallow. Also, presenting the bolus to the patient on a spoon and allowing the patient to place the bolus in his or her own mouth or giving the patient the food and spoon to feed himself or herself normally may facilitate oral activity. Refraining from giving any commands to swallow can also be helpful, because apraxia is usually worse when the target activity becomes highly volitional.

Tongue Moves Forward To Start Swallow—Tongue Thrust

Normally, when the bolus is on the tongue, the tongue tip remains anchored against the alveolar ridge and initiates the swallow by lifting the midline sequentially in an upward and backward direction against the palate. At times, neurologic impairment may cause the tongue to thrust forward toward the central incisors, sometimes pushing food from the mouth, as shown in Figure 4.5.

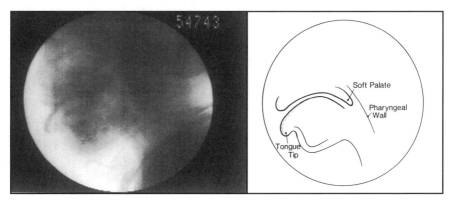

Figure 4.5. Lateral radiographic view of the oral cavity in a child with cerebral palsy showing a severe tongue thrust with the tongue protruding well out between the lips.

Usually, a tongue thrust is preceded by an abnormal hold position of the bolus against the central incisors, or inability to hold the bolus at all, as is seen in some individuals with cerebral palsy.

Residue in Anterior Sulcus—Reduced Labial Tension/Tone

If, during initiation of the oral phase of the swallow, the bolus lodges in the anterior sulcus, it is a symptom of reduced labial–buccal muscle tension or tone.

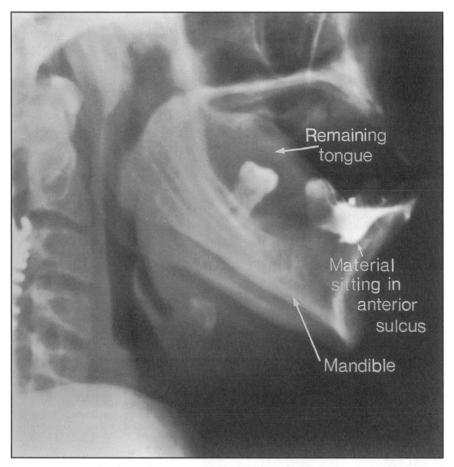

Figure 4.6. Lateral radiographic view of food collecting on the anterior floor of mouth and anterior sulcus in an oral cancer patient whose anterior floor of mouth was surgically resected.

Residue in the Lateral Sulcus—Reduced Buccal Tension/Tone

If, during initiation of the oral phase of the swallow, food falls or lodges in the lateral sulcus, as shown in Figure 4.3, it is an indication of reduced muscle tension or tone in the buccal musculature. Some investigators believe that buccal muscle tension plays a role in the backward movement of the bolus during oral transit by providing resistance or pressure in the lateral walls of the oral cavity (Shedd, Scatliff, & Kirchner, 1960).

Residue on the Floor of the Mouth—Reduced Tongue Shaping or Failure of the Peripheral Seal of the Tongue to the Anterior and Lateral Alveolus

If food falls onto the anterior or lateral floor of the mouth during attempts at oral transit, it is an indication of reduced ability to shape and coordinate the tongue around the bolus and/or to maintain contact of the tongue tip and sides of the tongue to the alveolus as the bolus moves posteriorly. Figure 4.6 illustrates residual food on the anterior floor of mouth in a surgically treated oral cancer patient, and Figure 4.7 illustrates residue on the lateral floor of mouth in another surgically treated oral cancer patient.

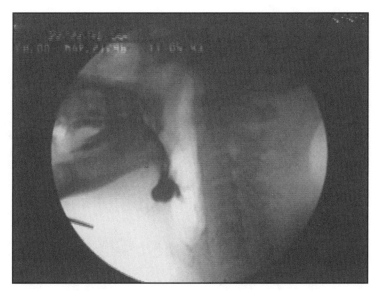

Figure 4.7. Lateral radiographic view illustrating residual food on the lateral floor of mouth in a surgically treated oral cancer patient. The patient also exhibits premature spillage from the mouth to the valleculae.

Residue in a Midtongue Depression—Tongue Scarring

If food tends to lodge in a depression in the tongue's surface, this usually indicates scar tissue in the tongue. Scar tissue can appear quite benign on anatomic examination (i.e., when the speech pathologist or physician does an oral examination of the tongue). However, scar tissue is usually tight and relatively immobile so that when the patient attempts to swallow, the normal tongue tissue surrounding the scar can elevate and move, but the scar tissue cannot, thus forming a deep crevice into which food will fall as the patient struggles to swallow. The greater the lingual struggle to swallow, the worse the effect of the scar tissue on the swallow, and the greater the amount of food that collects in the depression created by the scar tissue. Figure 4.8 illustrates residue in a midtongue depression in a surgically treated oral cancer patient. When scar tissue is present, it is usually the result of surgical treatment for oral cancer or some trauma to the mouth, such as a knife or gunshot wound.

Residue of Food on the Tongue—Reduced Tongue Range of Movement or Strength

If tongue range of movement is very poor, food may sit on the tongue surface or the hard palate and remain there despite numerous attempts to initiate a

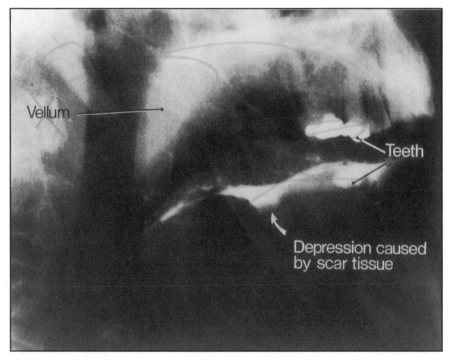

Figure 4.8. Lateral radiographic view of a collection of residual material in the midtongue depression created by a scar tissue in a surgically treated oral cancer patient.

swallow. This usually occurs with food of thicker consistency, since liquid tends to splash around the oral cavity and collect in the natural crevices in the oral cavity rather than on the tongue itself. Any stasis or residue of food on the tongue is an indication of reduced tongue range of movement. If the residue increases as food becomes more viscous, it is an indication of reduced tongue strength.

Disturbed Lingual Contraction (Peristalsis)—Lingual Discoordination

In normal swallowing, the tongue tip and sides remain in contact with the anterior and lateral alveolar ridge, while the front and center of the tongue envelop the bolus and then elevate and squeeze or roll the bolus along the hard palate until it reaches the back of the oral cavity or pharynx. Thus, the midline of the tongue is elevating sequentially while squeezing against the palate. This is done in a single organized action. If this sequential squeezing action is in any way disturbed (e.g., if the tongue moves in somewhat random, nonproductive motions), the normal smooth anterior–posterior movement becomes disorganized. This disturbed lingual contraction is to be distinguished from a repetitive kind of tongue movement pattern, such as the repetitive lingual rolling motion often seen in patients with Parkinson's disease, described later.

Incomplete Tongue–Palate Contact—Reduced Tongue Elevation

In the normal initiation of a swallow, sequential front-to-back tongue–palate contact is made as the bolus is moved backward. If tongue–palate contact is incomplete, it is an indication of reduced range of vertical tongue motion. This may also result in disturbances in lingual contraction, or struggling behavior of the tongue. If there is a great deal of lingual struggling action, the bolus may be spread throughout the mouth.

Adherence (Residue) of Food on the Hard Palate— Reduced Tongue Elevation or Strength

Normally, as the tongue propels the bolus posteriorly, only minimal food residue is left coating the oral structures. When food is observed to collect on the hard palate and to remain there after the swallow, it is an indication of reduced tongue elevation. If increased amounts of food collect on the palate as more viscous food is presented, it is an indication of reduced tongue strength, because increased lingual pressure is needed to propel more viscous food cleanly through the oral cavity. Figure 4.9 illustrates residual food collected on the palate in a patient with motor neuron disease.

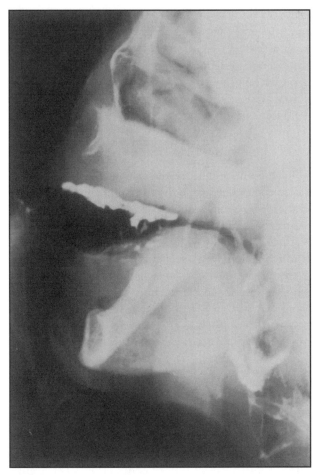

Figure 4.9. Lateral radiographic view of reduced tongue strength as indicated by the entire pudding bolus caught on the hard palate. The patient has adequate vertical motion to contact the palate but not adequate strength to move the material from the palate.

Reduced Anterior–Posterior Tongue Movement—Reduced Lingual Coordination

Normal lingual propulsion of the bolus involves smooth front-to-back action of the midline of the tongue with the sides and tip of the tongue maintaining contact with the lateral and anterior alveolar ridge. If this smooth front-to-back action is interrupted or broken into multiple small tongue movements in the presence of normal range of motion, it is a symptom of reduced lingual coordination.

Repetitive Lingual Rocking–Rolling Actions—Parkinson's Disease

In the normal swallow, the midline of the tongue produces a single upward and backward motion, propelling the bolus posteriorly. Patients with Parkinson's disease show a typical tongue movement pattern characterized by a repetitive upward and backward movement of the central portion of the tongue (Robbins, Logemann, & Kirshner, 1986). The posterior tongue, however, fails to lower at the appropriate time, so the bolus can move only to the region of the posterior hard palate before it rolls forward again. The front tongue activity then repeats itself in an attempt to reinitiate the swallow. This repetitive front-to-back rolling motion of the tongue often lasts 10 seconds or more before a full swallow is initiated in patients with Parkinson's disease.

Uncontrolled Bolus/Premature Loss of Liquid or Pudding Consistency into the Pharynx—Reduced Tongue Control; Reduced Linguavelar Seal

An uncontrolled bolus or premature loss of liquid or pudding into the pharynx indicates that, during the oral preparatory phase prior to initiation of the oral stage of swallow, or during the lingual initiation of the swallow, part or all of the bolus has already fallen over the base of the tongue, prematurely, into the pharynx. By definition, this occurs while the oral preparatory or oral stages of swallow are still under way, prior to the triggering of the pharyngeal swallow. When liquid or pudding boluses are placed in the mouth, the soft palate should be pulled down and anteriorly against the back of the tongue, sealing the bolus in the mouth posteriorly. If this seal fails, part or all of the bolus can be lost into the pharynx prematurely. On foods requiring chewing, premature loss of food into the valleculae is normal, because the contact of the soft palate to the back of the tongue is not maintained due to the vigorous chewing motions. Thus, during the radiographic study of oropharyngeal swallow, if premature loss of bolus is observed on liquid or pudding materials, it is abnormal; however, it is not an abnormal behavior during chewing, because the soft palate seal to the back of the tongue is broken by active tongue movement.

When part of the liquid or pudding bolus falls into the pharynx prematurely, it may lodge in the valleculae or the pyriform sinuses, or it may fall into the open airway. The exact path of the food when it lands in the pharynx depends on the patient's posture, the amount of food taken, and the consistency of the food. An uncontrolled bolus and premature loss indicate reduced lingual control during the oral preparatory or oral phase of the swallow. This may result in aspiration *before* the swallow since a part of the bolus is lost into the pharynx before the pharyngeal swallow is triggered and while the airway is open. It is important to note that the entry of this material into the pharynx does not trigger a pharyngeal swallow. In all probability, no pharyngeal swallow is triggered because the tongue has not yet completed its necessary movement in the oral stage of the swallow. The patient is barely initiating the oral phase of the swallow when part of the material falls into the pharynx in an uncontrolled manner. Until the tongue propels the remaining bolus to the point where a pharyngeal swallow would be triggered, the mere presence of this material in the pharynx will *not* trigger the pharyngeal swallow. It may be that this lack of initiation of the pharyngeal swallow in response to material in the pharynx indicates a neurological "priority" system. That is, as long as the patient is still in the oral preparatory or oral phases of the swallow, this voluntary motor activity may neurologically override the sensory input from the food in the pharynx, which might otherwise trigger a pharyngeal swallow. Figure 4.10 (A and B) illustrates premature loss of a bolus into the pharynx.

If food requiring chewing is given to the patient, premature loss of food into the pharynx (valleculae) is normal. It is most apt to occur when larger amounts of food requiring chewing are placed in the mouth. Premature loss of food is not normal on small (1- to 10-ml) measured amounts of liquid or pudding unless the material is masticated.

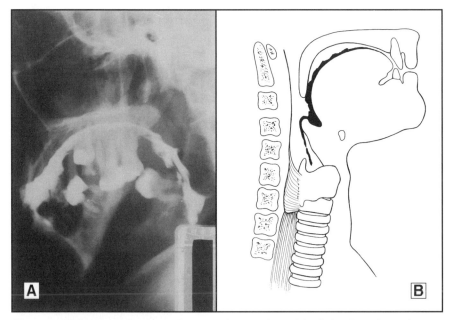

Figure 4.10. (A) Lateral radiographic view showing loss of the bolus from the oral cavity into the pharynx. In this case, the bolus is spread from the front of the oral cavity, over the back of the tongue, and into the vallecula. (B) Lateral diagram of the mechanism of aspiration in a patient who has lost bolus control because of poor tongue coordination or range of motion with bolus trickling from the oral cavity into the vallecula and then into the airway.

Piecemeal Deglutition

The term *piecemeal deglutition* indicates that, rather than swallowing the bolus in a single cohesive mass, the patient swallows only one portion or piece of the bolus at a time. Thus the patient requires two, three, or more repeated swallows to empty the oral cavity. This might be normal behavior if the bolus were very large (e.g., 20 to 30 ml); however, in the modified barium swallow, the patient is initially given only small amounts of food to swallow. These small amounts should be cleared from the oral cavity in a single swallow. Piecemeal deglutition may indicate a fear of swallowing, as the patient carefully meters out small amounts to be swallowed for fear of swallowing an entire bolus and aspirating.

Oral Transit Time (in Seconds)

As indicated earlier, oral transit time in normal individuals should last no more than 1 to 1.50 seconds and increases slightly as bolus viscosity increases. In subjects over age 60, oral transit also increases slightly (by approximately 0.25 seconds). The reason for abnormally slowed oral transit time should be defined according to the disorder observed in the oral phase of swallow. A slow oral transit time must be considered in combination with pharyngeal transit time to determine the full duration of the oropharyngeal swallow. The speed of the swallow through the oral and pharyngeal stages is one important factor in determining whether a patient is going to get sufficient nutrition and/or hydration by mouth.

Other

This space is provided on the worksheet for the clinician to note any other abnormal movement patterns or disorders that may be observed during the oral phase of the swallow in the lateral view. Specific abnormal patterns of tongue movement that are characteristic of specific types of patients may be noted here.

Posture/Treatment Introduced

Postural and treatment techniques introduced to mitigate oral phase disorders can be noted at the end of this worksheet section, as can the effectiveness of these intervention strategies.

Disorders in Triggering the Pharyngeal Swallow: Transition Between Oral and Pharyngeal Stages of Swallow

Delayed Pharyngeal Swallow

Normally, when the head (the leading edge) of the bolus passes the tongue base, the point where the lower edge of the mandible crosses the tongue base, as

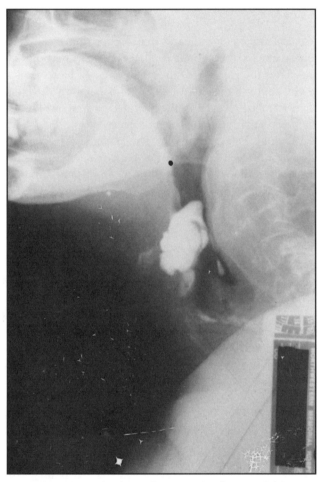

Figure 4.11. Lateral radiographic view of a pharyngeal delay on a pudding bolus that has lodged in the vallecula. The black dot indicates the trigger point, that is, the point where the pharyngeal swallow should trigger when the head of the bolus reaches it.

identified on Figures 4.11 and 4.12, the pharyngeal swallow should have begun. Delayed pharyngeal swallow occurs when the head of the bolus enters the pharynx and the pharyngeal swallow has not been triggered, as indicated by laryngeal elevation in the context of the rest of the pharyngeal swallow. The presence of the bolus head below the point where the tongue base crosses the lower edge of the mandible, increases the risk of aspiration as long as the pharyngeal swallow has not been initiated. Most patients with delay in triggering the pha-

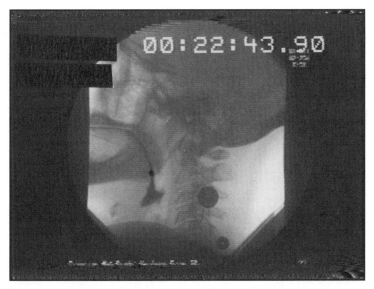

Figure 4.12. Lateral radiographic view of the pharynx with the bolus beginning to fall from the vallecula to the pyriform sinus during a pharyngeal delay.
The black dot indicates the trigger point. When the bolus head reaches this
point, the pharyngeal swallow should be seen to trigger.

ryngeal swallow complain of difficulty swallowing liquids. Thin liquids are usually swallowed in larger volumes (10 to 20 ml) and will splash into the pharynx
rapidly. If the pharyngeal swallow has not been initiated as the liquid passes the
tongue base, there is increased risk that the liquid will enter the open airway
before the pharyngeal swallow has been activated. During a pharyngeal swallow
delay, the bolus may land in the pyriform sinuses, the valleculae, or the open airway. Where the bolus rests during the delay is a result of gravity, head posture,
and food consistency, and is not the major symptom of a pharyngeal swallow
delay. The critical symptom of delay is the location of the bolus head—that is,
it has progressed too far down into the pharynx before the pharyngeal swallow
is activated. The bolus head must be differentiated from premature bolus loss.
The bolus head is the leading edge of the main portion of the bolus. Premature
bolus loss occurs during the oral preparatory or oral stages of the swallow as part
of the bolus breaks away from the main portion of the bolus and falls over the
tongue base. Premature bolus loss is not a delay in triggering the pharyngeal
swallow.

If the bolus reaches the pyriform sinuses, as shown in Figure 4.13, before the
pharyngeal swallow triggers, there is increased risk of aspiration as the pharyngeal swallow is activated because the pyriform sinuses are significantly shortened

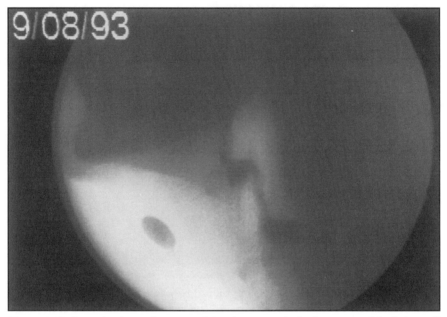

Figure 4.13. Lateral radiographic view of the pharynx with the large part of the bolus well into the pyriform sinus during a pharyngeal delay.

as the pharynx and larynx elevate during the pharyngeal swallow. If the pyriform sinuses fill with food or liquid during the delay in triggering the pharyngeal swallow, as the pharynx and larynx are initially elevating, the contents of the pyriform sinuses are at high risk of being dumped into the airway, as shown in Figure 4.14. In patients with a delayed pharyngeal swallow in whom the bolus falls to the pyriform sinuses, a chin-down posture may be less helpful (Shanahan, Logemann, Rademaker, Pauloski, & Kahrilas, 1993). The chin-down posture affects the anterior–posterior pharyngeal dimensions, that is, narrowing the laryngeal entrance and the distance between the epiglottis and the pharyngeal wall and the tongue base and the pharyngeal wall. These changes occur above the level of the pyriform sinuses. Chin-down posture neither changes the degree of pharyngeal shortening that occurs during swallow, nor prevents the contents of the pyriform sinus from emptying into the airway if the bolus reaches the pyriform sinuses.

Occasionally, the swallow in which the bolus falls to the pyriform sinus during the pharyngeal delay has been misdiagnosed as a cricopharyngeal disorder or "late opening" of the cricopharyngeus. This is not a cricopharyngeal disorder; the cricopharyngeal region is not dysfunctional. The sphincter is not opening because the *swallow center* or *central pattern generator* in the brainstem (the

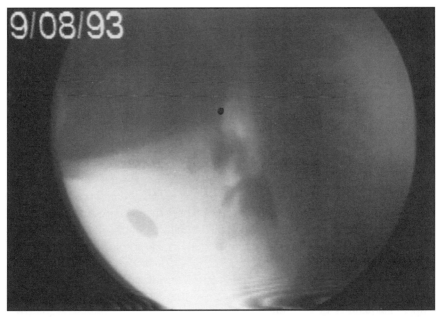

9/08/93

Figure 4.14. Lateral radiographic view of the pharynx immediately after pharyngeal swallow triggering, as the larynx begins its elevation. With laryngeal elevation, the pharynx is shortened and the contents of the pyriform sinus overflow into the larynx, as shown here. Again, the black dot is the trigger point.

medulla) has not programmed it to open (i.e., the entire pharyngeal swallow has not been triggered).

Timing the Pharyngeal Delay

In the report of the radiographic study, the duration of the pharyngeal delay should be noted. This serves as a baseline measure against which treatment effects can be defined. The delay is timed from the initial video frame showing the bolus head passing the point where the lower edge of the mandible crosses the tongue base (as illustrated in Figures 4.11 and 4.12) until the first frame where the pharyngeal swallow is initiated (where laryngeal and hyoid elevation begin as part of the pharyngeal swallow). In the pharyngeal swallow, elevation of the larynx and hyoid are the first events. These actions serve as a marker for triggering of the pharyngeal swallow, if they are followed by activation of the rest of the pharyngeal swallow. During a pharyngeal swallow delay, many patients struggle to stimulate a swallow, and in the struggle behavior, move their tongue base forward and backward and lift the larynx up and down. These movements are not the same as those seen during the pharyngeal swallow. When timing the pharyngeal swallow delay, these movements of the larynx up and down as the oral tongue and tongue base are moving to try to stimulate a swallow are not part of the pharyngeal swallow and should not be identified as such. It is easy to iden-tify the triggering of the pharyngeal swallow by watching the swallow as it pro-gresses and reversing the videotape in slow motion until the larynx first comes back to rest. Any laryngeal movements prior to the actual pharyngeal swallow should be considered part of the delay.

In normal young adult subjects, pharyngeal delay is minimal (0 to 0.2 sec-onds) and the pharyngeal swallow often triggers as the bolus head reaches the anterior faucial arch. In normal subjects over age 60, there is a statistically significant prolongation of the delay by approximately 0.4 to 0.5 seconds (Tracy et al., 1989). In these older normal subjects, the bolus head may reach the middle of the tongue base, or specifically the point where the lower rim of the mandible crosses the tongue base on a radiograph. A delay of more than 2 seconds, or an even shorter delay during which aspiration occurs, is considered an abnormal delay in adults, regardless of age.

The pharyngeal triggering and delay time in infants and young children is quite different from those in adults because the bolus may be collected in the valleculae before the pharyngeal swallow is triggered. In an infant, an abnormal delay is defined as more than 1 second between the last tongue pump and the onset of the pharyngeal swallow, or aspiration occurring during bolus collection.

Disorders in the Pharyngeal Stage of Deglutition

The pharyngeal phase of deglutition begins when the pharyngeal swallow is trig-gered as the bolus passes the anterior faucial arch or the back or base of tongue, and continues until the bolus passes through the cricopharyngeal region, also known as the upper esophageal segment (UES), or the pharyngoesophageal (PE) segment. Normal pharyngeal transit time is a maximum of 1 second, regardless of the patient's age or material swallowed. For small volume swallows, pharyngeal transit time is approximately 0.32 seconds and increases as volume increases. Disorders of the pharyngeal phase of the swallow include dysfunctions of any of the neuromuscular components that actualize the pharyngeal swallow or charac-terize the pharyngeal motor response.

Nasal Penetration During Swallow—Reduced Velopharyngeal Closure

When velopharyngeal closure is inadequate, material can backflow into the nose during swallow, as shown in Figure 4.15. However, it is important to note that velopharyngeal closure during the swallow lasts for only a fraction of a second as the bolus passes the velopharyngeal port. If nasal backflow occurs later in the

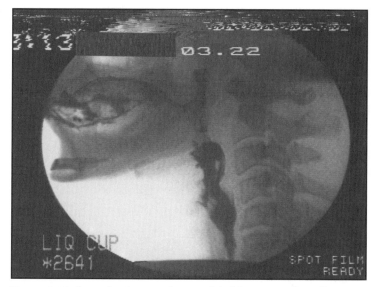

Figure 4.15. Lateral videoprint from modified barium swallow illustrating nasal regurgitation in a postsurgical oral cancer patient.

swallow, it may be the result of a dysfunction farther down in the pharynx. If the bolus cannot pass through the pharynx into the esophagus, food, especially liquid, will often move back upward, as a result of any struggling action in the pharynx, and at that moment the velopharyngeal port is normally open, since velopharyngeal closure is complete only as the bolus passes the nasopharynx. When a patient complains of nasal leakage of food, a complete examination of the pharynx during swallow is warranted.

Pseudoepiglottis (After Total Laryngectomy)

After total laryngectomy some patients exhibit a fold of mucosa at the base of the tongue. This fold of tissue forms what appears to be an epiglottis when viewed radiographically in the lateral plane (see Figure 4.16). This pseudoepiglottis can look quite benign when viewed anatomically at rest because it collapses against the base of the tongue and leaves an open pharynx posteriorly. However, when the patient attempts to swallow, whatever contraction occurs in the pharyngeal constrictors will pull the tissue fold posteriorly and narrow the pharynx so that the patient can barely move any food past the pseudoepiglottis. It is important to assess the effect of this tissue fold on swallow function physiologically through fluoroscopy, rather than depending only on an anatomic examination.

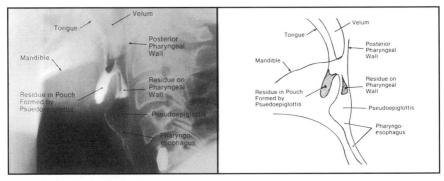

Figure 4.16. Lateral radiographic view of a pseudoepiglottis and the pouch formed by the pseudoepiglottis containing residual barium.

Bony Outgrowth from Cervical Vertebrae—Cervical Osteophytes

Bony outgrowths from the cervical vertebrae are known as cervical osteophytes (see Figure 4.17) (Blumberg, Prapote, & Viscomi, 1977). At times they can be large enough to interfere with the swallow by narrowing the pharynx, or they may direct the bolus toward the airway entrance (Parker, 1989; Saunders, 1971; Valadka, Kubal, & Smith, 1995). At other times they may simply cause patients to have the sensation of a swallowing disorder (i.e., the sense of "something there" when they swallow). During the radiographic study, the clinician should always scan the cervical vertebrae for any abnormalities.

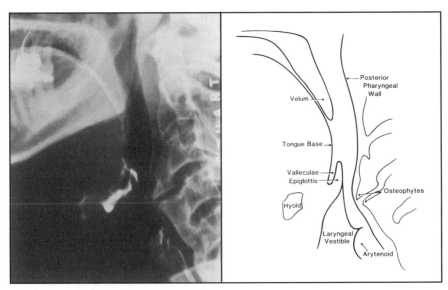

Figure 4.17. Lateral radiographic view of large cervical osteophytes.

Residue on One Side of Pharynx and in Pyriform Sinus—
Unilateral Pharyngeal Wall Weakness

If one side of the pharynx is weak, food tends to cling to that pharyngeal wall and collect in the pyriform sinus on that side. This is visible in the A–P view and is further discussed later in this chapter.

Coating on the Pharyngeal Walls After the Swallow—
Reduced Pharyngeal Contraction Bilaterally

After the swallow in normal individuals, only a minimal residue of material is left in the pharynx. In many normal subjects, no residue whatsoever remains. Older normal individuals exhibit only a slight increase in residue as compared with younger adults. Figures 4.18 and 4.19 illustrate the range of normal pharyngeal residue. To some extent, the amount of coating in the pharynx varies with the type of barium contrast given. Some types of barium contrast agents cause a greater amount of coating, even in normal individuals, than other types of barium. In general, if the pharyngeal structures are merely lightly coated with barium after the swallow, as if the barium has mixed with saliva or mucus, this is a normal amount of residue. If, however, a significant amount of residual material is on the pharyngeal walls, as judged by the apparent density of the material remaining, it would be considered abnormal and a symptom of reduced

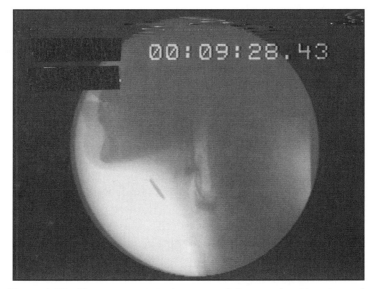

Figure 4.18. Illustrates a minimal amount of pharyngeal residue observed in normal individuals after the swallow. Some normal individuals have no residue.

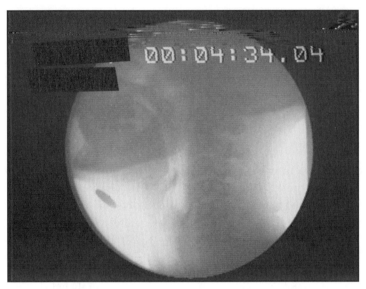

Figure 4.19. Lateral radiographic view of the pharynx illustrating maximum residue observed in normal swallowers after the swallow. Interestingly, Figure 4.18 is of a normal 32-year-old individual and Figure 4.19 is of a normal 74-year-old swallower.

pharyngeal contraction (peristalsis) bilaterally. A normal individual would dry swallow immediately after the food swallow to clear this residue. It is important to watch for the patient's reaction to any residue left in the pharynx after the swallow. Does he or she dry swallow or attempt to dry swallow, indicating awareness of the residue? Whenever any larger amount of residue remains in the pharynx after the swallow, the patient is at risk for aspiration following the swallow if he or she inhales any of the residue.

Vallecular Residue After Swallow—Reduced Tongue Base Posterior Movement

When the bolus tail reaches the tongue base and/or vallecular level during the normal swallow, the tongue base moves posteriorly to contact the anteriorly bulging pharyngeal wall. Approximately two thirds of the distance between the tongue base and the posterior pharyngeal wall at rest is encompassed by the posterior tongue base movement and one third by the anterior movement of the posterior pharyngeal wall (Kahrilas, Logemann, Lin, & Ergun, 1992). Clearance of the valleculae largely appears to be the result of the tongue base movement. When vallecular residue is noted, tongue base movement should be observed carefully, to determine if it is adequate and makes complete contact with the

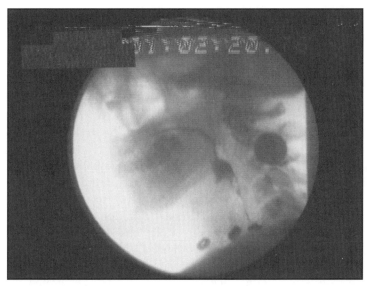

Figure 4.20. Lateral radiographic view of the pharynx illustrating significant residue of pudding in the vallecula after the swallow indicating reduced tongue base motion.

anteriorly bulging posterior pharyngeal wall. Figure 4.20 illustrates residue in the valleculae as the result of reduced posterior tongue base motion. If the residue in the valleculae is a large amount, the patient may be at risk of aspirating some or all of the residue during respiration after the swallow. Again, if the patient is aware of this residue, he or she should dry swallow in an attempt to clear this material.

Coating in a Depression on the Pharyngeal Wall—Scar Tissue; Pharyngeal Pouch

Collection of material in a depression on the pharyngeal wall may be an indication of the beginning of a pharyngeal pouch or scar tissue in the pharynx. If a patient has had a pharyngocutaneous fistula, the internal end of the fistula will often heal as a scar tissue depression, which will collect material during and after the swallow. As with any pharyngeal residue, the patient is at risk for aspiration *after* the swallow if the residue is a large amount.

Reduced Laryngeal Elevation—Residue at Top of Airway

In normal individuals, when the pharyngeal swallow is triggered, the larynx elevates and moves anteriorly to tuck itself under the base of the tongue, as a component of airway protection. During swallow, the larynx elevates approximately 2 cm in normal young adult men (Jacob, Kahrilas, Logemann, Shah, & Ha, 1989).

If laryngeal elevation during the swallow is mildly impaired, some residual material will remain on top of the larynx after the swallow. Pharyngeal contraction cannot completely clear material from the top of the airway when the larynx is in an abnormally lowered position. Thus, the patient is at risk for aspiration of the food sitting on top of the airway after the swallow, when he or she opens the larynx to inhale following deglutition.

As the larynx elevates, the arytenoid cartilage is brought to a level where it is closer to the base of the epiglottis and can tilt forward to contact the thickening base of the epiglottis and close the entrance to the airway (Logemann et al., 1992). Moderately reduced laryngeal elevation can, therefore, result in inability of the arytenoids to tilt anteriorly enough to make good contact with the epiglottic base, leaving the entrance to the airway slightly open, allowing penetration of the bolus *into* the airway entrance. If the larynx does not continue to lift to a normal degree and material has penetrated the airway entrance, this material will remain in the airway entrance and usually be aspirated after the swallow. Some patients can compensate for reduced laryngeal elevation by tilting the arytenoid more anteriorly than normal to close the airway entrance. These patients will not have penetration into the airway entrance, despite reduced laryngeal elevation. Sometimes, these patients begin arytenoid tilting before the swallow begins, thus closing the airway entrance preventatively before and during the swallow. This occurs more often with large volume swallows.

Laryngeal Penetration and Aspiration After the Swallow: Reduced Closure of the Airway Entrance (Arytenoid to Base of Epiglottis and False Vocal Folds)

Laryngeal penetration occurs when food or liquid enters the vestibule or entrance of the airway to any level but not below the superior surface of the true vocal folds. In contrast, aspiration involves entry of food into the airway below the true vocal folds. Both penetration and aspiration are symptoms of a variety of swallowing problems. Observation of penetration or aspiration on an X-ray study of swallow should cause the clinician to review the videotaped swallow carefully to identify the anatomic or physiologic cause of the penetration or aspiration.

Etiologies of Laryngeal Penetration

Laryngeal penetration can occur as a result of a variety of etiologies. The bolus may penetrate to a variety of levels, as shown in Figures 4.21, 4.22, and 4.23

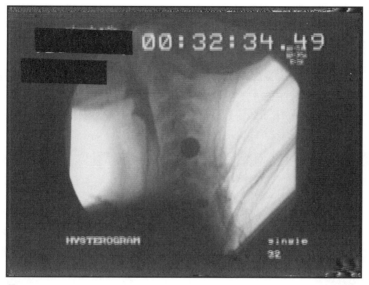

Figure 4.21. Lateral radiographic view of minimal bolus penetration into the airway entrance. There is a slight "hook" over the arytenoid.

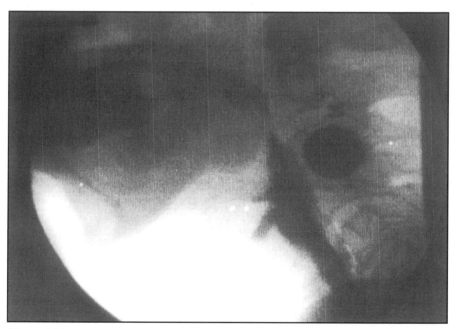

Figure 4.22. A lateral videoprint illustrating penetration of liquid into the airway entrance to the level of the false vocal folds because of moderately reduced laryngeal elevation.

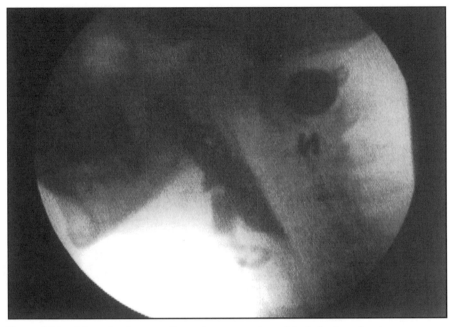

Figure 4.23. A lateral videoprint illustrating penetration of the bolus into the airway entrance to the level of the true vocal folds during a pharyngeal swallow delay, before the pharyngeal swallow was triggered. This 10-ml bolus has filled the pharynx and entered the laryngeal vestibule (airway entrance) to the surface of the true vocal folds.

(Rosenbek, Robbins, Roecker, Coyle, & Wood, 1996). The bolus may enter the airway to the level of the middle of the arytenoid cartilage, the level of the surface of the false vocal folds, or the level of the true vocal folds. Penetration can occur if the larynx lifts inadequately and thus leaves the airway entrance slightly open; or if the arytenoid cartilage fails to tilt forward adequately to close off the entrance to the airway; or if the larynx lifts too slowly during the swallow. If the larynx lifts too slowly but eventually lifts to its full range of motion, all of the penetrated material will usually be cleared from the airway entrance. Figures 4.24 and 4.25 illustrate penetration in supraglottic laryngectomees because of failure of the arytenoid to fully tilt and contact the tongue base.

In normal individuals, when laryngeal penetration occurs, the material in the airway is squeezed out during the swallow as the larynx continues to lift and close inferiorly to superiorly. Penetration is a problem only when the larynx fails to lift adequately during the course of the swallow, and the penetrated material remains in the larynx after the swallow, and is then aspirated as the individual inhales following the swallow. Penetration may also occur if the bolus falls into the airway entrance before the pharyngeal swallow triggers; that is, penetration

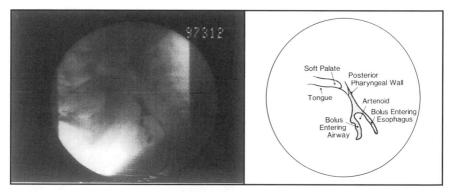

Figure 4.24. Penetration of a bolus into the airway to the level of the surface of the true vocal folds in a supraglottic laryngectomee.

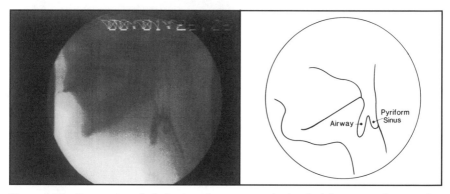

Figure 4.25. Penetration of a bolus into the airway to the level of the true cords in another supraglottic laryngectomee.

results from a delay in triggering the pharyngeal swallow, as shown in Figure 4.23. If the patient who has a delayed pharyngeal swallow has the vocal folds closed during the delay, food or liquid may enter the airway entrance but not proceed further than the surface of the true vocal folds. When the pharyngeal swallow triggers and the larynx lifts and closes from the level of the true vocal folds upward, this penetrated material is usually cleared efficiently from the airway, as shown in Figure 4.26.

Aspiration, like penetration, has a wide range of etiologies. When aspiration is seen on the videofluoroscopic study, the clinician should carefully review the videotaped swallow in slow motion and frame by frame to identify the etiology of the aspiration. The etiology for any aspiration should be clearly noted in the patient's report.

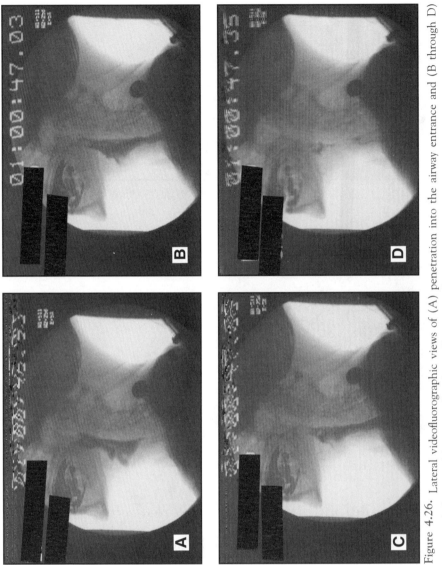

Figure 4.26. Lateral videofluorographic views of (A) penetration into the airway entrance and (B through D) sequential clearing of the material as the swallow proceeds.

Aspiration During Swallow—Reduced Laryngeal Closure

During the pharyngeal phase of the swallow, the larynx closes at three levels or valves: (1) the true vocal folds; (2) the arytenoid to base of epiglottis and false vocal folds (i.e., the airway entrance); and (3) the aryepiglottic folds and epiglottis. The true vocal folds close as the larynx elevates about 50% of its full distance. If the larynx does not close adequately from bottom to top *during* the swallow, material will enter the airway *during* the swallow. It will appear as if the larynx is offering no obstruction to the flow of material into the airway, as shown in Figure 4.27A–B. This is the only etiology for aspiration *during* the swallow.

Residue (Stasis) in Both Pyriform Sinuses—Reduced Anterior Laryngeal Motion; Cricopharyngeal Dysfunction; Stricture

Normally, little or no residual material is in the pyriform sinuses after the swallow. When significant residue is in both pyriform sinuses, it is a symptom of reduced anterior laryngeal movement and/or cricopharyngeal dysfunction (upper esophageal valve dysfunction) or stricture at the level of the opening of the esophagus (Calcaterra, Kadell, & Ward, 1975). All other aspects of the swallow, including the triggering of the pharyngeal swallow, should be normal. If the pharyngeal swallow has not triggered, a cricopharyngeal disorder cannot be diagnosed. Because anterior and vertical hyolaryngeal movement controls cricopharyngeal opening and relaxation of the cricopharyngeal muscle is an enabling event, failure of this upper sphincter opening must be investigated further to determine which component is disordered (Kahrilas, Dodds, Dent, Logemann, & Shaker, 1988). Usually, pharyngeal manometry must be combined with videofluoroscopy to assess these components (Kahrilas & Logemann, 1993). Figure 4.28 illustrates residue in the pyriform sinuses in a 3-year-old child with a head injury and a cricopharyngeal disorder related to reduced anterior laryngeal movement.

Residue Throughout the Pharynx

If residue in the pyriform sinuses is combined with residue in other parts of the pharynx (valleculae, pharyngeal walls), as shown in Figure 4.29, it is a symptom of generalized dysfunction in pharyngeal pressure generation during the swallow, not an isolated cricopharyngeal problem. Generalized pharyngeal dysfunction includes reduced posterior movement of the tongue base and reduced pharyngeal wall movement. Often, laryngeal elevation is also reduced.

Pharyngeal Transit Time (in Seconds)

Normally, pharyngeal transit time is less than 1 second regardless of patient age or food consistency. Slowed pharyngeal transit time must be considered in

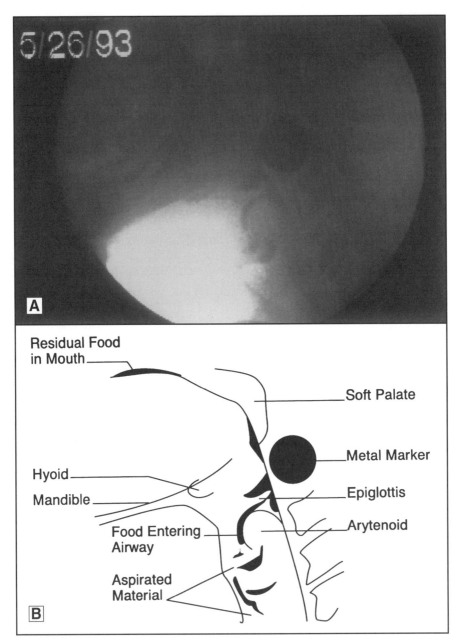

Figure 4.27. Aspiration during the swallow because of poor laryngeal closure at the entrance and the vocal folds. Figure B clarifies location of structures.

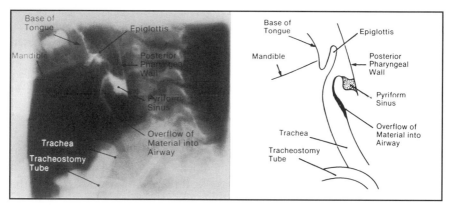

Figure 4.28. Lateral radiographic view of residue in the pyriform sinuses because of poor laryngeal anterior motion and resulting poor cricopharyngeal opening with overflow of the material into the airway in a 3-year-old child with a head injury.

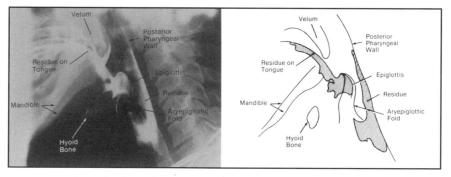

Figure 4.29. Lateral radiographic view of residue spread throughout the pharynx, down the tongue base, in the vallecula, on the posterior pharyngeal wall, and in the pyriform sinuses.

combination with oral transit time to determine the full duration of the oropharyngeal swallow. The speed of the swallow through the oral and pharyngeal stages is one important factor in determining whether a patient is going to get sufficient nutrition and hydration by mouth.

Other

This space on the worksheet is provided for the clinician to note any other abnormal movement patterns or structural problems that may be observed during the pharyngeal phase of deglutition in the lateral plane. An example of this would be a pharyngeal pouch.

Space is provided to note any treatment procedures introduced and evaluated during the radiographic study.

Disorders in the Cervical Esophageal Phase of Deglutition

The cervical esophageal phase of deglutition involves the initial peristaltic wave in the esophageal musculature. While the patient is being viewed radiographically in the lateral plane during the modified barium swallow, the cervical esophageal aspect of deglutition is observable. If there is any question about the patient's esophageal function, an esophageal study (traditional barium swallow) should be performed *after* the modified barium swallow is completed, or the patient should be referred to a gastroenterologist for assessment. In this way the patient's ability to swallow without aspiration will have been established and the barium swallow can be done safely. If the patient cannot swallow safely without aspiration, the esophageal examination can be postponed until the risk of aspiration is eliminated.

The esophageal stage of deglutition cannot be modified by therapy, although postural changes are sometimes helpful. It is, however, important that the swallowing clinician be aware of those esophageal disorders that can masquerade as pharyngeal phase swallowing disorders because they can cause backflow of the material out of the esophagus into the pharynx, thus also causing aspiration. A number of these disorders are defined here, particularly those that may present a diagnostic problem for the swallowing therapist and radiologist performing modified barium swallow procedures.

Esophageal-to-Pharyngeal Backflow

Esophageal-to-pharyngeal backflow of food is sometimes observed on a modified barium swallow and is a symptom of a number of esophageal disorders, including achalasia or failure of the lower esophageal sphincter to relax, reflux, tumor, stenosis, and so forth. Backflow of material out of the esophagus into the pharynx requires the upper esophageal sphincter to open, to allow this backflow to occur. Once material has come out of the esophagus into the pharynx, it may overflow into the airway, causing aspiration and possibly symptoms of a pharyngeal swallowing disorder. One cause of backflow is gastroesophageal reflux. Patients with reflux may exhibit redness in the arytenoid area of the larynx on indirect laryngoscopy because the material overflowing into the airway contains stomach acid. They may also complain of a burning sensation in their pharynx and/or esophagus, or frequent gagging or coughing. Aspirated material that contains any gastric acid is more irritating to the lungs than aspirated saliva or food.

Tracheoesophageal Fistula

Occasionally, a fistula (hole) can develop in the soft tissue common wall between the trachea and the esophagus. This fistula tract allows food entering the esophagus to flow back into the trachea. Patients with tracheoesophageal (TE) fistulae have symptoms similar to those of patients who aspirate after the swallow for other reasons (i.e., coughing after the swallow). Thus, they may be referred to a swallowing therapist for evaluation. Any time a patient with a history of possible aspiration is referred for a radiographic study, and the modified barium swallow results are normal, the radiographic study should be continued to evaluate the esophagus carefully to determine the presence or absence of a TE fistula. Because the fistula is usually located at the level of the 1st to 3rd thoracic vertebrae, the shoulders often shadow the radiographic image in the lateral plane. To improve visualization of this part of the esophagus and trachea, the patient's shoulders should be turned diagonally while the patient's head and body remain in the lateral view. Swallows should be repeated with the patient in this position and the fluoroscopic tube lowered to the base of the cervical esophagus in order to visualize the fistula tract.

Zenker's Diverticulum

A diverticulum is a side pocket that forms when pharyngeal or esophageal muscle herniates (Lund, 1968; Ponzoli, 1968). A Zenker's diverticulum occurs in the area of the cricopharyngeal region or upper esophageal sphincter. One theory of its genesis is that a hypertonic cricopharyngeus muscle requires the patient to increase pharyngeal pressures to push food through the upper esophageal sphincter, thus causing the tissue to herniate over time. On X-ray, the diverticulum appears as a round balloon that fills with radiopaque material as the patient swallows. After the swallow, the diverticulum usually empties of material. Upon emptying, this material may fall into the airway, causing aspiration after the swallow. Figure 4.30 presents a Zenker's diverticulum and the dynamics of the backflow.

Reflux or Gastroesophageal Reflux Disease (GERD)

The term *reflux* indicates a specific type of backflow—that is, backflow of food and stomach acid from the stomach to the esophagus because of a failure of the lower esophageal sphincter (LES) to keep food in the stomach (Henderson, Woolf, & Marryatt, 1976). In the modified barium swallow, reflux is usually not diagnosed because the study is not viewing the *lower* esophageal sphincter. If reflux is suspected from the patient's history, a consult to a gastroenterologist is indicated.

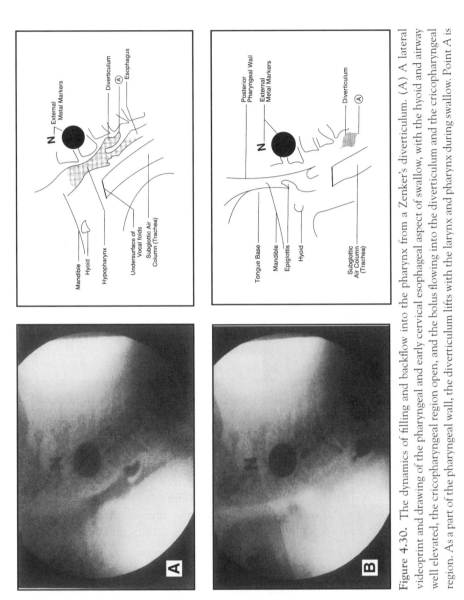

Figure 4.30. The dynamics of filling and backflow into the pharynx from a Zenker's diverticulum. (A) A lateral videoprint and drawing of the pharyngeal and early cervical esophageal aspect of swallow, with the hyoid and airway well elevated, the cricopharyngeal region open, and the bolus flowing into the diverticulum and the cricopharyngeal region. As a part of the pharyngeal wall, the diverticulum lifts with the larynx and pharynx during swallow. Point A is

(continued)

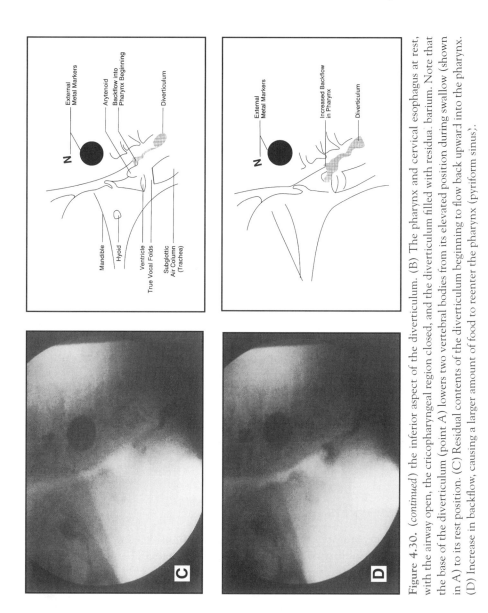

Figure 4.30. (*continued*) the inferior aspect of the diverticulum. (B) The pharynx and cervical esophagus at rest, with the airway open, the cricopharyngeal region closed, and the diverticulum filled with residual barium. Note that the base of the diverticulum (point A) lowers two vertebral bodies from its elevated position during swallow (shown in A) to its rest position. (C) Residual contents of the diverticulum beginning to flow back upward into the pharynx. (D) Increase in backflow, causing a larger amount of food to reenter the pharynx (pyriform sinus).

Other

This space on the worksheet is provided for the clinician to note any other abnormal movement patterns or structural problems that may be observed during the cervical esophageal aspect of the swallow.

Posture/Treatment Introduced

Space is provided to note any treatment procedures introduced and evaluated during the radiographic study. Generally, treatment for esophageal disorders is surgical or medical. However, there are times when a postural technique may facilitate swallow in these patients, such as in a Zenker's diverticulum when head rotation to one side or the other may close off the entry to the diverticulum.

The Posterior–Anterior View

The posterior–anterior radiographic view allows the clinician to examine the symmetry of structures and function in the oral cavity and pharynx during deglutition and in the larynx during phonation. In approximately 80% of normal individuals, the bolus divides fairly equally to pass down the two sides of the pharynx and into the esophagus; the other 20% swallow unilaterally (Logemann, Kahrilas, Kobara, & Vakil, 1989). The posterior–anterior plane also allows assessment of oral functions during mastication and preparation to swallow.

Oral Preparatory Phase

During the oral preparatory phase in the posterior–anterior view, the clinician can examine (1) the ability of the tongue to lateralize material and (2) the pattern of jaw motion in crushing the food during mastication. The shape of the tongue in holding the bolus prior to initiation of the swallow in the oral cavity can also be assessed. The sides of the tongue should be in contact with the lateral alveolus with a central groove down midline surrounding the bolus.

Unable To Align Teeth—Reduced Mandibular Movement

Some patients, particularly those who have had surgery to the lower jaw, will have difficulty putting the mandible into proper occlusion for chewing. This is an indication of reduced mandibular range of motion, and usually occurs when there has been removal of part of the mandible.

Unable To Lateralize Material with the Tongue—Reduced Tongue Lateralization

During chewing, the tongue lateralizes food or moves it to the side of the oral cavity, placing it onto the teeth. If the patient cannot lateralize food from the midline, it is an indication of reduced range of tongue movement laterally.

Unable To Mash Materials—Reduced Tongue Elevation

If a patient cannot lateralize food to the teeth for chewing, he or she may compensate or be asked to compensate by vertically crushing the food between the tongue and the palate. If the patient is unable to accomplish this mashing of food, it is an indication of reduced range of tongue elevation to the hard palate.

Material Falls into the Lateral Sulcus—Reduced Buccal Tension/Tone

If, as the patient is chewing, material falls into the lateral sulcus, it is an indication of reduced facial-buccal muscle tension or tone. It is facial-buccal muscle tension that closes the lateral sulcus and throws food medially to the tongue during mastication.

Material Falls to the Floor of the Mouth—Reduced Tongue Control

Food falling onto the floor of the mouth as the patient is chewing is a symptom of reduced tongue control, particularly in the seal of the lateral margins of the tongue to the lateral alveolus.

Bolus Spread Across Mouth—Reduced Lingual Shaping and Fine Tongue Control

When a liquid or paste bolus is placed into the oral cavity, the tongue normally shapes around the bolus to hold it in a cohesive ball. Also, after chewing, the tongue normally pulls the food together into a single bolus and shapes itself around the bolus so that the sides of the tongue are sealed to the superior lateral alveolar ridge. If the patient is unable to shape his or her tongue around the bolus (i.e., to elevate one or both sides of the tongue or form a central groove to contain the food), it is an indication of reduced fine control of the tongue.

Posture/Treatment Introduced

This space on the worksheet allows notation of postures or other treatment strategies introduced in the radiographic study and their effects.

Pharyngeal Phase

The pharyngeal phase of the swallow, as assessed in the posterior–anterior view, provides information on the unilateral nature of any pharyngeal swallowing disorder.

Unilateral Vallecular Residue—Unilateral Dysfunction
in Posterior Movement of the Tongue Base

When there is food left in the valleculae on only one side after the swallow, it indicates dysfunction of one side of the tongue base or the pharyngeal constrictors. This residue, if a large amount, may be aspirated *after* the swallow.

Residue in One Pyriform Sinus—Unilateral Dysfunction of Pharynx

Residue in only one pyriform sinus after the swallow indicates unilateral dysfunction of the pharyngeal walls. This may result from neurologic or structural damage. When a large amount of residue remains in the pharynx *after* the swallow, the patient is at risk for aspiration *after* the swallow should any of the residue be inhaled or fall into the airway. Figures 4.31 and 4.32 illustrate unilateral pharyngeal wall damage in an adult and a child, respectively. In contrast, Figure 4.33 illustrates bilateral pharyngeal wall impairment with residue on both sides of the pharynx.

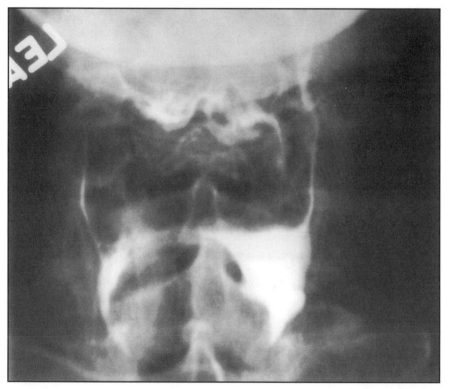

Figure 4.31. An anterior view of the pharynx illustrating unilateral pharyngeal wall damage with residue in one pyriform sinus. The pharyngeal wall on the damaged side enables the enlargement of the pyriform sinus on that side.

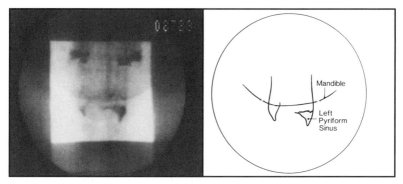

Figure 4.32. An anterior radiographic view of the pharynx showing an asymmetrical residue indicating unilateral pharyngeal wall impairment.

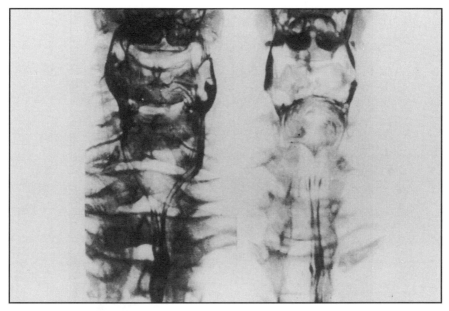

Figure 4.33. Anterior radiographic views showing fairly symmetrical residue in the vallecula, on the pharyngeal walls, and in the pyriform sinuses, indicating bilateral involvement of the pharyngeal walls.

Reduced Vocal Fold Adduction

With the patient's head tilted backward to get the mandible out of view, vocal fold adduction can be evaluated. The patient should be asked to repeat, "ah, ah, ah," rapidly to facilitate the clinician's localization of the vocal folds. When the vocal folds are identified, the patient should inhale, prolong "ah" for several seconds, inhale, then prolong "ah" for several seconds. This will reveal vocal fold abduction and adduction and allow the clinician to assess the symmetry of vocal fold movement, particularly on adduction. Reduced movement of one vocal fold indicates reduced laryngeal adduction and a possible unilateral adductor vocal fold paresis or paralysis. This may be a cause of aspiration *during* the swallow because the larynx may be unable to protect the airway *during* the pharyngeal swallow.

Unequal Height of the Vocal Folds

Occasionally, in partially laryngectomized patients, the reconstructed larynx on one side may be at a vertical position different from that of the vocal fold on the

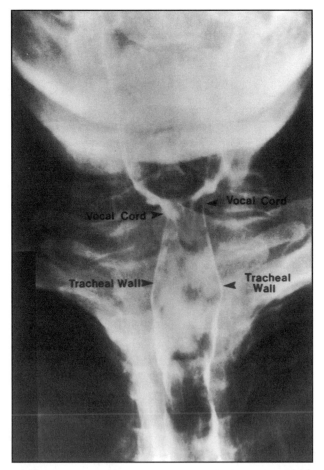

Figure 4.34. Anterior view of the airway illustrating vocal folds at unequal heights. The vocal folds and tracheal walls are coated with barium.

unoperated side. Thus, when the patient attempts to close his or her larynx to protect the airway during the swallow, even if both sides of the larynx move well, the two sides of the larynx do not meet each other and airway closure is incomplete, as shown in Figure 4.34. This is another cause of aspiration *during* the swallow, because the larynx is not closed sufficiently to protect the airway.

Other

Space is provided on the worksheet for the clinician to note any other abnormal radiographic symptoms that may be observed during the modified barium swallow.

Posture/Treatment Introduced

Space is provided on the worksheet to note any treatment procedures introduced and evaluated during the radiographic study.

Appendix 4A
Videofluorographic Examination
of Swallowing Worksheet

The purpose of the Videofluorographic Examination of Swallowing worksheet is to structure observations of anatomy and physiology made during modified barium swallow videofluorographic studies. The worksheet includes the most commonly seen anatomic and physiologic swallowing disorders, and leaves space for the examiner(s) to note other disorders seen during the radiographic study. The worksheet focuses on the oral, pharyngeal, and cervical esophageal examination using the modified barium swallow procedure (Logemann, 1983). This worksheet has been updated from that published in the first edition of this text (Logemann, 1983) so that it is easier to use and includes space for documenting data from posterior–anterior (P–A) views as well as lateral views.

At the top of the worksheet, the clinician notes the patient's name and age, the date of the radiographic study, the date when oral feeding was initiated (in part or totally), the apparent etiology of the patient's swallowing disorder (i.e., the underlying condition causing the swallowing problem, such as cerebrovascular accident or head trauma), the patient's current method of nutritional intake (i.e., oral feeding, nasogastric tube, gastrostomy, jejunostomy), the presence of a tracheostomy tube and the type (e.g., unplugged, cuffed), and the purpose of the radiographic study. The radiographic study may be done to examine the physiology of the swallowing mechanism, or to evaluate the effectiveness of a particular treatment strategy or the effects of recovery, and to identify the presence and cause of aspiration.

The worksheet is divided into two sections, the first for use during swallows of various volumes of liquid and the second for use during swallows of paste, cookie, and any other foods presented. Each section is divided into swallow symptoms and disorders viewed videofluorographically in the lateral plane and disorders visible videofluorographically in the posterior–anterior (P–A) plane. In each section, radiographic symptoms are listed in the left column from anterior to posterior and from superior to inferior.

Blanks are provided adjacent to each symptom, so that the clinician can check those symptoms observed during each swallow of a particular volume or consistency. Space is provided to record data from three swallows each of five liquid volumes and of other consistencies. Although liquid barium (as close to water as possible), pudding containing paste barium (Esophatrast), and cookie coated with barium pudding (representing masticated material) are usually used, the clinician may fill in the name of any other consistencies introduced. Clinicians may substitute other food consistencies or omit some consistencies from the evaluation, particularly if a patient is aspirating significantly, despite the introduction of treatment strategies.

Those symptoms that may result in aspiration before, during, or after the swallow are so indicated. Space is provided below each symptom on the sheet for clinical judgment of the amount of aspiration on each swallow.

At the end of each section of the sheet, space is provided to note whether any postural intervention or treatment strategy was introduced and its effect(s) on swallowing of various bolus types.

Physiologic disturbances in swallowing that correspond to radiographic symptoms are listed in the far right column, for consideration by the clinician in diagnosing the patient's swallowing disorder.

In the section of the form devoted to notation of observations in the P–A view, space is also provided for swallows of all bolus types. In fact, often only one or two swallows are repeated in this P–A view to identify structural or physiologic asymmetries, and at the same time minimize the risk of aspiration.

Videofluorographic Examination of Swallowing
Jeri A. Logemann, Ph.D., Northwestern University

Patient's name _____ Age _____

Date of study _____ Date oral feeding began _____

Etiology of patient's swallowing disorder _____

Status of nutritional intake _____ Tracheostomy tube _____

Purpose of study _____

LATERAL VIEW

Radiographic Symptoms	Liquids					Possible Swallowing Disorders
	1ml	3ml	5ml	10ml	Cup	
Preparation to Swallow						
Cannot hold food in mouth anteriorly	☐☐☐	☐☐☐	☐☐☐	☐☐☐	☐☐☐	Reduced lip closure
Cannot form bolus	☐☐☐	☐☐☐	☐☐☐	☐☐☐	☐☐☐	Reduced tongue movement range or coordination
Cannot hold bolus— premature bolus loss	☐☐☐	☐☐☐	☐☐☐	☐☐☐	☐☐☐	Reduced tongue shaping/coordination; reduced velar movement
Aspiration (%) before swallow	_____	_____	_____	_____	_____	
Material falls into anterior sulcus	☐☐☐	☐☐☐	☐☐☐	☐☐☐	☐☐☐	Reduced labial tension
Material falls into lateral sulcus	☐☐☐	☐☐☐	☐☐☐	☐☐☐	☐☐☐	Reduced buccal tension
Abnormal hold position	☐☐☐	☐☐☐	☐☐☐	☐☐☐	☐☐☐	Tongue thrust, reduced tongue control
Other _____	☐☐☐	☐☐☐	☐☐☐	☐☐☐	☐☐☐	Describe _____
Posture/treatment introduced	☐☐☐	☐☐☐	☐☐☐	☐☐☐	☐☐☐	Which one? _____
Oral Phase						
Delayed oral onset of swallow	☐☐☐	☐☐☐	☐☐☐	☐☐☐	☐☐☐	Apraxia of swallow; reduced oral sensation
Searching tongue movements	☐☐☐	☐☐☐	☐☐☐	☐☐☐	☐☐☐	Apraxia of swallow
Tongue moves forward to start swallow	☐☐☐	☐☐☐	☐☐☐	☐☐☐	☐☐☐	Tongue thrust

© 1998 by PRO-ED, Inc.

(continued)

LATERAL VIEW (continued)

Radiographic Symptoms	Liquids					Possible Swallowing Disorders
	1ml	3ml	5ml	10ml	Cup	

Oral Phase (continued)

Radiographic Symptoms	1ml	3ml	5ml	10ml	Cup	Possible Swallowing Disorders
Residue (stasis) in anterior sulcus	❏❏❏	❏❏❏	❏❏❏	❏❏❏	❏❏❏	Reduced labial tension; reduced lingual control
Residue (stasis) in lateral sulcus	❏❏❏	❏❏❏	❏❏❏	❏❏❏	❏❏❏	Reduced buccal tension
Residue (stasis) on floor of mouth	❏❏❏	❏❏❏	❏❏❏	❏❏❏	❏❏❏	Reduced tongue shaping or coordination
Residue in midtongue depression	❏❏❏	❏❏❏	❏❏❏	❏❏❏	❏❏❏	Tongue scarring
Residue (stasis) on tongue	❏❏❏	❏❏❏	❏❏❏	❏❏❏	❏❏❏	Reduced tongue movement; reduced tongue strength
Disturbed lingual contraction	❏❏❏	❏❏❏	❏❏❏	❏❏❏	❏❏❏	Disorganized A–P tongue movement
Incomplete tongue— palate contact	❏❏❏	❏❏❏	❏❏❏	❏❏❏	❏❏❏	Reduced tongue elevation
Residue on hard palate	❏❏❏	❏❏❏	❏❏❏	❏❏❏	❏❏❏	Reduced tongue elevation; reduced tongue strength
Reduced A–P tongue movement	❏❏❏	❏❏❏	❏❏❏	❏❏❏	❏❏❏	Reduced A–P lingual coordination
Repetitive lingual rolling actions	❏❏❏	❏❏❏	❏❏❏	❏❏❏	❏❏❏	Parkinson's disease
Uncontrolled bolus/ premature swallow	❏❏❏	❏❏❏	❏❏❏	❏❏❏	❏❏❏	Reduced tongue control; reduced linguavelar seal
Aspiration (%) before swallow	——	——	——	——	——	(Any reduced tongue control may cause aspiration before swallow)
Piecemeal deglutition	❏❏❏	❏❏❏	❏❏❏	❏❏❏	❏❏❏	
Oral transit time (in seconds)	——	——	——	——	——	
Other _____	❏❏❏	❏❏❏	❏❏❏	❏❏❏	❏❏❏	Describe _____
Posture/treatment introduced	❏❏❏	❏❏❏	❏❏❏	❏❏❏	❏❏❏	Which one? _____

(continued)

© 1998 by PRO-ED, Inc.

LATERAL VIEW (continued)

Radiographic Symptoms	Liquids					Possible Swallowing Disorders
	1ml	3ml	5ml	10ml	Cup	
Triggering the Pharyngeal Swallow						
Duration of delay (in sec)	⎯⎯	⎯⎯	⎯⎯	⎯⎯	⎯⎯	Delay in triggering pharyngeal swallow
Aspiration (%) before swallow	⎯⎯	⎯⎯	⎯⎯	⎯⎯	⎯⎯	
Pharyngeal Phase						
Nasal penetration	☐☐☐	☐☐☐	☐☐☐	☐☐☐	☐☐☐	Reduced velopharyngeal closure
Pseudoepiglottis (total laryngectomy)	☐☐☐	☐☐☐	☐☐☐	☐☐☐	☐☐☐	Fold of mucosa at base of tongue
Bony outgrowth from cervical vertebrae	☐☐☐	☐☐☐	☐☐☐	☐☐☐	☐☐☐	Cervical osteophytes
Coating on pharyngeal walls after swallow	☐☐☐	☐☐☐	☐☐☐	☐☐☐	☐☐☐	Reduced pharyngeal contraction
Vallecular residue (%) after swallow	⎯⎯	⎯⎯	⎯⎯	⎯⎯	⎯⎯	Reduced tongue base posterior movement
Aspiration (%) after swallow	⎯⎯	⎯⎯	⎯⎯	⎯⎯	⎯⎯	
Coating in depression on pharyngeal wall	☐☐☐	☐☐☐	☐☐☐	☐☐☐	☐☐☐	Scar tissue; pharyngeal wall/pharyngeal pouch
Aspiration (%) after swallow	⎯⎯	⎯⎯	⎯⎯	⎯⎯	⎯⎯	
Residue at top of airway	☐☐☐	☐☐☐	☐☐☐	☐☐☐	☐☐☐	Reduced laryngeal elevation
Aspiration (%) after swallow	⎯⎯	⎯⎯	⎯⎯	⎯⎯	⎯⎯	
Penetration into airway entrance	☐☐☐	☐☐☐	☐☐☐	☐☐☐	☐☐☐	Reduced laryngeal elevation/reduced closure of airway entrance
Aspiration (%) after swallow	⎯⎯	⎯⎯	⎯⎯	⎯⎯	⎯⎯	
Reduced laryngeal closure	☐☐☐	☐☐☐	☐☐☐	☐☐☐	☐☐☐	Reduced closure of airway entrance
Aspiration (%) after swallow	⎯⎯	⎯⎯	⎯⎯	⎯⎯	⎯⎯	

© 1998 by PRO-ED, Inc.

(continued)

LATERAL VIEW (continued)

Radiographic Symptoms	1ml	3ml	Liquids 5ml	10ml	Cup	Possible Swallowing Disorders
Pharyngeal Phase (continued)						
Aspiration during swallow	❑❑❑	❑❑❑	❑❑❑	❑❑❑	❑❑❑	Reduced laryngeal closure
Aspiration (%) during swallow	———	———	———	———	———	
Residue (stasis) in both pyriform sinuses	❑❑❑	❑❑❑	❑❑❑	❑❑❑	❑❑❑	Reduced anterior laryngeal motion; cricopharyngeal dysfunction, stricture
Aspiration (%) after swallow	———	———	———	———	———	
Residue throughout the pharynx	❑❑❑	❑❑❑	❑❑❑	❑❑❑	❑❑❑	Generalized reduced pressure during swallow
Aspiration (%) after swallow	———	———	———	———	———	
Pharyngeal transit time (in seconds)	———	———	———	———	———	
Other ———————	❑❑❑	❑❑❑	❑❑❑	❑❑❑	❑❑❑	Describe ———————
Posture/treatment introduced	❑❑❑	❑❑❑	❑❑❑	❑❑❑	❑❑❑	Which one? —————
Cervical Esophageal Phase						
Esophageal-to-pharyngeal backflow	❑❑❑	❑❑❑	❑❑❑	❑❑❑	❑❑❑	Esophageal abnormality—further assessment needed
Tracheoesophageal fistula	❑❑❑	❑❑❑	❑❑❑	❑❑❑	❑❑❑	Tracheoesophageal fistula
Zenker's diverticulum	❑❑❑	❑❑❑	❑❑❑	❑❑❑	❑❑❑	Zenker's diverticulum
Other ———————	❑❑❑	❑❑❑	❑❑❑	❑❑❑	❑❑❑	Describe ———————

POSTERIOR–ANTERIOR VIEW

Radiographic Symptoms	1ml	3ml	Liquids 5ml	10ml	Cup	Possible Swallowing Disorders
Preparation to Swallow						
Unable to align teeth	❑❑❑	❑❑❑	❑❑❑	❑❑❑	❑❑❑	Reduced mandibular movement
Unable to lateralize material	❑❑❑	❑❑❑	❑❑❑	❑❑❑	❑❑❑	Reduced tongue lateralization

(continued)

© 1998 by PRO-ED, Inc.

POSTERIOR–ANTERIOR VIEW (continued)

Radiographic Symptoms	1ml	3ml	Liquids 5ml	10ml	Cup	Possible Swallowing Disorders
Preparation to Swallow (continued)						
Unable to mash materials	☐☐☐	☐☐☐	☐☐☐	☐☐☐	☐☐☐	Reduced tongue elevation
Material falls into lateral sulcus	☐☐☐	☐☐☐	☐☐☐	☐☐☐	☐☐☐	Reduced buccal tension
Material falls to floor of mouth	☐☐☐	☐☐☐	☐☐☐	☐☐☐	☐☐☐	Reduced tongue control
Bolus spread across mouth	☐☐☐	☐☐☐	☐☐☐	☐☐☐	☐☐☐	Reduced fine tongue control
Posture/treatment introduced	☐☐☐	☐☐☐	☐☐☐	☐☐☐	☐☐☐	Which one?_____
Pharyngeal Phase						
Unilateral vallecular residue	☐☐☐	☐☐☐	☐☐☐	☐☐☐	☐☐☐	Unilateral dysfunction of tongue base
Residue in one pyriform sinus	☐☐☐	☐☐☐	☐☐☐	☐☐☐	☐☐☐	Unilateral dysfunction of pharynx
___ right left ___						
Aspiration (%) after swallow	____	____	____	____	____	
Reduced laryngeal movement medially	☐☐☐	☐☐☐	☐☐☐	☐☐☐	☐☐☐	Reduced adduction
___ right left ___						
Aspiration (%) during swallow	____	____	____	____	____	
Unequal height of vocal folds	☐☐☐	☐☐☐	☐☐☐	☐☐☐	☐☐☐	Unequal height of vocal folds
Aspiration (%) during swallow	____	____	____	____	____	
Other _____	☐☐☐	☐☐☐	☐☐☐	☐☐☐	☐☐☐	Describe _____
Posture/treatment introduced	☐☐☐	☐☐☐	☐☐☐	☐☐☐	☐☐☐	Which one? _____

··

LATERAL VIEW

Preparation to Swallow	1ml Paste	Cookie	Other ____	____	____	
Cannot hold food in mouth anteriorly	☐☐☐	☐☐☐	☐☐☐	☐☐☐	☐☐☐	Reduced lip closure

© 1998 by PRO-ED, Inc.   *(continued)*

LATERAL VIEW (continued)

Radiographic Symptoms	1ml Paste	Cookie	Other ___	___	___	Possible Swallowing Disorders
Preparation to Swallow (continued)						
Cannot form bolus	☐☐☐	☐☐☐	☐☐☐	☐☐☐	☐☐☐	Reduced tongue movement range or coordination
Cannot hold bolus—premature bolus loss	☐☐☐	☐☐☐	☐☐☐	☐☐☐	☐☐☐	Reduced tongue shaping/coordination; reduced palatal movement
Aspiration (%) before swallow	___	___	___	___	___	
Material falls into anterior sulcus	☐☐☐	☐☐☐	☐☐☐	☐☐☐	☐☐☐	Reduced labial tension
Material falls into lateral sulcus	☐☐☐	☐☐☐	☐☐☐	☐☐☐	☐☐☐	Reduced buccal tension
Abnormal hold position	☐☐☐	☐☐☐	☐☐☐	☐☐☐	☐☐☐	Tongue thrust, reduced tongue control
Other ___	☐☐☐	☐☐☐	☐☐☐	☐☐☐	☐☐☐	Describe ___
Posture/treatment introduced	☐☐☐	☐☐☐	☐☐☐	☐☐☐	☐☐☐	Which one? ___
Oral Phase						
Delayed oral onset of swallow	☐☐☐	☐☐☐	☐☐☐	☐☐☐	☐☐☐	Apraxia of swallow; reduced oral sensation
Searching tongue movements	☐☐☐	☐☐☐	☐☐☐	☐☐☐	☐☐☐	Apraxia of swallow
Tongue moves forward to start swallow	☐☐☐	☐☐☐	☐☐☐	☐☐☐	☐☐☐	Tongue thrust
Residue (stasis) in anterior sulcus	☐☐☐	☐☐☐	☐☐☐	☐☐☐	☐☐☐	Reduced labial tension; reduced lingual control
Residue (stasis) in lateral sulcus	☐☐☐	☐☐☐	☐☐☐	☐☐☐	☐☐☐	Reduced buccal tension
Residue (stasis) on floor of mouth	☐☐☐	☐☐☐	☐☐☐	☐☐☐	☐☐☐	Reduced tongue shaping or coordination
Residue in midtongue depression	☐☐☐	☐☐☐	☐☐☐	☐☐☐	☐☐☐	Tongue scarring
Residue (stasis) on tongue	☐☐☐	☐☐☐	☐☐☐	☐☐☐	☐☐☐	Reduced tongue movement; reduced tongue strength

(continued)

© 1998 by PRO-ED, Inc.

LATERAL VIEW (continued)

Radiographic Symptoms	1ml Paste	Cookie	Other ___	___	___	Possible Swallowing Disorders

Oral Phase (continued)

Radiographic Symptoms	1ml Paste	Cookie	Other			Possible Swallowing Disorders
Disturbed lingual contraction	□□□	□□□	□□□	□□□	□□□	Disorganized A–P tongue movement
Incomplete tongue–palate contact	□□□	□□□	□□□	□□□	□□□	Reduced tongue elevation
Residue on hard palate	□□□	□□□	□□□	□□□	□□□	Reduced tongue elevation; reduced tongue strength
Reduced A–P tongue movement	□□□	□□□	□□□	□□□	□□□	Reduced A–P lingual coordination
Repetitive lingual rolling actions	□□□	□□□	□□□	□□□	□□□	Parkinson's disease
Uncontrolled bolus/premature swallow	□□□	□□□	□□□	□□□	□□□	Reduced tongue control
Aspiration (%) before swallow	___	___	___	___	___	(Any reduced tongue control may cause aspiration before swallow)
Piecemeal deglutition	□□□	□□□	□□□	□□□	□□□	
Oral transit time (in seconds)	___	___	___	___	___	
Other _____	___	___	___	___	___	Describe _____
Posture/treatment introduced	□□□	□□□	□□□	□□□	□□□	Which one? _____

Triggering the Pharyngeal Swallow

Radiographic Symptoms						Possible Swallowing Disorders
Duration of delay (in seconds)	___	___	___	___	___	Delay in triggering pharyngeal swallow
Aspiration (%) before swallow	___	___	___	___	___	

	Liquids					
Pharyngeal Phase	1ml	3ml	5ml	10ml	Cookie	
Nasal penetration	□□□	□□□	□□□	□□□	□□□	Reduced velopharyngeal closure
Fold of mucosa at base of tongue	□□□	□□□	□□□	□□□	□□□	Pseudoepiglottis (total laryngectomy)

(continued)

© 1998 by PRO-ED, Inc.

LATERAL VIEW (continued)

Radiographic Syptoms	Liquids					Possible Swallowing Disorders
	1ml	3ml	5ml	10ml	Cookie	

Pharyngeal Phase (continued)

Radiographic Syptoms						Possible Swallowing Disorders
Bony outgrowth from cervical vertebrae	❏❏❏	❏❏❏	❏❏❏	❏❏❏	❏❏❏	Cervical osteophytes

	1ml Paste	Cookie	Other ___	___	___	
Coating on pharyngeal walls after swallow	❏❏❏	❏❏❏	❏❏❏	❏❏❏	❏❏❏	Reduced pharyngeal contraction
Vallecular residue (%) after swallow	___	___	___	___	___	Reduced tongue base posterior movement
Aspiration (%) after swallow	___	___	___	___	___	
Coating in depression on pharyngeal wall	❏❏❏	❏❏❏	❏❏❏	❏❏❏	❏❏❏	Scar tissue; pharyngeal wall/pharyngeal pouch
Aspiration (%) after swallow	___	___	___	___	___	
Residue at top of airway	❏❏❏	❏❏❏	❏❏❏	❏❏❏	❏❏❏	Reduced laryngeal elevation
Aspiration (%) after swallow	___	___	___	___	___	
Penetration into airway entrance	❏❏❏	❏❏❏	❏❏❏	❏❏❏	❏❏❏	Reduced closure of airway entrance
Aspiration (%) after swallow	___	___	___	___	___	
Reduced closure of airway entrance	❏❏❏	❏❏❏	❏❏❏	❏❏❏	❏❏❏	Reduced closure of airway entrance
Aspiration (%) after swallow	___	___	___	___	___	
Aspiration during swallow	❏❏❏	❏❏❏	❏❏❏	❏❏❏	❏❏❏	Reduced laryngeal closure
Aspiration (%) during swallow	___	___	___	___	___	
Residue (stasis) in both pyriform sinuses	❏❏❏	❏❏❏	❏❏❏	❏❏❏	❏❏❏	Reduced anterior laryngeal motion; cricopharyngeal dysfunction, stricture

© 1998 by PRO-ED, Inc.

(continued)

LATERAL VIEW (continued)

Radiographic Symptoms	1ml Paste	Cookie	Other ___	___	___	Possible Swallowing Disorders
Pharyngeal Phase (continued)						
Aspiration (%) after swallow	___	___	___	___	___	
Residue throughout pharynx	❑❑❑	❑❑❑	❑❑❑	❑❑❑	❑❑❑	Reduced tongue base movement and reduced laryngeal elevation
Aspiration (%) after swallow	___	___	___	___	___	
Pharyngeal transit time (in seconds)	___	___	___	___	___	
Other ___	❑❑❑	❑❑❑	❑❑❑	❑❑❑	❑❑❑	Describe ___
Posture/treatment introduced	❑❑❑	❑❑❑	❑❑❑	❑❑❑	❑❑❑	Which one? ___
Cervical Esophageal Phase						
Esophageal-to-pharyngeal backflow	❑❑❑	❑❑❑	❑❑❑	❑❑❑	❑❑❑	Esophageal abnormality—further assessment needed
Tracheoesophageal fistula	❑❑❑	❑❑❑	❑❑❑	❑❑❑	❑❑❑	Tracheoesophageal fistula
Zenker's diverticulum	❑❑❑	❑❑❑	❑❑❑	❑❑❑	❑❑❑	Zenker's diverticulum
Other ___	❑❑❑	❑❑❑	❑❑❑	❑❑❑	❑❑❑	Describe ___
Posture/treatment introduced	❑❑❑	❑❑❑	❑❑❑	❑❑❑	❑❑❑	Which one? ___

Posterior–Anterior View

Preparation to Swallow

Radiographic Symptoms	1ml Paste	Cookie	Other			Possible Swallowing Disorders
Unable to align teeth	❑❑❑	❑❑❑	❑❑❑	❑❑❑	❑❑❑	Reduced mandibular movement
Unable to lateralize material	❑❑❑	❑❑❑	❑❑❑	❑❑❑	❑❑❑	Reduced tongue lateralization
Unable to mash material	❑❑❑	❑❑❑	❑❑❑	❑❑❑	❑❑❑	Reduced tongue elevation
Material falls into lateral sulcus	❑❑❑	❑❑❑	❑❑❑	❑❑❑	❑❑❑	Reduced buccal tension

(continued)

© 1998 by PRO-ED, Inc.

Material falls to floor of mouth	❑❑❑	❑❑❑	❑❑❑	❑❑❑	❑❑❑	Reduced tongue control
Bolus spread across mouth	❑❑❑	❑❑❑	❑❑❑	❑❑❑	❑❑❑	Reduced fine tongue control
Posture/treatment introduced	❑❑❑	❑❑❑	❑❑❑	❑❑❑	❑❑❑	Which one?_____

Pharyngeal Phase

Unilateral vallecular residue	❑❑❑	❑❑❑	❑❑❑	❑❑❑	❑❑❑	Unilateral dysfunction of tongue base
Residue in one pyriform sinus	❑❑❑	❑❑❑	❑❑❑	❑❑❑	❑❑❑	Unilateral dysfunction of pharynx
___ right left ___ Aspiration (%) after swallow	_____	_____	_____	_____	_____	
Reduced laryngeal movement medially	❑❑❑	❑❑❑	❑❑❑	❑❑❑	❑❑❑	Reduced vocal fold adduction
___ right left ___ Aspiration (%) during swallow	_____	_____	_____	_____	_____	
Unequal height of vocal folds	❑❑❑	❑❑❑	❑❑❑	❑❑❑	❑❑❑	Unequal height of vocal folds
Aspiration (%) during swallow	_____	_____	_____	_____	_____	
Other _____	❑❑❑	❑❑❑	❑❑❑	❑❑❑	❑❑❑	Describe _____
Posture/treatment introduced	❑❑❑	❑❑❑	❑❑❑	❑❑❑	❑❑❑	Which one? _____

© 1998 by PRO-ED, Inc.

References

Blonsky, E., Logemann, J., Boshes, B., & Fisher, H. (1975). Comparison of speech and swallowing function in patients with tremor disorders and in normal geriatric patients: A cinefluorographic study. *Journal of Gerontology, 30,* 299–303.

Blumberg, P., Prapote, C., & Viscomi, G. (1977). Cervical osteophytes producing dysphagia. *Ear, Nose and Throat Journal, 56,* 15–21.

Calcaterra, T., Kadell, B., & Ward, O. (1975). Dysphagia secondary to cricopharyngeal muscle dysfunction. *Archives of Otolaryngology, 101,* 726–729.

Dodds, W. J., Taylor, A. J., Steward, E. T., Kern, M. K., Logemann, J. A., & Cook, I. J. (1989). Tipper and dipper types of oral swallows. *American Journal of Roentgenology, 153,* 1197–1199.

Henderson, R., Woolf, C., & Marryatt, G. (1976). Pharyngoesophageal dysphagia and gastroesophageal reflux. *Laryngoscope, 86,* 1531–1539.

Jacob, P., Kahrilas, P., Logemann, J., Shah, V., & Ha, T. (1989). Upper esophageal sphincter opening and modulation during swallowing. *Gastroenterology, 97,* 1469–1478.

Kahrilas, P., Dodds, W., Dent, J., Logemann, J., & Shaker, R. (1988). Upper esophageal sphincter function during deglutition. *Gastroenterology, 95,* 52–62.

Kahrilas, P. J., Lin, S., Logemann, J. A., Ergun, G. A., & Facchini, F. (1993). Deglutitive tongue action: Volume accommodation and bolus propulsion. *Gastroenterology, 104,* 152–162.

Kahrilas, P. J., & Logemann, J. A. (1993). Volume accommodations during swallowing. *Dysphagia, 8,* 259–265.

Kahrilas, P. J., Logemann, J. A., Lin, S., & Ergun, G. A. (1992). Pharyngeal clearance during swallow: A combined manometric and videofluoroscopic study. *Gastroenterology, 103,* 128–136.

Logemann, J. (1983). *Evaluation and treatment of swallowing disorders.* Austin, TX: PRO-ED.

Logemann, J. A. (1993). *Manual for the videofluoroscopic study of swallowing* (2nd ed.). Austin, TX: PRO-ED.

Logemann, J. A. (1997). Role of the modified barium swallow in management of patients with dysphagia. *Otolaryngology—Head and Neck Surgery, 116,* 335.

Logemann, J. A., Kahrilas, P. J., Cheng, J., Pauloski, B. R., Gibbons, P. J., Rademaker, A. W., & Lin, S. (1992). Closure mechanisms of the laryngeal vestibule during swallow. *American Journal of Physiology, 262 (Gastrointestinal Physiology, 25),* G338–G344.

Logemann, J., Kahrilas, P., Kobara, M., & Vakil, N. (1989). The benefit of head rotation on pharyngoesophageal dysphagia. *Archives of Physical Medicine and Rehabilitation, 70,* 767–771.

Lund, W. (1968). The cricopharyngeal sphincter: Its relationship to the relief of pharyngeal paralysis and the surgical treatment of the early pharyngeal pouch. *Journal of Laryngology and Otology, 82,* 353–367.

Mandelstam, P., & Lieber, A. (1970). Cineradiographic evaluation of the esophagus in normal adults. *Gastroenterology, 58,* 32–38.

Miller, A. (1972). Characteristics of the swallowing reflex induced by peripheral nerve and brain stem stimulation. *Experimental Neurology, 34,* 210–222.

Parker, M. D. (1989). Dysphagia due to cervical osteophytes: A controversial entity revisited. *Dysphagia, 3,* 157–160.

Pommerenke, W. (1928). A study of the sensory areas eliciting the swallowing reflex. *American Journal of Physiology, 84,* 36–41.

Ponzoli, V. (1968). Zenker's diverticulum: A review of pathogeneses and presentation of 25 cases. *Southern Medical Journal, 61*, 817–821.

Rademaker, A. W., Pauloski, B. R., Logemann, J. A., & Shanahan, T. K. (1994). Oropharyngeal swallow efficiency as a representative measure of swallowing function. *Journal of Speech and Hearing Research, 37*, 314–325.

Robbins, J., Logemann, J., & Kirshner, H. (1986) Swallowing and speech production in Parkinson's disease. *Annals of Neurology, 19*, 283–287.

Rosenbek, J. C., Robbins, J., Roecker, E. B., Coyle, J. L., & Wood, J. L. (1996). A Penetration–Aspiration Scale. *Dysphagia, 11*, 93–98.

Saunders, W. (1971). Cervical osteophytes and dysphagia. *Journal of Otology, Physiology and Laryngology, 79*, 1091–1097.

Shanahan, T. K., Logemann, J. A., Rademaker, A. W., Pauloski, B. R., & Kahrilas, P. J. (1993). Chin-down posture effect on aspiration in dysphagic patients. *Archives of Physical and Medical Rehabilitation, 74*, 736–739.

Shawker, T. H. Sonies, B. C., Stone, M., & Baum, B. (1983). Real-time ultrasound visualization of tongue movement during swallowing. *Journal of Clinical Ultrasound, 11*, 485–494.

Shedd, D., Scatliff, J., & Kirchner, J. (1960). The buccopharyngeal propulsive mechanism in human deglutition. *Surgery, 48*, 846–853.

Tracy, J., Logemann, J., Kahrilas, P., Jacob, P., Kobara, M., & Krugler, C. (1989). Preliminary observations on the effects of age on oropharyngeal deglutition. *Dysphagia, 4*, 90–94.

Valadka, A. B., Kubal, W. S., & Smith, M. M. (1995). Updated management strategy for patients with cervical osteophytic dysphagia. *Dysphagia, 10*, 167–171.

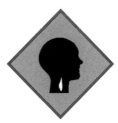

EVALUATION OF
SWALLOWING DISORDERS

This chapter reviews the process of evaluation, beginning with screening procedures and moving to a full bedside or clinical examination and then to the radiographic study. The bedside or clinical and radiographic evaluations are selected for in-depth discussion because they are the most frequently used procedures and provide the greatest amount of information on the patient's eating behavior, language, cognition, and oromotor function (the bedside examination), as well as the patient's oral and pharyngeal physiology (the X-ray study). Usually the bedside or clinical examination precedes the videofluorographic (modified barium swallow) procedure; this order ensures that the patient is appropriate for the modified barium swallow.

Screening Procedures

Screening procedures provide the clinician with some indirect evidence that the patient has a swallowing disorder but do not provide information on the physiology of that disorder. For example, a procedure may identify that the patient is aspirating but does not provide the physiologic information as to *why* the patient is aspirating. Screening procedures tend to identify the signs and symptoms of dysphagia, such as coughing behaviors, history of pneumonia, particular diagnoses at greatest risk, food squirting out the tracheostomy indicating aspiration, penetration, or the presence of residual food in the mouth. Screening procedures are generally performed at the patient's bedside or in a home or school environment and provide the clinician with increased evidence that the patient needs an in-depth physiological assessment. In some situations, screening is limited to chart review and perhaps observation of eating if the patient is being orally fed or observations of saliva management. In all situations, screening should be quick, low risk, and low cost. Its purpose is to identify the highest risk patients who require further assessment.

In recent years, there has been increased interest in refining screening procedures, with the goal of eliminating the need for a videofluoroscopic study or other instrumental procedures (DePippo, Holas, & Reding, 1992; Hamlet, Nelson, & Patterson, 1990; Hamlet, Patterson, Fleming, & Jones, 1992; Nathadwarawala, McGroary, & Wiles, 1994; Nathadwarawala, Nicklin, & Wiles, 1992; Zenner, Losinski, & Mills, 1995). However, screening procedures answer a very different set of questions than does a diagnostic procedure such as videofluoroscopy. Screening procedures ask and attempt to answer the question, Is the patient dysphagic? They do not answer the question, What is the nature of the patient's physiology during swallowing? The latter question is answered by a diagnostic procedure. Some of the newly developed screening procedures involve continuous swallowing of larger amounts of liquid (the 3-oz water test and the timed swallowing test) (DePippo et al., 1992; Nathadwarawala et al., 1992; Nathadwarawala et al., 1994). These should be used very judiciously, if at all, in patients at any significant risk for aspiration, as the patient could develop significant immediate or delayed pulmonary reaction (Batchelor, Neilson, & Sexton, 1996).

In general, when a screening procedure is examined for its accuracy in identifying the presence of a dysphagia symptom, two characteristics are statistically examined. First, the procedure should correctly identify those individuals who are actually aspirating or have residue (true positives), known as procedural *sensitivity*, and those who have none of these symptoms (true negatives), known as procedural *specificity*. Second, the procedure should not generate many false positives (i.e., those who are identified as aspirating but are not actually aspirating) or false negatives (i.e., those who are aspirating but are identified as not aspirating). The ability of a screening procedure to identify the presence of a symptom, such as aspiration or residual food in the pharynx, has not nearly reached 100% accuracy in any of the studies that have been completed to date with any of the screening procedures (DePippo et al., 1992; Nathadwarawala et al., 1992; Nathadwarawala et al., 1994; Zenner et al., 1995). Those procedures with a higher rate of correct identification of aspirators also usually have a higher rate of false positives; that is, they overidentify patients as aspirating who actually are not aspirating. At this time, it is suggested that the swallowing therapist use a noninvasive, low-risk procedure that is quick and easy. We have found that using the checklist in Table 5.1 results in sensitivity and specificity equal to that of other procedures. It is simple to use, involving chart review and observation of the patient eating, if he or she is orally fed, or swallowing saliva

Table 5.1
Checklist of Items for Dysphagia Screening

Screening should be quick (less than 15 minutes), easy, and inexpensive.

Check appropriate box for each item.

Yes   No

☐	☐	1. History of recurrent pneumonia
		2. Diagnosis of
☐	☐	• partial laryngectomy
☐	☐	• oral resection
☐	☐	• full course radiation to head or neck
☐	☐	• anoxia
☐	☐	• Parkinson's disease
☐	☐	• motor neuron disease (e.g., Werdnig–Hoffmann disease)
☐	☐	• myasthenia gravis
☐	☐	• bulbar polio
☐	☐	• anterior cervical spinal fusion
☐	☐	• brainstem stroke
☐	☐	• Guillain-Barré
☐	☐	• laryngeal trauma
☐	☐	3. History of prolonged or traumatic intubation or emergency tracheostomy
☐	☐	4. Severe respiratory problems
☐	☐	5. Gurgly voice, cry
☐	☐	6. Coughing before, during, and/or after swallowing
☐	☐	7. Poor awareness and poor control of secretions
☐	☐	8. Infrequent swallowing (less than one saliva swallow in 5 minutes)
☐	☐	9. Constant copious chest secretions
		10. If patient is eating, observe eating. If patient is not eating, observe saliva swallowing. Identify any of these, particularly if they change during or immediately after a meal:
☐	☐	• breathing difficulty
☐	☐	• increased secretions
☐	☐	• voice changes (gurgly sound)
☐	☐	• multiple swallowing per bolus
☐	☐	• reduced laryngeal lifting on swallow
☐	☐	• throat clearing
☐	☐	• coughing
☐	☐	• significant fatigue

Note. Items 1 through 4 should be obtained from brief chart review. Items 5 through 10 require brief patient observation.

if nonorally fed, and meets the criteria for a noninvasive screening procedure. If the patient exhibits any one or more of these characteristics, a more in-depth physiologic assessment is needed.

In infants, children, and developmentally delayed adults, certain abnormal behaviors observed during eating are important indicators of the need for an in-depth physiologic study:

- *Rejection of Food*—If a child (or developmentally delayed adult) rejects oral intake, a physiologic swallow assessment is critical. In that nutritional intake is critical to survival, rejection of all intake is frequently an indication that eating is perceived as more dangerous than safe and is a major indicator of chronic aspiration. These individuals should receive a modified barium swallow.

- *Food Selectivity*—Some children limit their oral intake to only selected foods, rejecting all others. Often there is preference for a specific taste, such as salty or sweet. The clinician should test the child's reactions to various taste, temperature, and texture combinations, as described in Chapter 6. The need for a radiographic study should be determined after this additional testing.

- *Gagging*—Gagging during eating may indicate several different abnormalities. Gagging as food is placed in the mouth is often an indication of oral hypersensitivity or abnormal oral sensation. In normal young children (6 to 12 months of age approximately), the gag is triggered forward in the mouth. All of the play activity that involves placing toys, fingers, and toes in the mouth desensitizes the gag in the front of the oral cavity, moving it back to the pharynx where it triggers in the normal adult. Children with neuromotor involvement often do not have the ability to bring toys or other objects to the mouth and therefore they are hypersensitive to oral stimulation. Gagging may also result from a tactile agnosia (i.e., inability to recognize food as food rather than a foreign body). If food is not recognized as food, the gag is triggered to push this foreign body out of the mouth and pharynx. A radiographic study is usually indicated if the gagging occurs very frequently at every feeding attempt.

- *Open-Mouth Posture*—If the child displays an open-mouth posture during eating, the upper airway should be assessed to define whether the child has an adequate upper airway to allow nasal breathing during swallowing. Dental structure should also be assessed to assure that the dental alignment allows lip closure. Normally, the child should be able to maintain lip closure from the time the food is placed in the mouth until the pharyngeal stage of swallow is over.

Following completion of the screening procedure, the clinician should indicate whether the patient is a normal swallower or whether the risk of dysphagia is high and further diagnostic assessment is needed.

The Bedside or Clinical Examination

The bedside or clinical examination of swallowing is designed to provide the clinician with the following data for use in dysphagia diagnosis and treatment planning: (1) information on the current medical diagnosis and patient's medical history and the history of the patient's swallowing disorder, including the person's awareness of his or her swallowing disorder and indications of the localization and nature of the disorder; (2) the patient's medical status, including nutritional and respiratory status (i.e., presence of a nasogastric feeding tube or gastrostomy and placement of a cuffed or uncuffed tracheostomy tube); (3) the patient's oral anatomy; (4) the patient's respiratory function and its relationship to swallow; (5) the patient's labial control, as this may affect keeping food in his or her mouth; (6) the patient's lingual control, as it may affect oral manipulation of food and the posterior transit of food through the oral cavity; (7) the patient's palatal function, as it may affect entrance of food into his or her nose during the swallow; (8) the patient's pharyngeal wall contraction, as it may affect movement of food through the pharynx and may cause aspiration after the swallow; (9) the patient's laryngeal control, as it may affect airway protection and aspiration during the swallow; (10) the patient's general ability to follow directions and monitor and control his or her behavior; (11) the patient's reaction to oral sensory stimulation, including taste, temperature, and texture; and (12) the patient's reactions and symptoms during attempts to swallow (K. Griffin, 1974; Linden & Siebens, 1980). The bedside or clinical examination can be divided into two parts: the preparatory examination, with no actual swallows, and the initial swallowing examination, when actual swallowing may be attempted and some aspects of physiology observed.

Preparatory Examination

The preparatory examination begins with collection of information from the patient's chart and includes a complete examination of vocal tract control (K. Griffin, 1974).

Patient Chart Review

Initially, the swallowing therapist should carefully examine the patient's medical chart to determine the individual's respiratory status, including any reports or comments on recent pneumonia and on pulmonary function and/or the presence of a tracheostomy tube (cuffed or uncuffed) or history of mechanical ventilation and intubation. Also, information on the history of the patient's swallowing problem, including duration, the patient's general medical status, ability to follow directions, motivation, and other aspects of the patient's general behavior, is helpful to the therapist prior to beginning the bedside examination. The nutritional status (oral feeding vs. nonoral nutrition and type) should also be determined from the patient's medical chart.

Specifically, the chart review and history should identify (1) current and past medical problems, focusing on those that may cause dysphagia; (2) current and immediate past medications, particularly those causing dry mouth (xerostomia), reduced alertness, or delayed reaction time, as these are likely to cause swallowing problems; (3) history of the swallowing disorder, including time and nature of its onset, symptoms such as coughing or food "catching" in the pharynx, difficult and easy foods, and the patient's general perception or awareness of the problem; (4) presence, type, duration, and method of placement (emergency or planned) of any airway device (tracheostomy, mechanical ventilation, intubation); and (5) presence, type, duration of placement, adequacy, and complications of oral and nonoral nutrition.

Observations upon Entering the Patient's Room

As the clinician enters the patient's room, several observations should be made: the patient's posture in bed, his or her alertness and reaction to the clinician's entrance, the presence or absence of a tracheostomy tube and its status (cuff inflated or deflated), and the patient's general awareness and handling of his or her own secretions and management of the tube itself. During the initial part of the bedside examination, as the history is being taken, the clinician should be making informal observations on the patient's ability to follow directions and answer questions, as well as the individual's general alertness. Throughout this time, the clinician should also be observing the patient's management of secretions and of the tracheostomy tube, if present.

Respiratory Status

In assessing dysphagic patients, it is critical that the clinician examine the upper aerodigestive tract according to its physiologic hierarchy: respiration, which must be maintained at all costs for survival; swallowing; and speech. There is slowly increasing evidence that a significant respiratory problem can affect swallowing because the mechanism will naturally make shifts to keep respiration at a functional level (Loughlin & Lefton-Greif, 1994; Martin, Corlew, et al., 1994).

In the bedside clinical assessment, the clinician should observe the patient's respiratory rate at rest. If the patient is in any degree of respiratory distress, it may be inappropriate to begin swallowing therapy or to proceed with assessment that may place additional stress on respiration. Even normal swallowing stresses the respiratory status because it requires some degree of airway closure and cessation of breathing, even for a fraction of a second (0.3 to 0.5 seconds, depending on the volume swallowed) (Logemann et al., 1992; Martin, Logemann, Shaker, & Dodds, 1994). Some therapy procedures, notably swallowing maneuvers, require or result in longer periods of apnea (i.e., cessation of breathing) and may be inappropriate for a patient with respiratory problems.

In addition to observing respiratory rate, the clinician should make the following observations:

1. The timing of the patient's saliva swallows in relation to the phases of the respiratory cycle (i.e., inhalation and exhalation). Studies of normal swallow indicate that most food swallows (60% to 80%, depending on the study) interrupt exhalation (Martin, Logemann, et al., 1994) and that most adult swallowers return to exhalation after the swallow. The clinician should observe the phase of respiration in which the patient swallows and in which he or she returns to respiration.

2. The timing of any coughing in relation to respiration–swallow coordination. Those swallows that are followed by inhalation may put the patient at aspiration risk.

3. The duration of comfortable breath hold if feasible. The clinician should determine whether the patient can hold his or her breath comfortably for 1 second, 3 seconds, and 5 seconds.

4. The patient's rest breathing pattern, oral or nasal. If the patient is mouth breathing, the clinician should observe whether the patient can comfortably breathe through his or her nose as is usual during chewing and the oral stages of swallow.

Tracheostomy Tubes, Intubation, and Mechanical Ventilation

Tracheostomy tubes are normally placed for (1) upper airway obstruction at or above the level of the true vocal folds; (2) potential upper airway obstruction, such as may be created by edema following oral, pharyngeal, or laryngeal surgery; and/or (3) provision of respiratory care. The tube is generally inserted into the trachea through a surgical incision made between the third and fourth tracheal rings. This placement well below the true vocal cords avoids damage to the larynx. Occasionally, in emergency situations, tracheostomas are placed higher than the second tracheal ring and may cause laryngeal scarring. Tubes are usually left in place until the airway obstruction or the potential for airway obstruction is past and until the need for respiratory care is completed. Occasionally, tracheostomy tubes remain permanently.

Tracheostomy tubes generally have three parts, as illustrated in Figure 5.1: an outer cannula, an inner cannula, and an obturator. In normal use, the outer cannula always stays in place; the inner cannula remains in the tube except for cleaning; and the obturator is inserted only to provide a smooth, rounded tip for

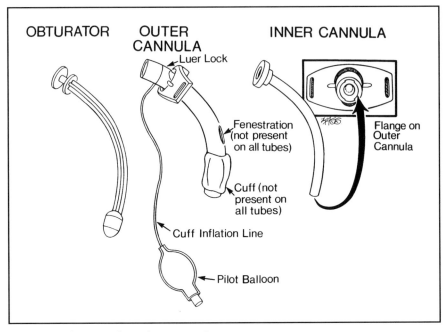

Figure 5.1. The parts of a tracheostomy tube.

the initial insertion of the tracheostomy tube. The outer cannula remains in place to hold the tracheostomy site open until it can be allowed to close. When patients are being weaned from tracheostomy tubes, two procedures may be used. First, the tube (in adults, most often a size 8) will be changed to a smaller size to encourage oral–nasal breathing in combination with breathing through the tracheostomy site. If the smaller tube (often a size 6 or 4) is tolerated well, it will be plugged with the obturator or a cork for periods of time to assess the patient's ability to maintain oral–nasal breathing without distress before the tube is removed altogether.

Normally, there is a small amount of space between the tracheostomy tube and the walls of the trachea, as seen in Figure 5.2A. When the patient inhales and occludes the outer end of the tracheostomy tube with a finger, air can pass around the tube and through the larynx, and produce voice (Figure 5.2B). Because the amount of air passing between the tube and the walls of the trachea is reduced from normal, voice will often be softer and more breathy in quality than normal.

There are two important variations in tracheostomy tubes. A tracheostomy tube may be cuffed or uncuffed, and fenestrated or unfenestrated.

Cuffed Tracheostomy Tubes. A cuffed tracheostomy tube (shown in Figure 5.3) is sometimes placed when there is (1) need for respiratory treatment or (2) poten-

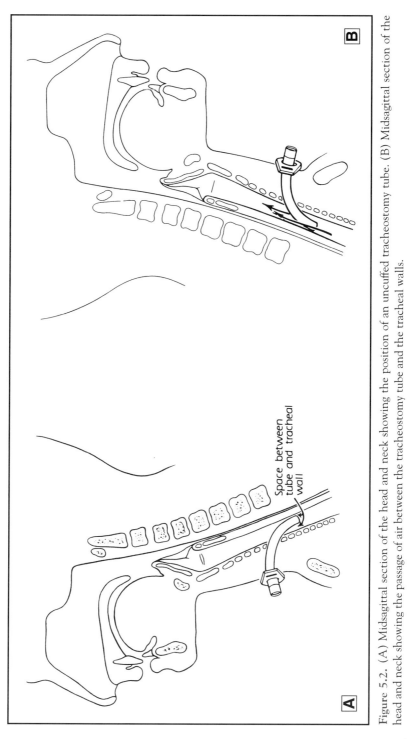

Figure 5.2. (A) Midsagittal section of the head and neck showing the position of an uncuffed tracheostomy tube. (B) Midsagittal section of the head and neck showing the passage of air between the tracheostomy tube and the tracheal walls.

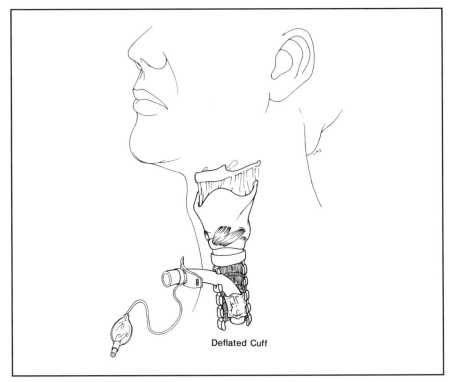

Deflated Cuff

Figure 5.3. Drawing of the head and neck showing the position of a cuffed tracheostomy tube, with the cuff deflated.

tial for the patient to aspirate material. The cuff surrounds the lower portion of the tracheostomy tube like a balloon. When the cuff is deflated, as in Figure 5.3, the tracheostomy tube is the same as if it had no cuff; that is, space between the tracheal wall and the tube allows air to pass upward, as indicated by the arrow in Figure 5.4. When fully inflated, as in Figure 5.5, however, the cuff contacts the tracheal wall, preventing air from passing upward and sealing the lower airway from secretions from above. Thus, with the cuff fully inflated, no material from above the larynx can pass through into the trachea and bronchi. The cuff must remain inflated if a patient is on mechanical ventilation that operates on positive pressure principles. The cuff may also be temporarily inflated to deliver respiratory therapy to the patient. The cuff is sometimes fully inflated for patients who are aspirating their saliva, to prevent aspiration pneumonia. Saliva and other secretions then collect above the cuff. When the cuff is deflated in this situation, therefore, thorough suctioning is necessary to catch material draining around the tube into the lower airway. Fully inflated cuffed tracheostomy tubes are generally not left in place for a long time, as the pressure of the cuff contacting the tracheal wall can create tracheal irritation, unless the patient is terminal

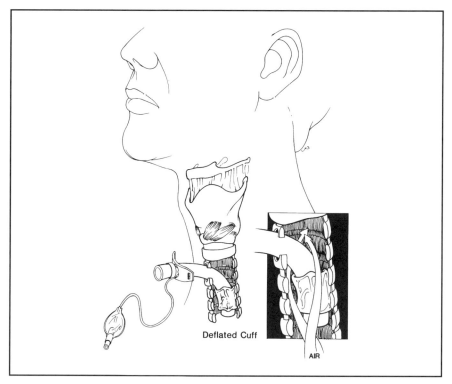

Figure 5.4. Drawing of the head and neck showing the passage of air between the tracheostomy tube, with the cuff deflated, and the tracheal walls.

and long-lasting effects are not relevant. This irritation can occur even though cuffs are designed to create minimal pressure against the tracheal wall. If the cuff is fully inflated and contacting the tracheal walls, it can cause ischemia in the tracheal wall and lead to tracheal stenosis, a problem that is difficult to manage (Miller & Sethl, 1970).

For this reason, many respiratory therapy departments manage cuffed tracheostomy tubes using the "minimal leak technique." This technique involves inflating the cuff until the patient can no longer pass air around the tube, then taking 1 to 2 cc of air out of the cuff so there is a minimal leak around the cuff, thereby preventing tracheal stenosis but allowing some leakage of material (aspiration) around the cuff. Also, an inflated tracheostomy cuff may inhibit a patient's relearning to swallow by restricting laryngeal elevation (Bonanno, 1971), reducing laryngeal sensitivity (Feldman, Deal, & Urquhart, 1966), or placing pressure on the esophagus via the common posterior wall between the trachea and the esophagus. If tracheostomy is done in an emergency situation or is constructed with sutures attaching the superficial tissues to the trachea, it is

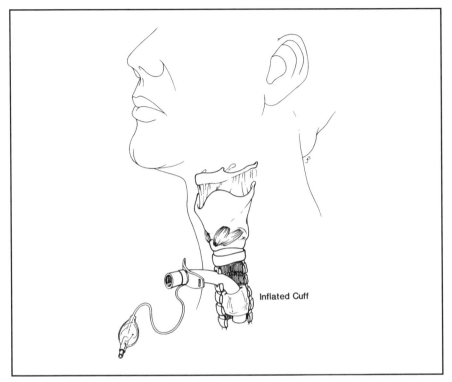

Inflated Cuff

Figure 5.5. Drawing of the head and neck showing the cuffed tracheostomy tube in place with the cuff inflated and in contact with the tracheal walls.

likely that these effects will worsen (Paloschi & Lynn, 1965). If the tracheostomy has been present for more than 6 months, there may be greater scar tissue and reduced closure of the vocal folds because of reduced stimulation of the sensory receptors under the vocal folds (Buckwalter & Sasaki, 1984; Sasaki, Suzaki, Horiuchi, & Kirchner, 1972). It should also be noted that occasionally an inflated or cuffed tracheostomy tube will not completely occlude the trachea because of tracheal wall deviations or misfit tubes, resulting in some aspiration past the inflated cuff.

Fenestrated Tracheostomy Tubes. If a patient is having difficulty producing voice with a normal tracheostomy tube, a fenestration, or window, may be cut into the tube to allow for greater airflow, as shown in Figures 5.6 and 5.7. Often this fenestration is made only in the outer cannula so, when the patient wants to talk, the inner cannula is removed. When the inner cannula is placed into the tracheostomy tube, the fenestration is closed. Fenestrated tubes may be used in patients who are close to being weaned from the tracheostomy tube or in

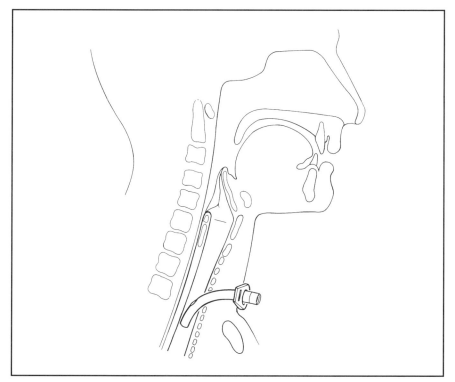

Figure 5.6. Midsagittal section of the head and neck with a fenestrated tracheostomy tube in place.

patients whose communication is ineffective with the small amount of airflow generally possible with an unfenestrated tube. It is rare for a cuffed tracheostomy tube to be fenestrated, as the fenestration would negate the occlusive effects of the inflated cuff. A fenestration might be made in a cuffed tube, however, if a patient no longer needs the cuff inflated.

Management of the Tracheostomized Patient During
Swallowing Assessment and Treatment

At the beginning of bedside–clinical or radiographic study, the clinician should examine the tracheostomy tube of tracheotomized patients to determine the presence of a cuff and the status of the cuff (inflated or deflated), the size of the tracheostomy tube, and the presence of a fenestration. The clinician should also review the patient's chart to determine the length of time the tracheostomy has been in place. If the tracheostomy tube has been in place more than 6 months, scar tissue may have formed that can restrict laryngeal elevation. A tracheostomy tube in place for more than 6 months will also result in reduced airflow

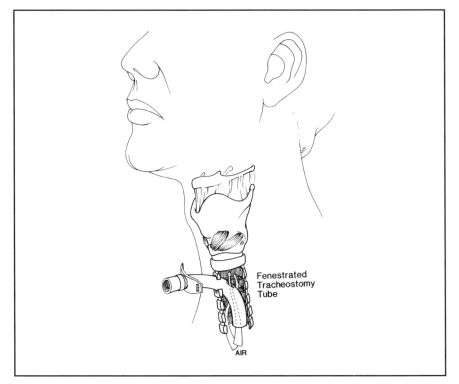

Figure 5.7. Midsagittal section of the head and neck with a fenestrated tracheostomy tube in place, with arrows showing the path of airflow between the tracheostomy tube and tracheal wall and through the tube and fenestra (window).

and stimulation to subglottic sensory receptors that play a role in vocal fold closure. Patients with this long-term tracheostomy may have reduced vocal fold closure for swallowing and vocalization. Tracheostomy tubes in place for a shorter time may have little effect on laryngeal elevation if the cuff is deflated. *If medically feasible*, the tracheostomy cuff should be deflated during the bedside or radiographic study, because an inflated cuff can reduce laryngeal elevation by creating friction against the tracheal wall. However, the tracheostomy cuff should not be deflated until medical clearance is given. If the tracheostomy cuff is inflated during the bedside or radiographic study, the clinician should note this in the report.

The patient with a tracheostomy tube may be taught to lightly cover the external end of the tube with a gauze pad or gloved finger during the moment of the swallow and for several seconds after the swallow, if this is found to improve the swallow when later examined on the radiographic study. In this way, increased airflow is directed through the larynx, which stimulates subglottic sensory receptors before the swallow and may improve vocal fold closure. Most swallows occur during the exhalatory phase of the respiratory cycle, with exhalation temporarily stopped by the swallow (Martin, Logemann, et al., 1994). Exhalation usually resumes after the swallow. Thus, if the patient's tracheostomy is occluded during and immediately after the swallow, the small exhalatory air-flow after the swallow may potentially contribute to clearance of residual food away from the top of the airway, lessening the chance of aspiration after the swallow. It is also thought that covering the tracheostomy tube helps to restore more normal subglottic pressures during swallowing and thus also helps to improve closure of the vocal folds during swallow (Shin, Maeyama, Morikawa, & Umezaki, 1988). Several reports indicate reduction or elimination of aspiration with the tube covered (Muz, Hamlet, Mathog, & Farris, 1994; Muz, Mathog, Nelson, & Jones, 1989). Other studies and my own experience indicate variable or less consistently positive results from tube occlusion (Leder, Tarro, & Burrell, 1996). A recent study completed in our laboratory has found that the tube occlusion digitally does not negatively affect swallowing and, in fact, may result in improvements in laryngeal elevation (Logemann, Pauloski, & Colangelo, in press). However, such effects are not universal and need to be examined during the radiographic study.

Use of a one-way valve on the patient's tracheostomy tube may be helpful in place of light digital occlusion if the patient's respiratory status is stable and can tolerate the valve comfortably. This may also facilitate speech production. The one-way valve is open during rest breathing and closes when exhalatory pressure increases for speech. With the valve closed, air is directed up and around the tracheostomy tube. The patient's tolerance for a valve should be determined by the respiratory service in conjunction with the swallowing therapist. Like digital occlusion, the effects of the valve on the patient's swallow should be examined radiographically. Although one report (Dettelbach, Gross, Mahlmann, & Eibling, 1995) indicates uniformly positive effects of one-way valves with dysphagic, tracheotomized patients, I have found variable effects in my clinical experience, making it necessary for the clinician to define the effects for each patient radiographically.

Ventilator-Dependent Patients

Often, patients on a ventilator complain that their swallowing worsened when they went onto the ventilator. Swallowing and respiration are reciprocal. Because the ventilator controls the respiratory cycle, the patient cannot lengthen the exhalation to allow for the swallow. If the patient has slightly slow oral or pharyngeal stages of swallow, which cannot be completed in the time period allocated for exhalation by the ventilator, the swallow may be further disrupted by the restart of inhalation. Also, ventilator-dependent patients normally have a tracheostomy tube in place with the cuff inflated. The inflated cuff on the tracheostomy tube may reduce laryngeal elevation and thus reduce closure of the entrance of the airway, which, in turn, may allow food to enter or penetrate the entrance of the airway and be aspirated after the swallow. Because normal swallowing usually occurs toward the beginning of exhalation, it is usually helpful to present food to the patient during the bedside study at the beginning of the exhalation phase of the respiratory cycle.

The blue dye test may be used at the bedside for a tracheotomized patient (Thompson-Henry & Braddock, 1995; Tippett & Siebens, 1995). This test is a screening test for the presence of aspiration. The patient can be given measured amounts of blue-dyed foods and the tracheostomy suctioned immediately after the swallow for the presence of the blue-dyed foods, indicating aspiration. The test does not reveal the anatomic or physiologic cause(s) of aspiration, but, if the result is clearly positive (i.e., the blue-dyed material is coughed and/or suctioned from the tracheostomy), the clinician should recommend a radiographic study. If blue-tinged secretions are later suctioned from the tracheostomy, the conclusion should not necessarily be that the patient is aspirating. Normal secretion flow is down from the mouth and pharynx, and it is quite normal for blue dye to mix with secretions and gradually coat the trachea. Also, unless a variety of food consistencies are presented, the patient may not aspirate on the food consistency tested but may aspirate on other food consistencies.

Intubation

In contrast to tracheostomy, intubation usually involves placing a tube through the mouth or nose, through the pharynx and larynx, to the lower trachea, as shown in Figure 5.8. Intubation is often placed in an emergency situation and usually considered a more stable airway. Intubation may be maintained for hours, days, or weeks, depending on the nature and severity of the patient's damage. If the placement of the tube is traumatic, there may be damage to the patient's larynx. If the tube is in place for days or weeks, a variety of types of laryngeal tissue damage that may affect laryngeal closure during swallow may result, including redness, edema, nodule or polyp formation, and unilateral adductor paresis or paralysis. In addition, the bottom edge of the tube may rub and irritate the soft-tissue, posterior common wall of the trachea, causing tissue breakdown and the formation of a tracheoesophageal (TE) fistula (DeVita & Spierer-Rundback, 1990; Gallivan, Dawson, & Robbins, 1989).

At some point, when the patient's respiratory status is stabilized, a tracheostomy may replace the intubation. Until the intubation is removed, no swallowing therapy is appropriate. When intubation is removed, there may be reduced range of motion of the lips, tongue, pharynx, and larynx for speech and swallowing,

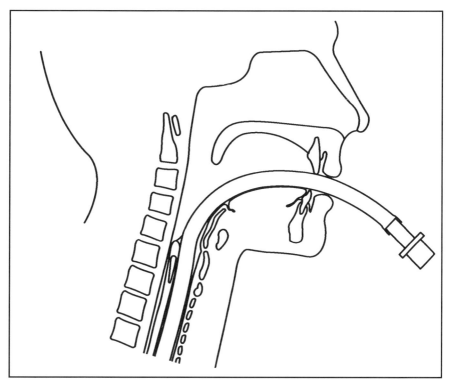

Figure 5.8. A midsagittal drawing of the head and neck showing the placement of a tube for oral intubation.

which may last up to a week (DeLarminat, Montravers, Dureuil, & Desmonte, 1995). Gentle range-of-motion exercises may be needed.

History

It is important to gather information from the patient if possible, or from the family or nursing staff if the patient is unable to give a sufficient report, regarding the exact nature of the patient's symptoms indicative of a possible swallowing disorder (Dobie, 1978; Donald & Dawes, 1977; Edwards, 1970; J. Griffin & Tollison, 1980; K. Griffin, 1974; Kirchner, 1967; McConchie, 1973; O'Connor & Ardran, 1976; Phillips & Hendrix, 1971; Pitcher, 1973). When did the disorder begin? Did it worsen gradually or rapidly? How does the problem vary with different consistencies of food (i.e., liquid, pudding, and solid food, particularly meat or bread)? What specifically happens when the patient tries to swallow? Does material stop somewhere along the way? If so, where (i.e., high or low in the throat)? Does the patient cough and choke? If food collects, can the patient point to the spot in his or her mouth or throat where he or she feels material collect?

Radiographic studies have shown that patients who are aware that an oropharyngeal swallowing disorder is present are highly reliable in their identification and description of the swallowing disorder. However, if a patient denies having a swallowing disorder, the individual is frequently in error and often has a swallowing problem, sometimes severe in nature, to which he or she is oblivious. Typically, if a patient points to the base of the tongue area or the epiglottis and indicates that material has collected at that point, or the individual feels material "stuck" in his or her throat at that point, the material is likely to be hesitating in the valleculae at the base of the tongue. If, however, the patient points lower on the neck, just below the larynx, and indicates that material is sticking there, material is usually collecting in the pyriform sinuses. Coughing and choking, when present, generally indicate aspiration or entry of material into the patient's airway, but are obviously nonspecific signs of the cause(s) of aspiration. Over 50% of patients who aspirate do not cough.

The pattern of the patient's swallowing difficulty with particular consistencies of food is also helpful information for the clinician. Because in therapy it is generally best to start with easiest consistencies, it is important to know which consistency the patient feels is easiest to swallow. Particular swallowing disorders present differing symptoms as related to consistency of material. For example, patients with difficulty in oral transit because of poor control of the tongue may find liquids easiest to swallow, but pastes and thicker materials very difficult. Conversely, patients who have very delayed or absent triggering of the pharyngeal swallow generally do best with materials of a thicker consistency that tend to cling to the tongue base and the valleculae until the pharyngeal swallow triggers, and have greater difficulty with thin liquids because these splash into the pharynx and the airway before the pharyngeal swallow has triggered. There are no hard and fast rules, however, that tell the clinician that a particular disorder always presents with a particular pattern of difficulty with particular food consistencies. This is especially true for patients with multiple swallowing disorders that affect both the oral and the pharyngeal stages of the swallow.

In many cases, when the patient describes a problem with swallowing, it is important to ask the patient to demonstrate what he or she did when starting to swallow. In these demonstrations it often becomes clear that the patient took too much material, positioned it inappropriately in the mouth, or used an instrument or utensil that he or she could not manage well. The patient does not actually need to swallow the food or liquid. Simply repeating the motions leading to the swallow will give the clinician much information.

On the basis of a careful history, the swallowing therapist may have information on (1) the localization of the disorder in terms of the oral or pharyngeal stage of the swallow, or both; (2) the easiest and most difficult types of material for the patient to swallow; and (3) the nature of the swallowing disorder.

The Examination of Oral Anatomy

The examination of oral anatomy should include careful observation of lip configuration, hard palate configuration (height and width), soft palate and uvular dimensions relative to the distance to the posterior pharyngeal wall, intact nature of the faucial arches (both anterior and posterior), lingual configuration, and adequacy of the sulci at the sides and front of the mandible. Any scarring in the oral cavity or on the neck and any asymmetries in structures should be examined very carefully. The status of dentition and oral secretions should be assessed. Is the mouth moist or dry? If dry, a dampened gauze should be placed in the mouth to gently loosen these secretions and wipe them from the mouth prior to proceeding with the assessment. When the anatomical examination has been completed, the functional assessment should begin.

Oral-Motor Control Examination

The oral-motor control examination should include evaluation of the range, rate, and accuracy of movements of the lips, tongue, soft palate, and pharyngeal walls during speech, reflexive activity, and swallowing (Dobie, 1978). The clinician should always follow universal precautions when doing this examination.

Ability to Open the Mouth Voluntarily. For some patients with head injury or other severe neurologic impairment, voluntary mouth opening is difficult and slow, taking 3 to 5 minutes (Logemann, 1989). These patients may benefit most from bedside assessment with oromotor stimulation, including work on control of mouth opening, rather than an immediate radiographic study. The radiographic study can be scheduled when the patient is able to open the mouth more easily.

There are times when the clinician may wish to do a radiographic study in a patient with very slow mouth opening in order to determine that the pharyngeal swallow is triggered normally and has normal neuromotor control. Knowing this, the clinician can do more aggressive therapy in the oral cavity using food, if desired, without worry that the patient may aspirate.

These patients usually need oral massage to achieve mouth opening. In general, a combination of rotary massage of the cheek (masseter) on one side, with firm downward pressure on the chin, and continual verbal reinforcement over several minutes, will enable the patient to achieve mouth opening. As the patient's mouth opens, the clinician should determine whether a bite reflex is present. This can be done by using a 4″ × 4″ gauze roll to touch the teeth and alveolar ridge. Using the gauze roll prevents the patient from breaking a tooth or biting off a piece of the gauze, if a bite reflex is present. For patients with a bite reflex, a spoon that does not break or splinter easily should be used to place food in the patient's mouth. If possible, the clinician should avoid touching the spoon against the patient's teeth or alveolar ridge. In some cases, this is difficult because the patient can achieve only a limited mouth opening. Usually, however, with massage and verbal reinforcement to provide the patient with feedback regarding his or her success in achieving mouth opening, and time allocated for the patient to attain mouth opening, the patient can achieve mouth opening.

Identification of Optimal Oral-Sensory Stimuli and Bolus Types. Some patients with cognitive impairments produce most oral activity in response to particular combinations of taste, texture, and temperature. At the bedside, the clinician can use 4″ × 4″ pieces of cloth, such as gauze, burlap, and satin, rolled around a flexible, disposable plastic straw, to present various textures in the mouth. One end of these rolled materials can be dipped into liquid of various temperatures (cold, room temperature) and flavors (sour, sweet, bitter, salty) to present a variety of stimuli in the patient's oral cavity. Excess liquid can be squeezed from the cloth before presenting it to the patient's mouth. Using a variety of combinations of taste, temperature, and texture, the clinician can identify the particular combination of stimuli that elicits the most oral movements that are characteristic of chewing or a normal oropharyngeal swallow. These stimuli (mixed with barium) can then be introduced as one of the boluses during X-ray. In this way, during the radiographic study, the clinician can assess the patient's reaction to the stimuli identified at the bedside as optimal, in addition to presenting as many of the calibrated boluses included in the standard radiographic protocol as possible.

Identification of and Compensation for Swallowing Apraxia. A patient with swallowing apraxia usually performs best at the bedside when no verbal directions are given regarding eating or swallowing (Tuch & Neilsen, 1941). When a food tray is presented to the patient without verbal instruction, the patient often picks up the fork or spoon and begins eating normally with apparently normal swallowing. In contrast, when this patient is brought to X-ray, he or she often has severe difficulty initiating the oral stage of swallow because verbal commands are given regarding when to swallow. The more consciously this patient focuses on the swallowing act, the more difficulty the patient has in producing a swallow. If a patient shows only apraxia and no symptoms of any other swallowing disorder, particularly in the pharynx, a radiographic study is not needed.

Identification of and Compensation for Abnormal Oral Reflexes. Some patients with neurologic impairments exhibit abnormal oral reflexes, such as a hyperactive gag, tongue thrusting, or tonic bite (Logemann, 1989). These reflexes are usually counterproductive to the acceptance of food in the mouth and the production of a normal swallow. At the bedside, these abnormal reflexes can be identified, and techniques to avoid eliciting these reflexes or to desensitize these reflexes can be introduced prior to radiographic study. Identification of the location in the mouth where these reflexes are triggered and the nature of the stimuli that trigger them is important, so they can be avoided during the X-ray protocol.

LABIAL FUNCTION. To examine labial function, the clinician should have the patient spread the lips as widely as possible on the vowel /i/, round them as much as possible on the vowel /u/, rapidly alternate these two postures (/i/ and /u/) approximately 10 times, rapidly repeat the syllable *pa* to determine a diadochokinetic rate, and close the mouth tightly so as to observe the patient's labial closure during rest and during saliva swallowing. The clinician should also ask the patient to repeat a sentence that includes a large number of bilabial stop phonemes (e.g., "Put the papers by the back door"), and examine the completeness of bilabial closure on each articulation.

For chewing, the clinician should be concerned about the patient's ability to maintain lip closure despite changes in head posture and movements of the jaw in manipulating food. The clinician may ask the patient to move his or her jaw and maintain lip closure, or may ask the patient to shape his or her lips around a straw, spoon, or fork. The clinician should always check the patient's ability to tolerate nasal breathing comfortably.

LINGUAL FUNCTION. Lingual function should be assessed both anteriorly and posteriorly. For *anterior tongue examination*, the patient should be asked to (1) extend the tongue out of the mouth as far forward as possible and retract it as far backward as possible; (2) touch each corner of his or her mouth and then rapidly alternate the lateral movements; (3) attempt to clear the lateral sulcus on each side of the mouth as if it were full of food; (4) open the mouth widely and with the mouth in this position elevate the tongue tip to the alveolar ridge, and rapidly alternate elevation and depression of the tongue tip while maintaining an open mouth; (5) rapidly repeat the syllable /ta/ to determine a diadochokinetic rate; and (6) repeat a sentence containing a number of tip–alveolar stop consonants (e.g., "Take time to talk to Tom") and assess the completeness of tongue tip to alveolar ridge contact during these productions, including lateral seal on the lateral alveolus. The patient should also be asked to slide his or her tongue along the palatal vault from the very front near the alveolar ridge toward the back and to rub the tongue against the palate, as if clearing food from the palate.

Posterior tongue function can be assessed by asking the patient to (1) open the mouth and lift the back of the tongue as if saying a /k/ and hold the back of the tongue elevated in this position for several seconds; (2) repeat the syllable /ka/ as rapidly as possible to assess a diadochokinetic rate; and (3) repeat a sentence containing a number of back velar stop phonemes (e.g., "Can you keep the kitchen clean?") to determine the completeness of tongue–palate contact during these productions.

CHEWING FUNCTION. Assessment of chewing is most safely done with gauze rather than food. At the bedside, it is difficult to determine when chewing ends and the oral stage of swallow begins. Therefore, food chewing is not recommended for a bedside assessment. To assess chewing, a 4″ × 4″ gauze pad should be rolled into a 4″ roll and one end dipped into a pleasant tasting liquid. Excess liquid should be squeezed from the gauze and the damp end of the gauze placed on the midline of the patient's tongue, with the dry end of the gauze protruding from the mouth. The patient can then be asked to move the gauze onto the teeth, chew on it, move it to the other side, chew on it, and so on. The gauze is as flexible as food but cannot be lost in the mouth. If it becomes "stuck" so the patient cannot move it, the clinician can remove it from the patient's mouth (as the dry end of the gauze will be outside of the mouth) and replace the damp end of the gauze at midline of the tongue. The gauze provides the flexibility of food with none of the risk. Thus, this assessment of chewing can be done safely. If the patient has difficulty with this task, it can become a therapy exercise.

SOFT PALATE FUNCTION AND ORAL REFLEXES. Function of the soft palate can be examined by asking the patient to produce a strong, loud /a/ and to sustain that sound for several seconds (Dobie, 1978). The patient may also rapidly repeat the /a/. The clinician should note the action of the levator muscle in elevation of the palate and the palatopharyngeus muscle in retraction of the palate, as well as any observable lateral or posterior wall movement and soft palate movement. Velopharyngeal closure may not be as strong on this task as it is on swallow, however. The palatal and gag reflexes should also be tested. To elicit the palatal reflex, a cold instrument, such as the head of a size 00 laryngeal mirror (¼″ diameter) may be contacted against the juncture of the hard and soft palates or the inferior edge of the soft palate and uvula (DeJong, 1967), as shown in Figure 5.9. This contact should elicit an upward and backward movement of the soft palate, but no reaction in the pharyngeal walls. The palatal reflex stimulates soft palate movement but does not generate the total pharyngeal response of a gag reflex. In my experience, the palatal reflex is the least stable of the oral reflexes, often requiring two strokes to elicit it. Neurologically, the afferent portion of the reflex seems to be carried through the glossopharyngeal (and possibly the vagus) nerve, while the efferent portion of the reflex seems to be carried through the vagus (and possibly the glossopharyngeal) nerve. The trigeminal nerve, which also innervates part of the palate, may be involved in this reflex.

The gag reflex should be elicited by contacting a tongue blade or the head of a laryngeal mirror against the base of the tongue or the posterior pharyngeal wall. A strong, symmetrical contraction of the entire pharyngeal wall and soft palate should be observed as a result of this contact. If there is any asymmetry in the pharyngeal wall contraction, the clinician may suspect a unilateral pharyngeal weakness which is likely to affect swallowing. Despite the fact that many individuals with normal swallowing ability demonstrate reduced or absent

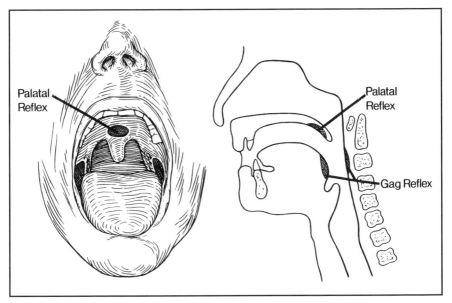

Figure 5.9. Frontal and lateral views of the oral cavity and pharynx with areas sensitive to triggering of the palatal and gag reflexes identified.

gag reflexes (Davies, Kidd, Stone, & MacMahon, 1995; DeJong, 1967; Leder, 1996, 1997), many health care professionals erroneously consider the presence or absence of a gag reflex in neurologically impaired patients to be an indication of the patient's ability to swallow. No data support this relationship, and an increasing number of investigators have confirmed no relationship (Davies et al., 1995; Leder, 1996, 1997). The afferent impulses for the gag reflex are carried mainly by cranial nerve X, although IX may be involved (DeJong, 1967). The gag reflex is triggered by a noxious stimulus, such as vomit or reflux, and the motor response is designed to squeeze the material up and out of the pharynx. This is in contrast to a swallow, which is an organized set of motor actions to take food safely and efficiently from the mouth to the stomach, thus clearing the noxious material from the pharynx. In addition, the gag is triggered from surface tactile receptors, whereas the swallow is triggered from deep proprioceptive receptors.

ORAL SENSITIVITY EXAMINATION. The oral sensitivity examination should include an assessment of light touch. The clinician needs to identify any areas in the mouth that have reduced sensitivity. There are no clear guidelines for interpretation of oral sensitivity testing; thus, the clinician can only compare the various areas of the patient's oral cavity to identify locations with greatest and least sensitivity. With a cotton swab, the clinician can make light contact at various points along the tongue, from anterior to posterior, along the buccal mucosa, and at the base and up the faucial arches, to determine the patient's awareness of light touch. If no gag is elicited, similar testing should be conducted on the posterior pharyngeal wall. This information will have an impact on the clinician's placement of food in the oral cavity, as all food should be positioned at the point of maximum sensitivity. Lack of awareness of light touch in the pharynx may indicate a patient who will have poor awareness of any pharyngeal residue remaining after a swallow.

MANAGEMENT INFORMATION TO BE COLLECTED FROM THE ORAL EXAMINATION. The results of the labial assessment should alert the clinician to any facial paralysis and any problem the patient may have in maintaining lip closure when food is placed in the mouth. The lingual function examination should identify any limitation in tongue function that may affect ability to propel food posteriorly or to hold food in a cohesive bolus, therefore identifying the area in the oral cavity where food can be positioned for best tongue control (K. Griffin, 1974). Similarly, identification of impairments in tongue function will help the clinician to select the particular consistencies of material that the patient can best manage.

Laryngeal Function Examination

Examination of *laryngeal function* should begin with assessment of voice quality (Dobie, 1978). Gurgly voice has been associated with aspiration and is an important enough sign of possible aspiration to warrant referral for a radiographic examination. A patient with hoarseness should be suspected of having reduced laryngeal closure during the swallow. This is not to say that patients who are hoarse automatically have swallowing problems, but patients with swallowing disorders whose vocal quality is hoarse should have a careful laryngeal examination. Referral to an otolaryngologist for indirect laryngoscopy is warranted. In addition, the swallowing therapist should examine laryngeal diadochokinetic rates (i.e., rapid repetition of the syllable /ha/, listening for clear production of the vowel and voiceless production of the h). Patients with some types of neurologic impairments tend to produce a single intermediate adduction of the larynx with a continuous breathy /ha/ instead of individual ha syllables. The patient should also be asked to cough as hard as possible and to clear the throat as strongly as possible. During these tasks, the therapist should evaluate the apparent strength and quality of the cough to determine its potential for expectorating aspirated material. The strength of a voluntary cough or throat clearing does not necessarily indicate that the patient will have a reflexive cough in response to aspiration or that the reflexive cough, if present, will be productive. Asking the patient to slide up and down a vocal scale enables the clinician to evaluate the function of the cricothyroid muscle and intrinsic muscles of the vocal cords, and test the superior laryngeal nerve as it innervates the cricothyroid muscle. Because the pharyngeal swallow may trigger from the superior laryngeal nerve, as may the cough reflex, inability to change pitch may imply reduced sensitivity within and surrounding the larynx. Phonation time tasks—that is, asking the patient to take a breath and prolong a /z/ for as long as possible on the subsequent exhalation or to prolong an /s/ on the subsequent exhalation—can provide some information on the relative control of the larynx. Phonation time is also a test of respiration, so during these prolonged articulations, the clinician should observe chest wall and abdominal movement during the exhalation.

Management Information to be Collected from the Laryngeal Examination. On the basis of the laryngeal control examination, the clinician should have some suspicion about the involvement of laryngeal function in the swallowing disorder. If laryngeal function appears to be borderline, the clinician may decide to teach the patient the supraglottic or super-supraglottic swallow in an attempt to increase the patient's airway protection prior to initiating any swallows. This technique is discussed in Chapter 6.

Pulmonary Function Testing

Pulmonary function testing helps the clinician determine whether the patient can tolerate any amount of aspiration. This test battery is ordered and interpreted by a physician. The information provided should be used when contemplating oral feeding regimens that may involve some small degree of aspiration. There are still no data that indicate how much aspiration a patient may tolerate before contracting aspiration pneumonia. There are also no guidelines on the level of pulmonary function that must be present in order for a patient to tolerate some degree of aspiration. Thus, each physician must establish his or her own guidelines to determine when oral feeding in the presence of aspiration is acceptable. Many physicians have found pulmonary function data helpful in making this determination. Patients who are observed to aspirate on a radiographic study have been found to be at significantly higher risk for developing pneumonia in the next 6 months than patients who exhibit no aspiration (Holas, DePippo, & Reding, 1994; Taniguchi & Moyer, 1994). Some patients who aspirate may not cough immediately but may cough within the next half hour and clear all of the aspirated material. This may be one reason why every patient who aspirates does not get pneumonia.

Information Collected from the Preparatory Examination

On the basis of the preparatory portion of the bedside clinical examination, the swallowing therapist should have the following information: (1) the posture that *may* result in best swallowing; (2) the best position for food in the mouth; (3) the potentially best food consistency; and (4) some indication of the nature of the patient's swallowing disorder.

Should Trial Swallows at the Bedside Be Attempted?

The swallowing therapist should consider the risk–benefit ratio in determining whether trial swallows should be attempted at the bedside. If the patient is acutely ill, has significant pulmonary complications, has a weak voluntary cough, is over 80 years old, and/or cannot follow directions and is suspected of having a pharyngeal swallowing disorder, the risk is high and the benefit is low. Because the patient needs a radiographic study to assess the pharyngeal swallowing dysfunction, little is likely to be gained from attempting swallows at the bedside. In contrast, if the patient can follow directions, cough on command, and has good pulmonary function, the risk is low and a few trial swallows can be assessed.

To date, there are no firm guidelines in this regard. The swallowing therapist must look at all aspects of the patient's function and determine the best course of action in regard to trial swallows. If the patient is being orally fed, the clinician should observe feeding to note (1) the patient's reaction to food; (2) oral movements in food manipulation and chewing; (3) any coughing, throat clearing, or struggling behaviors or changes in breathing and their frequency relative to swallowing and their occurrence during the meal (beginning, middle, or end); (4) changes in secretion levels throughout the meal; (5) duration of the meal and total intake; and (6) coordination of breathing and swallowing.

Decisions on Potentially Best Posture

Posture can be of great assistance in the management of swallowing disorders. The evaluation may have indicated poor tongue control, with the patient having difficulty maneuvering the bolus in his or her mouth, or the bolus trickling over the base of the tongue and into the pharynx before the voluntary swallow is initiated. In such a case, it may be best to ask the patient to tilt his or her head downward as food is introduced in the mouth and then throw his or her head backward to drain material from the mouth when the patient is ready to initiate the swallow, as shown in Figure 5.10.

Tilting the head backward is an entirely safe technique if the patient has normal pharyngeal and laryngeal control. Under those circumstances, airway protection will be adequate. If, on the basis of the careful history, the patient is known to have had a hemilaryngectomy, or any reason for a delay in triggering of the pharyngeal swallow, it may be helpful to tilt his or her head downward so that the vallecular space is widened, the airway entrance is narrowed, and the epiglottis is positioned more posteriorly, as shown in Figure 5.11 (Shanahan, Logemann, Rademaker, Pauloski, & Kahrilas, 1993; Welch, Logemann, Rademaker, & Kahrilas, 1993). With this position, material is more likely to rest in the valleculae long enough for the pharyngeal swallow to trigger, and the valleculae and epiglottis will divert material away from the airway. Similarly, if

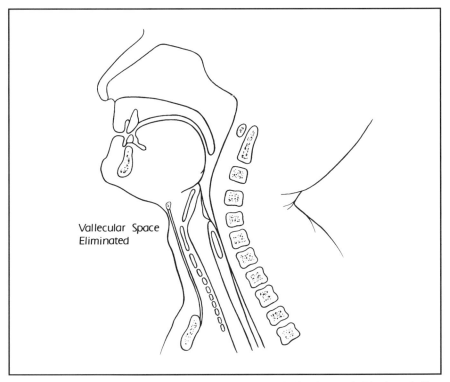

Figure 5.10. Midsagittal view of the head and neck with the head extended backward, illustrating the disappearance of the vallecular space in this position.

patients have slightly inadequate laryngeal closure, the forward tilting of the head may result in greater protection of the airway by the overhanging epiglottis. If, according to the history and medical examination, the patient exhibits a unilateral pharyngeal paralysis, as in a medullary stroke, it may be helpful to turn the patient's head toward the affected side to close the pyriform sinus on that side, directing material down the more functional side (Kirchner, 1967). If, on the other hand, a patient has a lingual hemiparesis or reduction in oral function on one side, in addition to involvement of the pharynx on that same side, tilting the head toward the stronger side may result in directing the material down that side, in both the oral and the pharyngeal stages of the swallow. If that technique is necessary, the patient will generally need to tilt his or her head before food is placed in the mouth. Otherwise, with the head in the normal position, material will tend to fall toward the affected side. These postural decisions should be made prior to attempting any swallows at the bedside with the patient, and should be based on the information collected in the preswallowing evaluation, including careful history taking and chart review.

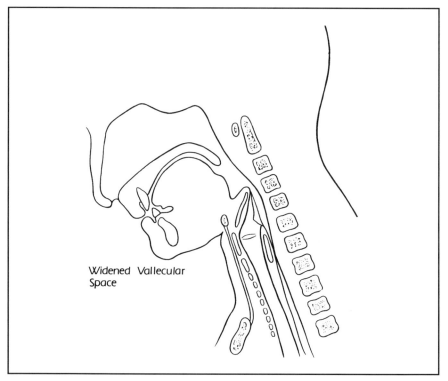

Figure 5.11. Midsagittal view of the head and neck, with the head down, illustrating the enhancement of the vallecular space in this position and the posterior positioning of the epiglottis, closer to the pharyngeal wall.

Selection of Optimal Food Position in the Mouth

Positioning food in the mouth should depend on information on oral sensitivity and oral function. In general, food should be positioned on the side of best function and best sensitivity. If liquid must be placed posteriorly in the oral cavity, a straw used as a pipette, or a syringe may be used. A tongue blade is often helpful in positioning thicker foods in particular places on the tongue.

Selection of Possible Best Food Consistency

Selection of food texture to use in the actual swallowing evaluation should depend on (1) information collected in the history, (2) data on oral control, and (3) information on pharyngeal and laryngeal control. In general, patients with poor oral control will do best with thickened liquid first, then moving toward materials of thin consistency; patients with a delayed pharyngeal swallow will do best with materials of a thicker consistency, such as applesauce or mashed potatoes; patients with reduced tongue base or pharyngeal wall contraction will do best with liquids; patients with reduced laryngeal elevation or reduced upper esophageal sphincter opening will do better with liquids; and patients with reduced closure of the laryngeal entrance will do best with materials of a thicker consistency. Combinations of disorders, however, make selection of material more difficult. For example, a patient with a disturbance in oral function and delayed pharyngeal swallow may do best with a consistency somewhere between liquid and paste. Thus, gravity can assist oral propulsion of the bolus during the oral phase of the swallow, but material will tend to cling to the valleculae and epiglottis while waiting for the pharyngeal swallow to trigger, rather than splashing into the pharynx and the larynx. The swallowing therapist should give careful consideration to selection of consistency of materials prior to initiating any swallows at the bedside.

Selection of Optimum Swallowing Instructions

When a patient is first asked to swallow, he or she should be given a series of instructions designed to elicit the most normal swallow possible. The sequence of swallowing instructions should be based on information collected in the preparatory examination. Posture or sequence of postures should be carefully noted, as should the need for voluntary protection of the airway during the swallow. For example, the patient with slightly reduced tongue control and reduced laryngeal control may need to begin by tilting his or her head downward while putting food in his or her mouth, then tip his or her head backward when he or she is going to swallow, and hold his or her breath during the swallow to voluntarily protect the airway. There may be a total of five or seven steps in a sequence of swallowing instructions. Details of this sequence will vary from patient to patient and are entirely dependent on results of the preparatory clinical examination. Clearly, this is not possible when patients have significant cognitive deficits or dementia.

Utensils To Be Used in the Initial Swallowing Evaluation

The clinician should bring a number of utensils into the patient's room for the swallowing evaluation. These include (1) a size 0 or 00 laryngeal mirror; (2) a tongue blade for wiping material onto the posterior tongue; (3) a cup to give the patient a small amount of material; (4) a spoon for presenting liquids and paste material; (5) a straw to be used as a pipette for placing liquid in the back of the mouth; and (6) a syringe to squirt small amounts (1 ml) of liquid into the posterior oral cavity.

The Swallowing Examination

Prior to initiating any actual swallows, the patient's preparation is most important. If the patient is exhibiting any excess secretions, suctioning should be completed both orally and transtracheostomy, if a tracheostomy tube is present.

Management of the Tracheostomy Tube

When working with swallowing, it is generally best to *deflate the tracheostomy cuff prior to attempting any swallows*. An inflated cuff may irritate the trachea as the larynx elevates during swallowing, or it may restrict laryngeal elevation. However, before proceeding with swallowing or with deflating the cuff, the clinician should *check with the patient's physician* and obtain his or her assessment of the advisability of deflating the cuff, as well as the patient's tolerance for possible aspiration, even in small amounts.

It is important to remember to *suction the patient well both orally and via the tracheostomy* to assure a clear oral cavity and airway prior to beginning therapy. It is particularly necessary to *suction the patient well immediately after the cuff is deflated* so that any secretions sitting above the cuff will be cleared away as they drain around the tube and into the trachea. This suctioning is usually best done by nursing staff, trained in suction techniques, rather than by the swallowing therapist. However, for emergencies and when nursing staff are not available, the swallowing therapist should know how to suction orally and transtracheostomy. If the nurse participates in this procedure, he or she will be able to observe the patient's swallowing training and can then reinforce the process with the patient throughout the day.

During each swallow, the patient should gently *occlude his or her tracheostomy* tube with a gloved finger or gauze pad to establish as near-normal tracheal pressure during swallowing as possible. This step should be incorporated into the sequence of instructions for swallowing until videofluoroscopy can verify whether or not this is helpful.

There are several advantages to initiating swallowing therapy with a tracheostomy tube in place. First, the swallowing therapist can observe aspiration more directly (but not perfectly) by examining any expectoration through the tube. At the same time, elimination of aspirated material by coughing or suction is accomplished more easily. Several authors have reported specific but infrequently occurring problems related to the presence of tracheostomy tubes during swallowing therapy: (1) restriction of upward laryngeal movement to protect the airway by anchoring the trachea to the strap muscles and skin of the neck along a tract of cicatrix or scar tissue, thus increasing the chances of aspiration (Bonanno, 1971; Pinkus, 1973); (2) compression of the esophagus by the tube pushing posteriorly on the common wall between the trachea and the esophagus (particularly true of cuffed tracheostomy tubes) (Betts, 1965; Pinkus, 1973); and (3) the change in intratracheal pressure because of the presence of the tube. Of the over 2,000 patients treated at Northwestern University for swallowing problems in the first 10 years of swallowing work at our center, only 1 patient's swallowing disorder could be attributed to the tracheostomy tube. For the majority of patients in swallowing therapy, the advantages of a tracheostomy outweigh the disadvantages. However, swallowing problems related directly to tracheostomy do occur occasionally and should be considered in tracheotomized patients with dysphagia, particularly if the tracheostomy has been in place 6 months or longer.

Prior to actually asking the patient to swallow, the clinician should review with the patient and write down his or her particular set of directions. The patient should be given an opportunity to practice several dry swallows according to this sequence. In general, patients do best if they are given adequate time to absorb the instructions and review them with the therapist before actually trying to swallow any food or liquid. Coaching by the therapist as the patient proceeds through the sequence is very helpful. Once the patient has demonstrated an ability to follow the outlined instructions, several actual swallows can be tried. It is usually advisable to assure the patient that the amount he or she will be given to swallow will be minimal. The patient should be encouraged to cough whenever necessary but to do the best he or she can throughout the swallowing sequence. It is also helpful to reassure the patient that the small amount of material to be swallowed should prevent difficulty with breathing during or after the swallow. Also, again, coughing should be reinforced as it clears the airway. Occasionally, patients feel that coughing indicates poor performance and try to consciously inhibit coughing to show how well they are doing.

When ready to check the patient's swallow, the clinician should use approximately ⅓ teaspoon for both the liquid and the paste or pudding-like consistencies. These small amounts of material are not sufficient to block a patient's airway and, if aspirated, should cause minimal difficulty.

Observations During the Trial Swallows

During the swallow, it is helpful for the clinician to place his or her hand under the patient's chin with fingers spread and making light contact, as illustrated in Figure 5.12. The index finger should be lightly positioned immediately behind the mandible anteriorly, the middle finger at the hyoid bone, the third finger at the top of the thyroid cartilage, and the fourth finger at the bottom of the thyroid cartilage. In this way, submandibular movement, hyoid movement, and laryngeal movement can be assessed during the swallow. No pressure should be placed on the tissue, but merely a light touch used to identify and assess the strength of movement (K. Griffin, 1974). The patient should then be asked to

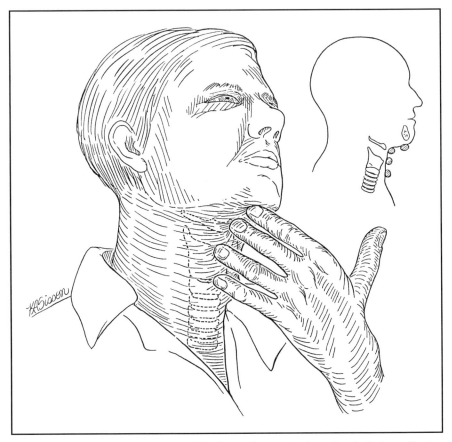

Figure 5.12. The correct positioning of the fingers during the clinical or bedside swallowing examination.

follow the sequence and swallow the material positioned in his or her mouth. As the patient swallows, the clinician's fingers on the patient's neck can assess initiation of tongue movement on the basis of movement felt by the index finger at the submandibular area immediately behind the anterior mandible. The second finger can perceive hyoid bone movement, and the third and fourth fingers can define laryngeal movement when the pharyngeal swallow triggers. Comparing the time elapsed between initiation of tongue movement and initiation of hyoid and laryngeal movement can provide the clinician with a very rough estimate of oral transit time and pharyngeal delay time, or the time taken from initiation of the swallow by the tongue until the pharyngeal swallow triggers. The major limitation to this technique is that, if the pharyngeal swallow does not trigger in a normal length of time (less than 1 second), the clinician at the bedside cannot assess what is occurring physiologically during the time delay. The exact duration of oral transit time and delay time cannot be separately defined. However, the clinician can follow the initial swallow with a swallow preceded by thermal–tactile stimulation to assess the difference in timing as a result of the thermal–tactile stimulation. This technique is described in Chapter 6. If the total time is reduced by several seconds on the swallow after thermal–tactile stimulation, the clinician may hypothesize that the time reduction was part of the pharyngeal delay. Movement of the bolus into the pharynx or into the airway cannot be assessed. Thus, only a very gross estimate of oral transit time and pharyngeal delay time can be identified, and no real information on the pharyngeal stage of the swallow can be collected.

It is often helpful in assessing aspiration if the patient is asked to perform several additional tasks after the swallow. First, immediately after the swallow, the patient should be asked to phonate *ah* for several seconds. The swallowing therapist can then examine the vocal quality for any signs of "gargling," indicative of material sitting on the vocal cords. Immediately after the vocalization, the patient should be asked to pant for several seconds. In this way, if material is residing in the pharyngeal recesses (valleculae or pyriform sinuses), it will be shaken loose and tend to fall into the airway. After panting, the patient should be asked to vocalize again so the therapist can again evaluate vocal quality.

The clinician can then ask the patient to turn his or her head to each side or encourage it by standing to each side of the patient and asking him or her to vocalize with the head turned to each side. This head rotation results in pressure on each pyriform sinus and may squeeze any residual material from the pyriform sinus into the pharynx causing the voice to become gurgly. If the voice is clear during these tasks, then the clinician can ask the patient to lift the chin up and hold it there for a few seconds. Then the patient should again vocalize. The chin-up posture will cause the tongue base to push on the vallecular space and result in clearing material from the valleculae which may then cause gurgly voice.

If the patient coughs during any part of this sequence and expectorates any material or if gargling vocal quality is heard, aspiration can be suspected. However, many patients are silent aspirators; that is, they aspirate material past the true vocal cords into the airway without responding in any of the usual ways, such as coughing. Thus, the clinician has no way of examining aspiration definitively at the bedside. It is important for the clinician to remember that 50% to 60% of patients who aspirate do not cough. If a patient aspirates and does not cough or give visible symptoms of aspiration, the clinician will be unaware of entry of material into the airway. Our study of the accuracy of bedside clinical examination of swallowing indicated that clinicians do not identify the presence of aspiration during clinical examinations approximately 40% of the time for patients who are actually aspirating. Others have found similar error rates (Linden & Siebens, 1983; Splaingard, Hutchins, Sulton, & Chauhuri, 1988). This is strong evidence for a radiographic approach to the examination of swallowing and the assessment of pharyngeal physiology during deglutition in order to identify patients who are aspirating, and the reason and amount of their aspiration.

Videofluoroscopic Procedure— The Modified Barium Swallow

Because swallowing is a dynamic and rapid process, fluoroscopy is particularly well suited to the study of this physiologic function (Dobie, 1978; Dodds, Logemann, & Stewart, 1990; Dodds, Stewart, & Logemann, 1990; Kirchner, 1967; Linden & Siebens, 1980; Logemann, 1983, 1993; O'Connor & Ardran, 1976; Palmer, Kuhlemeier, Tippett, & Lynch, 1993; Palmer, Rudin, Lara, & Crompton, 1992; Pitcher, 1973; Sloan, 1977). The fluoroscopic image is usually recorded on videotape for permanent storage. Although cinefluoroscopy, or the recording of the fluoroscopic image on movie film, had the advantage of permitting frame-by-frame analysis of the movement patterns of various structures and of the bolus of food or liquid (Kelley, 1970; Phillips & Hendrix, 1971; Scatliff, 1963; Schultz, Niemtzow, Jacobs, & Naso, 1979; Sloan, 1977), radiation exposure during cinefluoroscopy is greater than the alternative method of recording (i.e., videofluoroscopy) and has been eliminated in most hospitals. Also, no voice recordings can be placed on the cine film. In contrast, recording the fluoroscopic image on videotape (videofluoroscopy) permits voice recording simultaneously with the fluoroscopic image and requires less radiation exposure (O'Connor & Ardran, 1976). However, videofluoroscopy is more difficult to frame than cinefluoroscopy. Framing is possible, nonetheless, using a video counter timer, which places a number in the corner of the videoscreen, each number reflecting one frame of the videotape. Because video is framed at 30 frames with 60 fields per second, numbers are placed at the rate of 30 or 60 per second. Several videocassette recorder (VCR) players, both ½ and ¾ inch, are capable of slow-motion, frame-by-frame or stop-motion tape advance. Thus, when a tape with numbered frames is played on one of these recorders, frame-by-frame analysis of the movement of structures and the bolus is possible, similar to analysis of motion picture film. An additional advantage to videofluoroscopy in the analysis of deglutition is the ease of patching any video recorder player into the fluoroscopic equipment by attaching a cable from the back of the fluoroscopy monitor to the VCR. Such a hookup is not permanent, and, in fact, video equipment from the education department of a hospital may be borrowed for the time required (30 to 60 minutes) to complete two to three videofluoroscopic studies. Such equipment is generally available in all hospitals, and fluoroscopic units are among the most common types of radiographic equipment. Thus, even many smaller hospitals have the capability to do detailed videofluoroscopic studies of deglutition. Recently, mobile fluoroscopy units have been designed for use in rehabilitation centers and nursing homes, enabling access to fluoroscopic studies for most dysphagic patients needing them.

The fluoroscopic procedure designed to examine the details of oral, pharyngeal, and cervical esophageal physiology during swallowing is a modified barium swallow procedure. This is sometimes called a "cookie swallow" test because of the kinds of materials given to the patient. The methodology differs from the traditional upper gastrointestinal, or barium swallow, in several ways: purposes of the study, type and amount of material used in the study, and procedures used, including rehabilitation strategies introduced (Mandelstam & Lieber, 1970).

Purposes of the Study

The modified barium swallow has two purposes: (1) to define the abnormalities in anatomy and physiology causing the patient's symptoms and (2) to identify and evaluate treatment strategies that may immediately enable the patient to eat safely and/or efficiently. Oral and pharyngeal transit times are assessed during deglutition. The functioning of the valves in the system (the velopharynx, larynx, and cricopharyngeal or pharyngoesophageal region) is examined, as is cervical esophageal peristalsis. In contrast, the barium swallow gives information on structural competence of the esophagus, particularly the lower two thirds of the esophagus, with little attention paid to details of swallowing physiology in the oral cavity and pharynx. The modified barium swallow is designed to assess not only *whether* the patient is aspirating, but also *why*, so appropriate and efficient treatment can be initiated. Aspiration may occur for a number of reasons, as defined in Chapter 4, including reduced tongue function, delayed or absent pharyngeal swallow, reduced laryngeal closure at the entrance or at the vocal folds, cricopharyngeal dysfunction, and so forth. Each of these etiologies requires a different treatment.

Placement of Food in the Patient's Mouth

Generally, food is placed in the patient's mouth on a disposable plastic spoon. However, if a patient has a bite reflex, a heavier plastic spoon is more appropriate. At other times, for example with infants, a bottle and nipple may be used. Weathers, Becker, and Genieser (1974) described a special device to present the barium liquid to infants. It is a plastic tube with an end for attachment of an ordinary bottle nipple. A 50-cc syringe or a plastic bag with a 450-cc volume capacity is attached to the open end. The infant can then suck the liquid without the swallowing therapist's or the radiologist's hand entering the field of exposure.

Alternatively, the infant can be given formula mixed with barium and placed in a bottle, the end of which is held with a lead-gloved hand.

Types and Amounts of Materials Used

At least three consistencies of material are used in the modified barium swallow to investigate patient complaints of variable swallowing ability: thin liquid barium (as close to water as possible), barium paste (chocolate pudding mixed with Esophatrast), and material requiring mastication (a cookie coated with pudding mixed with Esophatrast). If the patient complains of difficulty swallowing particular foods, or if particular food consistencies are routinely given to the patient, or if the patient responded well to a particular taste, temperature, and texture combination in the bedside testing, this material should be provided during the radiographic study. At least two swallows of each material are given in the following amounts: 1 ml, 3 ml, 5 ml, 10 ml, and cup drinking of thin liquid; ⅓ teaspoon of pudding; and a fourth of a small Lorna Doone cookie coated with barium (Logemann, 1993). If the patient progresses through all of the volumes of liquid, the pudding, and the Lorna Doone cookie with no apparent difficulty, the clinician should proceed to give more foods of different types mixed with barium. The patient should be allowed to feed himself or herself as appropriate. In this way, normal eating can be observed radiographically. If the patient has a complaint, or if the staff in the patient's facility observe behaviors not seen during the radiographic study, it is the responsibility of the clinician conducting the radiographic study to try to simulate the same conditions under which the patient eats.

Volume of liquid is increased until or unless the patient aspirates. Once the reason for the aspiration is determined, intervention strategies are introduced to eliminate the aspiration. Intervention strategies are selected based on those that have been found to be effective with the swallowing disorder observed in the patient. Also, if it is thought that a patient can swallow other consistencies, such as honey-thickened or nectar-thickened liquids, without aspiration, these materials are also given in 1-ml, 3-ml, 5-ml, and 10-ml amounts and cup drinking as tolerated. Only liquids are given in various volumes because, as viscosity of the food increases, the volume normally swallowed decreases. Therefore, there is little need to increase volumes of pudding or cookie. However, it is valuable to have the patient self-feed so the clinician can see the amount the patient places in the mouth, as the patient may "overstuff" the mouth with food. In general, compensatory strategies, including postural changes, procedures for heightening sensory input, and changes in the way the patient is fed, are attempted first, followed by therapy procedures such as swallow maneuvers. Each of these procedures is described in Chapter 6. Compensatory procedures are used first because they require minimal direction following and little, if any, increased muscle effort. My colleagues and I have had no pulmonary problems result from this protocol, although a patient may aspirate on one or two more swallows if all treatment procedures fail (Logemann, Rademaker, Pauloski, & Kahrilas, 1994; Rasley et al., 1993).

The importance of *initially* giving the patient only *very* small amounts of material cannot be overstressed. In many cases, the patients referred for video-fluoroscopic study are ill, have poor respiratory status, and are aspirating. If any large amount (more than 1 teaspoon) of barium enters their airway, complications can result, including respiratory arrest. Only a small amount of material is needed initially to make an accurate diagnosis (Rossato & Wrightson, 1977; Schultz et al., 1979). This technique differs significantly from the traditional barium swallow, which is designed to diagnose structural lesions and anatomic deformities in the esophagus. During the barium swallow, the goal is to fill the esophagus with material and thus outline the structure and observe peristaltic contraction (Bachman, 1963; Haubrich, 1977). Unfortunately, if this technique were used with oropharyngeal dysphagic patients, they could aspirate a larger amount of material.

Beginning with liquids in the modified barium swallow ensures that the material will not block the airway, if aspirated. There is also some evidence that pneumonia is less likely from aspiration of liquids than from aspiration of thicker foods (Holas et al., 1994). The lungs may be better able to clear liquids from the tracheobronchial tree by a cough or ciliary action.

Positioning the Patient

Often the most difficult and time-consuming part of the radiographic procedure is positioning the patient. Optimally, the patient should be seated and initially viewed in the lateral plane. A number of chairs for positioning patients during the radiographic study have been designed and are commercially available (Logemann, 1993). A patient who is mobile and able to sit without a back rest can be seated on the horizontal platform attached to the fluoroscopy table, as shown in Figure 5.13, and raised or lowered to the desired height. Most fluoroscopy machines are fitted with handles so the patient can grip to stabilize his or her position. Initially, then, the patient is seated so that his or her side rests against the table of the fluoroscopy machine and the vocal tract is viewed laterally (Kirchner, 1967; Rossato et al., 1977).

Some fluoroscopy machines will not accommodate a patient unable to sit unassisted, who needs to sit in a wheelchair or lie on a cart. Because of the design of many types of fluoroscopy equipment, the distance between the tube and the table is not wide enough to fit a wheelchair or cart. However, with a

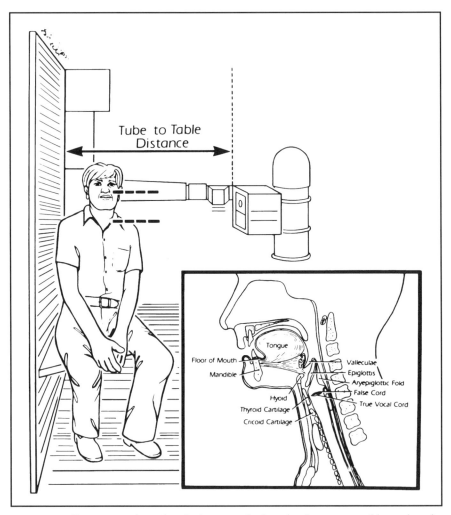

Figure 5.13. Patient seated on the platform attached to the fluoroscopy table so that the upper aerodigestive tract can be viewed laterally, as shown in the inset in the lower right-hand corner.

narrow back support attached to the cart, as shown in Figure 5.14, any fluoroscopy machine can accommodate the patient (T. Slominski, personal communication, June 10, 1993). Also, many fluoroscopy machines have limited vertical tube movement and can be lowered only a limited distance, usually not low enough to view the patient's laryngopharynx if he or she is seated in a wheelchair. If the fluoroscopy machine accommodates a cart as shown in Figure 5.15, even patients who are unable to walk or sit up independently can be examined

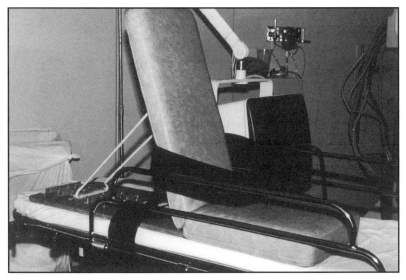

Figure 5.14. The attachment of a narrow back support to a cart or gurney in order to fit the fluoroscopy machine.

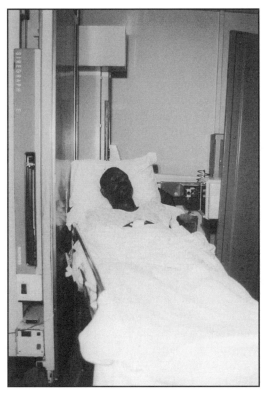

Figure 5.15. Patient lying on a cart with the head elevated so that the upper aerodigestive tract can be viewed laterally.

fluoroscopically when they are positioned on a cart with the head of the cart elevated to at least a 90° angle.

Focus of the Fluoroscopic Image

The fluoroscopy tube should focus on the lips anteriorly, the hard palate superiorly, the posterior pharyngeal wall posteriorly, and the bifurcation of the airway and the esophagus inferiorly. Many fluoroscopy machines permit image magnification. If a patient is suspected of aspirating, it is sometimes helpful to magnify the area around the bifurcation of the airway and the esophagus to get a clear picture of the amount of the aspiration on the first swallow or two. Then the image can be reduced to include the entire vocal tract on the remaining swallows to identify the reason for the aspiration, if it has not already been defined. The patient's arms should hang at his or her sides and not rest on the arms of a chair, which will elevate the shoulders. It is important to get the patient's shoulders as low as possible so they do not shadow or cover the pharynx.

Measures and Observations To Be Made

Lateral View

The lateral view permits a number of measures and observations critical to the identification of the patient's anatomic or physiologic swallowing disorder. First, the oral and pharyngeal transit times can be measured. *Oral transit time* is defined as the time taken for the movement of the bolus through the oral cavity from the initiation of posterior movement of the bolus by the tongue until the leading edge of the bolus passes the point where the mandible crosses the tongue base (see Figure 5.16). The pharyngeal phase of the swallow begins when the pharyngeal swallow triggers and terminates when the bolus tail passes through the cricopharyngeal juncture. *Pharyngeal transit time* is defined as the time elapsed as the bolus moves between these two points. Pharyngeal delay time is the time interval from the end of oral transit time until the pharyngeal swallow triggers, as indicated by hyolaryngeal elevation followed by the other muscular actions comprising the pharyngeal stage of swallow.

Esophageal transit time can also be measured, but is not usually included in this study because exercise programs for swallowing disorders are generally not effective in remediating esophageal disorders. Esophageal disorders are usually treated medically or surgically. It is generally not a good idea to attempt to assess the esophagus on the same swallows in which the pharyngeal and oral aspects are examined. The fluoroscopic tube should remain focused on the oral cavity and pharynx throughout the entire modified barium swallow. The fluoroscopic tube should not follow the bolus down through the esophagus on the same swallows on which the oral and pharyngeal function are assessed (Dodds, Logemann,

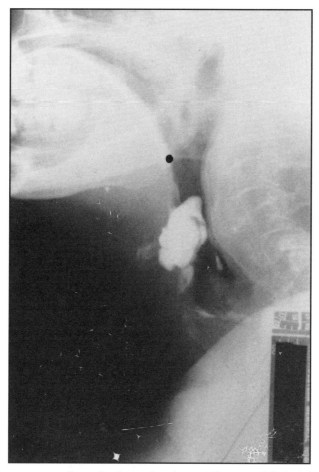

Figure 5.16. Lateral radiographic showing the point (black dot where the shadow of the mandible crosses the tongue base) where the oral transit time terminates and the pharyngeal delay time begins. If the pharyngeal swallow triggers on time, the point at the base of the tongue where the mandible shadow crosses is also the onset of pharyngeal transit time.

& Stewart, 1990; Dodds, Stewart, & Logemann, 1990).

In addition to definition of oral and pharyngeal transit times, the lateral view permits identification of the location of the bolus as it moves along the upper aerodigestive tract from anterior superior to posterior inferior. It permits analysis of patterns of lingual movement, gross estimate of the amount of vallecular residue after the swallow, and an estimate of the amount of material aspirated per bolus, as well as the anatomic or physiologic reason for the aspiration. The timing of aspiration relative to the triggering of the pharyngeal swallow

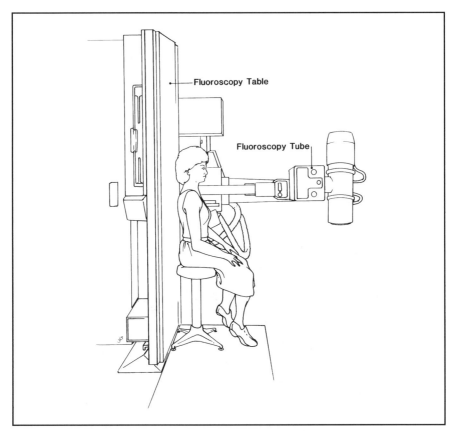

Figure 5.17. Patient seated on the platform attached to the fluoroscopy table so that the upper aerodigestive tract can be viewed in the posterior–anterior plane.

(i.e., before, during, or after the swallow) is also best examined in the lateral view.

Posterior–Anterior View

When the desired number of swallows of various materials has been completed in the lateral view, the patient can be turned and viewed in the posterior–anterior (P–A) plane, as shown in Figure 5.17 (Ardran & Kemp, 1951). In the P–A view, as the bolus of food or liquid enters the pharynx, it fills the valleculae, giving a scalloped appearance because of the hyoepiglottic ligament at midline, which subdivides the valleculae. Then the bolus divides and goes around the airway into the pyriform sinuses. Usually, the bolus divides fairly equally between the two sides, coming together at about the level of the opening into the esophagus (Ardran & Kemp, 1951). Approximately 20% of normal swallowers swallow down only one side, however (Logemann, Kahrilas, Kobara, &

Vakil, 1989). The P–A view is helpful in looking at asymmetries in function, particularly of the pharyngeal walls and vocal folds, and in viewing residues of material in the valleculae and in one or both pyriform sinuses. It is more difficult to measure transit times and to observe aspiration in the P–A view than in the lateral view. In the P–A view, it is usually best to repeat only swallows of particular materials that exhibit the most severe disturbance(s) in swallowing. This assures that the patient receives a minimal amount of radiation exposure, eliminating repetition of materials that elicit more normal swallows. In the P–A view, it is important to examine the residue in the pharynx after the swallow, comparing the two sides. It is also helpful to tilt the patient's head backward and ask him or her to vocalize a continuous *ah* and a rapidly repetitive /a/ to provide a clear picture of vocal fold movement. Although details of vocal fold movement cannot be examined in this manner, a gross judgment about relative movement of the two cords on adduction and abduction can be made (Bachman, 1963; Maguire, 1966). This is often helpful to the clinician in assessing the patient's ability to close his or her vocal folds during the swallow.

Instructions to the Patient

When the patient is positioned, the clinician should explain that the patient will be asked to swallow several different kinds of foods, and that only small amounts of each food will be given at first. All patients should be shown the small amount (1 ml) of material on the spoon before placing this into the mouth. Patients should be told that, if they have difficulty, they should feel free to cough and/or spit out the material if necessary. However, it should be emphasized that the patient should try his or her best throughout the examination.

Procedure To Be Followed with the Various Materials To Be Swallowed

Liquid barium in measured amounts is generally the first material used. First, 1 ml of liquid barium is measured in a syringe and placed in a teaspoon. The patient is asked to hold the material in his or her mouth until the examiner says to swallow the material when ready. Liquid is the first material presented, even if the patient is known to aspirate, because it is usually best to define the reason for aspiration and the amount of aspiration during the first several swallows. Liquids may be, but are not always, the most easily aspirated and yet are least apt to block the airway, reducing the patient's fear of swallowing. After two 1-ml swallows are completed, two 3-ml liquid swallows should be given, also on a teaspoon. Then two 5-ml swallows are given via the syringe placed gently in the mouth or placed in an empty cup and given to the patient in that manner. If no aspiration occurs at 5 ml, 10 ml should be given. Changing volume allows observation of the mechanism's ability to modulate volume (Cook, Dodds, Dantas, et al., 1989; Jacob, Kahrilas, Logemann, Shah, & Ha, 1989; Kahrilas, Lin, Logemann, Ergun, & Facchini, 1993; Kahrilas, Logemann, Krugler, & Flanagan, 1991; Kahrilas, Logemann, Lin, & Ergun, 1992; Lazarus, Logemann, Rademaker, et al., 1993). Finally, the patient can be given a cup and told to swallow normally. If the patient aspirates on a particular volume of liquid, the examiner should attempt treatment strategies to eliminate aspiration on the same volume, as described later in this chapter. If aspiration is eliminated on several swallows of that volume as a result of the intervention, the volume should be increased as far as tolerated, the goal being to allow the patient to take thin liquids orally of as many volumes as possible (Logemann et al., 1994; Rasley et al., 1993).

Second, swallows of thicker foods should be given. Again, if aspiration occurs, therapeutic strategies should be introduced to stop the aspiration. Chocolate pudding is mixed with Esophatrast to provide the pudding consistency but to maintain a good taste. If the patient is unable to take paste material or liquid from a spoon, a tongue blade can be used to wipe material of a thicker consistency onto the back of the tongue.

The third material used is one fourth of a Lorna Doone cookie with a light coating of the Esophatrast pudding as a contrast medium. On these last two swallows, the patient is asked to chew the material well and to initiate the swallow when he or she is ready. The directions are slightly different from the previous swallows in which the patient was asked to wait for the investigator's command to begin the swallow. In the case of the masticated material, the patient is told to go ahead and swallow as soon as he or she has completed chewing. If the patient cannot follow directions, the clinician can place the piece of cookie in the patient's mouth and observe the patient's spontaneous chewing and swallowing.

If the patient does well with the various foods presented using interventions or not, the clinician should also observe the patient's self-feeding radiographically to assure that he or she follows the same procedure and is equally successful in the self-feeding situation.

Patients with dementia or severe cognitive problems can be successfully assessed with the modified barium swallow. Food can be placed in their mouth and the clinician's hand removed quickly from the radiographic field so that the fluoroscopy can be activated and the pharyngeal swallow viewed. In some cases, the patient may swallow quickly, not understanding the clinician's directions, and the oral stage may be missed. However, the pharyngeal stage of the swallow, which is the most critical part of the study, will still be seen.

Trial Therapy

When the patient aspirates or has significant residue in the pharynx after the swallow, the clinician should decide on the nature of treatment for the patient's specific swallowing disorder and attempt trial therapy in the presence of video-fluoroscopy (Logemann, 1993; O'Connor & Ardran, 1976). If intervention strategies cannot be done, this should be noted along with the reason(s) why. The clinician can ask the patient to position his or her head or body in a particular way (or the clinician can position the patient who cannot follow directions), present sensory-enhancing boluses (cold, sour, larger volumes, etc.) or procedures to heighten oral sensory awareness prior to swallow or ask the patient to follow specific instructions (swallow maneuvers) while swallowing, and examine the results on videofluoroscopy, comparing the swallow physiology to the physiology observed on earlier swallows. Often, postural changes or other compensatory strategies can result in dramatic changes in physiology, as described further later in this chapter and in Chapter 6, and may permit the patient to begin oral intake (Logemann et al., 1994; Rasley et al., 1993). Therefore, it is very helpful when these changes are documented using videofluoroscopy. This is also the cost-effective part of the procedure because some patients will be able to return to oral intake quickly. Even with these added intervention swallows, the exposure time is generally less than 5 minutes and presents less radiation exposure to the patient than would be received during a standard radiographic procedure, such as a barium swallow or lower gastrointestinal series.

Guidelines for Videofluoroscopy Referral

In general, any patient who is suspected of aspirating, whose swallowing disorder is suspected to be of pharyngeal origin, or who has a pharyngeal component to the disorder should be referred for a videofluoroscopic study. At this time, pharyngeal physiology cannot be defined at the bedside. Therefore, therapy planning and implementation for pharyngeal dysphagia cannot be done without a radiographic study. Many patients who aspirate will not be identified at bedside because they give no sign of the aspiration. Most important, however, the anatomic or physiologic *cause* of the aspiration cannot be identified. Several studies have compared the results of the bedside examination of swallowing with the data from videofluoroscopic examinations of deglutition on the same patients (Splaingard et al., 1988). Approximately 40% of the patients who aspirated regularly during the videofluoroscopic study were not identified as aspirating when examined at the bedside, because they did not cough or give any other outward sign of aspiration. This is particularly true of neurologic patients, whose pharyngeal and/or laryngeal sensitivity may be reduced (Aviv et al., 1996).

Who Should Do the Videofluoroscopic Study?

Typically, it is best if the swallowing therapist and the radiologist collaborate in performing the videofluoroscopic study. Each brings particular expertise to the analysis of the swallowing disorder. The radiologist is trained to identify structural abnormalities but typically has minimal knowledge of the details of oral

and pharyngeal movement patterns during deglutition. The swallowing therapist is familiar with these movement patterns and the therapeutic regimens to
treat particular disorders. The combination of skills of the two professionals
results in optimum diagnosis and management decisions.

The Dysphagia Diagnostic Procedure as a Treatment Efficacy Trial

The purpose of any imaging assessment in most cases is not merely to determine
whether a patient aspirates, which is already suspected, but rather to define the
swallow physiology causing the aspiration. Equally important is the patient's
swallow efficiency or ability to move food quickly and cleanly through the mouth
and pharynx to the esophagus. Imaging procedures for the evaluation of swallowing are normally done as a part of a swallowing rehabilitation program, with
the ultimate goal of restoring the patient's full oral intake. Thus, the clinician
should take the opportunity during the imaging study to examine the effectiveness of at least some selected treatment options that fit the patient's oropharyngeal swallowing abnormalities, with the goal of establishing some safe, efficient
oral feeding immediately.

Order of Interventions Introduced

In general, the introduction of treatment strategies in the diagnostic study
begins with use of postural techniques; followed by introduction of techniques
to increase oral sensation, when appropriate; followed by swallowing maneuvers; and, finally, diet (food consistency) changes, if needed (Logemann, 1993).
The rationale for this sequencing of interventions is based on the muscle effort
required by patients and the ease of application and learning of the various
procedures. In general, postural techniques are easily used by a wide range of
patients, even those with reduced cognition, children, and patients with some
degree of restricted physical mobility. Procedures designed to increase oral sensation can also be used with a wide range of patients, as these procedures are
clinician controlled and do not require the patients to actively cooperate, other
than allowing the clinician to place something into their mouths. Swallow
maneuvers, on the other hand, require ability to actively follow directions
and voluntarily manipulate the oropharyngeal swallow as it is ongoing. Swallow
maneuvers also involve increased work or muscular effort in most cases, thus
increasing the patient's potential for fatigue. However, some patients cannot
swallow successfully without swallow maneuvers (Lazarus, Logemann, & Gibbons, 1993; Logemann & Kahrilas, 1990). Each of these techniques is described
briefly and documented with research studies. Also, methods are described for
measurement or observation of the success of the various techniques.

Postural Techniques

Postural techniques have been demonstrated to effectively eliminate aspiration on liquids and other foods in a wide range of patients (Horner, Massey, Riski, Lathrop, & Chase, 1988; Logemann et al., 1989; Rasley et al., 1993; Shanahan et al., 1993; Welch et al., 1993) when the postures were selected to match the patient's anatomic or physiologic swallowing disorder. Postural techniques redirect food flow and change pharyngeal dimensions. Table 5.2 presents the postures currently used and their effects on specific swallowing disorders and pharyngeal

Table 5.2
Rationale for Application of Postural Techniques
to Various Swallowing Disorders

Disorder Observed on Fluoroscopy	Posture Applied	Rationale
Inefficient oral transit (Reduced posterior propulsion of bolus by tongue)	Head back	Utilizes gravity to clear oral cavity
Delay in triggering the pharyngeal swallow (Bolus past ramus of mandible, but pharyngeal swallow not triggered)	Head down	Widens valleculae to prevent bolus entering airway; narrows airway entrance
Reduced tongue base posterior motion (Residue in valleculae)	Head down	Pushes tongue base backward toward pharyngeal wall
Unilateral laryngeal dysfunction (Aspiration during swallow)	Head down	Places epiglottis in more posterior protective position; narrows laryngeal entrance
	Head rotated to damaged side	Increases vocal fold closure by applying extrinsic pressure; narrows laryngeal entrance
Reduced laryngeal closure (Aspiration during swallow)	Head down	Places epiglottis in more protective position; narrows airway entrance
Reduced pharyngeal contraction (Residue spread throughout pharynx)	Lying down on one side	Changes direction of gravitational effect on pharyngeal residue
Unilateral pharyngeal paresis (Residue on one side of pharynx)	Head rotated to damaged side	Twists pharynx; eliminates damaged side of pharynx from bolus path
Cricopharyngeal dysfunction (Residue in pyriform sinuses)	Head rotated	Pulls cricoid cartilage away from posterior pharyngeal wall, reducing resting pressure in cricopharyngeal sphincter

dimensions. In general, postural techniques work equally well with neurologically impaired individuals, in patients who have experienced head and neck cancer resections or other structural damage, and in patients of all ages (Logemann et al., 1994; Rasley et al., 1993).

The best measure of postural effectiveness is the judgment of the amount of aspiration with and without the posture (Horner et al., 1988; Logemann et al., 1994; Rasley et al., 1993). Postures may also improve oral and pharyngeal transit times. In general, postural effects can best be observed and measured using videofluoroscopy (Shanahan et al., 1993; Welch et al., 1993). Occasionally, postural effects on residue and aspiration can be observed from endoscopy before or after, but not during, the swallow. Scintigraphy could be used to measure the effects of postural changes on residue and aspiration.

Techniques To Improve Oral Sensory Awareness

Techniques to improve oral sensory awareness are generally used in patients with swallow apraxia, delayed onset of the oral swallow, or delayed triggering of the pharyngeal swallow. These procedures all involve providing a preliminary sensory stimulus prior to the patient's initiation of the oral stage of swallow. Sensory techniques include (1) increasing downward pressure of the spoon against the tongue in presenting food in the mouth; (2) presentation of a sour bolus (50% lemon juice, 50% barium); (3) presentation of a cold bolus; (4) presentation of a bolus requiring chewing; (5) presentation of a larger volume bolus (3 ml or more); and (6) thermal–tactile stimulation (Lazzara, Lazarus, & Logemann, 1986; Ylvisaker & Logemann, 1986). In some patients with swallow apraxia, increasing oral sensation by a preliminary stimulus, such as the downward pressure of a spoon or the presentation of a bolus with increased volume, taste, or temperature characteristics, may facilitate the oral onset and oral transit. Thermal–tactile stimulation involves vertically rubbing the faucial arch firmly with a size 00 laryngeal mirror, which has been held in crushed ice for several seconds, in advance of the presentation of a bolus. This technique is designed to heighten oral awareness and provide an alerting sensory stimulus to the cortex and brainstem such that, when the patient initiates the oral stage of swallow, the pharyngeal swallow will trigger more rapidly. This technique has been demonstrated to facilitate faster triggering of the pharyngeal swallow after the stimulation and reducing the delay for several swallows thereafter (Lazzara et al., 1986).

Measures of the effectiveness of these procedures to increase oral sensory input include (1) duration of time from command to swallow until initiation of the oral stage of swallow; (2) oral transit time; and (3) pharyngeal delay time. These can be measured from videofluoroscopy. Oral onset time and oral transit time can be measured from ultrasonography. In some patients, pharyngeal delay time can be measured from videoendoscopy. However, if a patient exhibits premature spillage of a bolus because of oral abnormalities, videoendoscopy will not be capable of defining pharyngeal delay time with the same accuracy as videofluoroscopy, since the oral stage of swallow cannot be visualized with videoendoscopy.

Swallow Maneuvers

Swallow maneuvers are designed to place specific aspects of pharyngeal swallow physiology under voluntary control. Four swallow maneuvers have been developed to date: (1) the supraglottic swallow, designed to close the airway at the level of the true vocal folds before and during the swallow; (2) the super-supraglottic swallow, designed to close the airway entrance before and during the swallow; (3) the effortful swallow, designed to increase tongue base posterior motion during the pharyngeal swallow and thus improve bolus clearance from the valleculae; and (4) the Mendelsohn maneuver, designed to increase the extent and duration of laryngeal elevation and thereby increase the duration and width of cricopharyngeal opening. This latter maneuver can also improve the overall coordination of the swallow. During the videofluorographic study, if postural techniques and oral sensory facilitation techniques do not improve swallow physiology sufficiently to allow the patient to begin some oral intake, voluntary swallow maneuvers may be appropriate. However, these maneuvers require careful direction following ability and are not feasible in patients who have cognitive or significant language impairment. These maneuvers also require increased muscular effort and are not appropriate in patients who fatigue easily. However, there are patients who can swallow safely and efficiently only using a voluntary maneuver (Lazarus, Logemann, & Gibbons, 1993; Logemann & Kahrilas, 1990). Combinations of maneuvers and postures may need to be assessed in some patients (Logemann, 1993).

Food Consistency (Diet) Changes

Generally, elimination of certain food consistencies from the diet should be the last strategy examined. Restricting oral intake to certain food consistencies can be difficult for the patient. This should be done only if other therapy strategies are not feasible, as in a patient with a movement disorder whose posture changes continuously, who cannot follow directions and use swallow maneuvers, and for whom oral sensory procedures are inappropriate. Table 5.3 presents the easiest food consistencies and the food consistencies to be avoided for each swallowing disorder.

In some cases, introduction of therapy procedures into the diagnostic procedure can immediately enable the patient to begin eating. In other cases, evaluation of the effectiveness of the therapy procedure can validate its appropriateness for use with a patient in building the neuromuscular control necessary to return to oral intake.

Table 5.3
Easiest Food Consistencies and Foods To Be Avoided by Patients with Each Swallowing Disorder[a]

Swallowing Disorder	Easiest Food Consistencies	Food Consistencies to Avoid
Reduced range of tongue motion	Thick liquid	Thick foods
Reduced tongue coordination	Thick liquid	Thick foods
Reduced tongue strength	Liquid	Thick, heavy foods
Delayed pharyngeal swallow	Thick liquids and thicker foods	Thin liquids
Reduced airway closure	Pudding and thick foods	Thin liquids
Reduced laryngeal movement contributing to cricopharyngeal dysfunction	Liquid	Thicker, higher viscosity foods
Reduced pharyngeal wall contraction	Liquid	Thick, higher viscosity foods
Reduced tongue base posterior movement	Liquid	Higher viscosity foods

[a]These consistency categories are necessarily rather gross as we still do not have any definitions of the viscosity ranges that delineate the various food consistencies.

Not all therapy procedures can be introduced into the diagnostic setting, however, because not all therapy procedures result in immediate effects. For example, range-of-motion exercises for the lips, tongue, and/or jaw do not have an immediate effect, but typically show an effect after 2 to 3 weeks (see Chapter 6). However, the clinician can still quantify the effects of range-of-motion exercises by measuring the patient's structural movement at each therapy session. When a second assessment is completed, change in range of motion of the target structure can be assessed by comparing the first and second studies. Introducing treatment techniques into the diagnostic swallowing assessment requires the clinician to read the results of the radiographic study or other imaging procedure immediately and identify the physiologic dysfunction so that appropriate therapy procedures can be selected and introduced. Because videofluorography involves X-ray exposure to the patient, not all possible treatment techniques can be attempted while in X-ray to look at their relative value. Rather, the clinician must select those treatment techniques believed to be most appropriate for that patient's anatomy and swallowing physiology.

When effective techniques are identified, the videotape of the diagnostic procedure can be used as an educational tool with the patient, the family, nurses, physicians, and others, to educate and counsel them regarding the rationale for use of particular procedures with the patient, including introduction of particular posture, diets, and so forth. This type of visual evidence often improves the patient's and family's compliance with therapy recommendations.

Videofluoroscopic Study Report

The report of the study should be written and signed by all professionals involved. Typically, the report begins with a description of the patient's symptoms or complaints. Then, measures of oral transit time should be given for each material swallowed, followed by a description of any neuromuscular or anatomic problems observed in the oral phase of the swallow. Any variability in deglutition with the various food consistencies presented should be noted. If the patient aspirates because of a disorder in the oral stage of deglutition, this should be described. The duration of any delay in triggering the pharyngeal swallow and its variation with bolus volume or viscosity should be indicated and the location of the bolus during the delay should be identified. If aspiration occurs during the delay, this should be described and the approximate amount of the bolus aspirated noted.

Pharyngeal transit times should then be specified, noting variations with consistency of material. Any anatomic or neuromuscular problems observed in the pharyngeal phase of the swallow should be described. The approximate amount of aspiration on particular food consistencies, and the etiology of the aspiration should be noted. Approximate amounts of vallecular and pyriform residue should also be defined. If aspiration or significant residue is observed, the intervention strategies should be attempted and their results reported. If there is a reason that no strategies can be introduced, this should be explained.

Finally, recommendations should be outlined regarding (1) management of nutritional intake (i.e., nonoral feeding, oral feeding, or a combination) and any swallow management strategies to be used at meals; (2) results of the interventions and therapy used in the study; (3) procedures for swallowing therapy; and (4) reevaluation. These should include any recommendations for consultation(s) by other professionals. If the report does not contain the anatomic or physiologic reason for the aspiration or residue *and* the interventions attempted to reduce or eliminate these symptoms and their effects, or reasons why they could not be attempted, *the study is incomplete*.

References

Ardran, G., & Kemp, F. (1951). The mechanism of swallowing. *Proceedings of the Royal Society of Medicine, 44*, 1038–1040.

Aviv, J. E., Martin, J. H., Sacco, R. L., Zagar, D., Diamond, B., Keen, M. S., & Blitzer, A. (1996). Supraglottic and pharyngeal sensory abnormalities in stroke patients with dysphagia. *Annals of Otology, Rhinology, and Laryngology, 105,* 92–97.

Bachman, A. (1963). Methodology in the radiographic examination of the larynx and hypopharynx. *New York State Journal of Medicine, 63,* 1155–1163.

Batchelor, B., Neilson, S., & Sexton, K. (1996). Issues in maintaining hydration in nursing home patients with aspirated thin liquids. *Journal of Medical Speech-Language Pathology, 4,* 217–221.

Betts, R. (1965). Post-tracheostomy aspiration. *New England Journal of Medicine, 273,* 155.

Bonanno, P. (1971). Swallowing dysfunction after tracheostomy. *Annals of Surgery, 174,* 29–33.

Buckwalter, J. A., & Sasaki, C. T. (1984). Effect of tracheostomy on laryngeal function. *Otolaryngology Clinics of North America, 17,* 41–48.

Cook, I. J., Dodds, W. J., Dantas, R. O., et al. (1989). Opening mechanism of the human upper esophageal sphincter. *American Journal of Physiology, 257,* G748–G759.

Davies, A. E., Kidd, D., Stone, S. P., & MacMahon, J. (1995). Pharyngeal sensation and gag reflex in healthy subjects. *Lancet, 345*(8948), 487–488.

DeJong, R. (1967). *The neurologic examination.* New York: Hoeber Medical Division—Harper & Row.

DeLarminat, V., Montravers, P., Dureuil, B., & Desmonte, J. M. (1995). Alteration in swallowing reflex after extubation in intensive care unit patients. *Critical Care Medicine, 23,* 486–488.

DePippo, K. L., Holas, M. A., & Reding, M. J. (1992). Validation of the 3-ounce water swallow test for aspiration following stroke. *Archives of Neurology, 49,* 1259–1261.

Dettelbach, M. A., Gross, R. D., Mahlmann, J., & Eibling, D. E. (1995). Effect of the Passy-Muir valve on aspiration in patients with tracheostomy. *Head & Neck, 17,* 297–302.

DeVita, M. A., & Spierer-Rundback, L. (1990). Swallowing disorders in patients with prolonged orotracheal intubation or tracheostomy tubes. *Critical Care Medicine, 18,* 1328–1330.

Dobie, R. (1978). Rehabilitation of swallowing disorders. *American Family Physician, 27,* 84–95.

Dodds, W. J., Logemann, J. A., & Stewart, E. T. (1990). Radiological assessment of abnormal oral and pharyngeal phases of swallowing. *American Journal of Roentology, 154,* 965–974.

Dodds, W. J., Stewart, E. T., & Logemann, J. (1990). Physiology and radiology of the normal oral and pharyngeal phases of swallowing. *American Journal of Roentology, 154,* 953–963.

Donald, A., & Dawes, J. (1977). A case of dysphagia. *British Medical Journal, 30,* 1139–1141.

Edwards, D. (1970). Flow charts, diagnostic keys, and algorithms in the diagnosis of dysphagia. *Scottish Medical Journal, 15,* 378–385.

Feldman, S., Deal, C., & Urquhart, W. (1966). Disturbance of swallowing after tracheostomy. *Lancet, 1,* 954–955.

Gallivan, G., Dawson, J., & Robbins, L. D. (1989). Videolaryngoscopy after endotracheal intubation: Implications for voice. *Journal of Voice, 3*(1), 76–80.

Griffin, J., & Tollison, J. (1980). Dysphagia. *American Family Physician, 22,* 154–160.

Griffin, K. (1974). Swallowing training for dysphagic patients. *Archives of Physical Medicine and Rehabilitation, 55,* 467–470.

Hamlet, S. L., Nelson, R. J., & Patterson, R. L. (1990). Interpreting the sounds of swallowing: Fluid flow through the cricopharyngeus. *Annals of Otology, Rhinology, and Laryngology, 99,* 749–752.

Hamlet, S. L., Patterson, R. L., Fleming, S. M., & Jones, L. A. (1992). Sounds of swallowing following total laryngectomy. *Dysphagia, 7,* 160–165.

Haubrich, W. (1977). In defense of the radiographic diagnosis of dysphagia. *Gastrointestinal Endoscopy, 23*, 214.

Holas, M. A., DePippo, K., & Reding, M. J. (1994). Aspiration and relative risk of medical complications following stroke. *Archives of Neurology, 51*, 1051–1053.

Horner, J., Massey, E. W., Riski, J. E., Lathrop, D., & Chase, K. N. (1988). Aspiration following stroke: Clinical correlates and outcomes. *Neurology, 38*, 1359–1362.

Jacob, P., Kahrilas, P., Logemann, J., Shah, V., & Ha, T. (1989). Upper esophageal sphincter opening and modulation during swallowing. *Gastroenterology, 97*, 1469–1478.

Kahrilas, P. J., Lin, S., Logemann, J. A., Ergun, G. A., & Facchini, F. (1993). Deglutitive tongue action: Volume accommodation and bolus propulsion. *Gastroenterology, 104*, 152–162.

Kahrilas, P. J., Logemann, J. A., Krugler, C., & Flanagan, E. (1991). Volitional augmentation of upper esophageal sphincter opening during swallowing. *American Journal of Physiology, 260 (Gastrointestinal Physiology, 23)*, G450–G456.

Kahrilas, P. J., Logemann, J. A., Lin, S., & Ergun, G. A. (1992). Pharyngeal clearance during swallow: A combined manometric and videofluoroscopic study. *Gastroenterology, 103*, 128–136.

Kelley, M. (1970). Evaluation of the patient with dysphagia. *Modern Treatment, 7*, 1087–1097.

Kirchner, J. (1967). Pharyngeal and esophageal dysfunction: The diagnosis. *Minnesota Medicine, 50*, 921–924.

Lazarus, C., Logemann, J. A., & Gibbons, P. (1993). Effects of maneuvers on swallowing function in a dysphagic oral cancer patient. *Head & Neck, 15*, 419–424.

Lazarus, C. L., Logemann, J. A., Rademaker, A. W., Kahrilas, P. J., Pajak, T., Lazar, R., & Halper, A. (1993). Effects of bolus volume, viscosity and repeated swallows in non-stroke subjects and stroke patients. *Archives of Physical and Medical Rehabilitation, 74*, 1066–1070.

Lazzara, G., Lazarus, C., & Logemann, J. A. (1986). Impact of thermal stimulation on the triggering of the swallowing reflex. *Dysphagia, 1*, 73–77.

Leder, S. B. (1996). Gag reflex and dysphagia. *Head & Neck, 18*, 138–141.

Leder, S. B. (1997). Videofluoroscopic evaluation of aspiration with visual examination of the gag reflex and velar movement. *Dysphagia, 12*, 21–23.

Leder, S. B., Tarro, J. M., & Burrell, M. I. (1996). Effect of occlusion of a tracheotomy tube on aspiration. *Dysphagia, 11*, 254–258.

Linden, P., & Siebens, A. (1980, November). *Videofluoroscopy: Use in evaluation and treatment of dysphagia*. A miniseminar presented at the American Speech-Language-Hearing Association annual meeting, Detroit.

Linden, P., & Siebens, A. (1983). Dysphagia: Predicting laryngeal penetration. *Archives of Physical and Medical Rehabilitation, 64*, 281–283.

Logemann, J. A. (Ed.). (1989). Swallowing disorders and rehabilitation. *Journal of Head Trauma Rehabilitation, 4*(4).

Logemann, J. A. (1983). *Evaluation and treatment of swallowing disorders*. Austin, TX: PRO-ED.

Logemann, J. A. (1993). *Manual for the videofluoroscopic study of swallowing*. Austin, TX: PRO-ED.

Logemann, J. A., & Kahrilas, P. J. (1990). Relearning to swallow post CVA: Application of maneuvers and indirect biofeedback—A case study. *Neurology, 40*, 1136–1138.

Logemann, J. A., Kahrilas, P. J., Cheng, J., Pauloski, B. R., Gibbons, P. J., Rademaker, A. W., & Lin, S. (1992). Closure mechanisms of the laryngeal vestibule during swallowing. *American Journal of Physiology, 262*, G338–G344.

Logemann, J., Kahrilas, P., Kobara, M., & Vakil, N. (1989). The benefit of head rotation on pharyngoesophageal dysphagia. *Archives of Physical Medicine and Rehabilitation, 70*, 767–771.

Logemann, J. A., Rademaker, A. W., Pauloski, B. R., & Kahrilas, P. J. (1994). Effects of postural change on aspiration in head and neck surgical patients. *Otolaryngology—Head and Neck Surgery, 110*, 222–227.

Loughlin, A. M., & Lefton-Greif, M. A. (1994). Dysfunctional swallowing and respiratory disease in children. *Advances in Pediatrics, 41*, 135–161.

Maguire, G. (1966). The larynx: Simplified radiological examination using heavy filtration and high voltage. *Radiology, 87*, 102–110.

Mandelstam, P., & Lieber, A. (1970). Cineradiographic evaluation of the esophagus in normal adults. *Gastroenterology, 58*, 32–38.

Martin, B. W., Corlew, M. M., Wood, H., Olson, D., Gallipol, L. A., Wingbowl, M., & Kirmani, N. (1994). The association of swallowing dysfunction and aspiration pneumonia. *Dysphagia, 9*, 1–6.

Martin, B. J. W., Logemann, J. A., Shaker, R., & Dodds, W. J. (1994). Coordination between respiration and swallowing: Respiratory phase relationships and temporal integration. *Journal of Applied Physiology, 76*(2), 714–723.

McConchie, L. (1973). Dysphagia: General principles of management. *Australian New Zealand Journal of Surgery, 42*, 358–359.

Miller, D., & Sethl, G. (1970). Tracheal stenosis following prolonged cuffed intubation: Cause and prevention. *Annals of Surgery, 171*, 283–293.

Muz, J., Hamlet, S., Mathog, R., & Farris, R. (1994). Scintigraphic assessment of aspiration in head and neck cancer patients with tracheostomy. *Head & Neck, 16*, 17–20.

Muz, J., Mathog, R., Nelson, R., & Jones, L. A., Jr. (1989). Aspiration in patients with head and neck cancer and tracheostomy. *American Journal of Otolaryngology, 10*, 282–286.

Nathadwarawala, K. M., McGroary, A., & Wiles, C. M. (1994). Swallowing in neurological outpatients: Use of a timed test. *Dysphagia, 9*, 120–129.

Nathadwarawala, K. M., Nicklin, J., & Wiles, C. M. (1992). A timed test of swallowing capacity for neurological patients. *Journal of Neurology, Neurosurgery and Psychiatry, 55*, 822–825.

O'Connor, A., & Ardran, G. (1976). Cinefluorography in the diagnosis of pharyngeal palsies. *Journal of Laryngology and Otology, 90*, 1015–1019.

Palmer, J. B., Kuhlemeier, K. V., Tippett, D. C., & Lynch, C. (1993). A protocol for the videofluorographic swallowing study. *Dysphagia, 8*, 209–214.

Palmer, J. B., Rudin, N. J., Lara, G., & Crompton, A. W. (1992). Coordination of mastication and swallowing. *Dysphagia, 7*, 187–200.

Paloschi, G., & Lynn, R. (1965). Observations upon elective and emergency tracheostomy. *Surgery, Gynecology and Obstetrics, 120*, 356–358.

Phillips, M., & Hendrix, T. (1971). Dysphagia. *Postgraduate Medicine, 50*, 81–86.

Pinkus, N. (1973). The dangers of oral feeding in the presence of cuffed tracheostomy tubes. *Medical Journal of Australia, 1*, 1238–1240.

Pitcher, J. (1973). Dysphagia in the elderly: Causes and diagnosis. *Geriatrics, 28*, 64–69.

Rasley, A., Logemann, J. A., Kahrilas, P. J., Rademaker, A. W., Pauloski, B. R., & Dodds, W. J. (1993). Prevention of barium aspiration during videofluoroscopic swallowing studies: Value of change in posture. *American Journal of Roentgenology, 160*, 1005–1009.

Rossato, R., & Wrightson, P. (1977). Dionosil swallow: A test of laryngeal protection. *Surgical Neurology, 17*, 24.

Sasaki, C. T., Suzaki, M., Horiuchi, M., & Kirchner, J. A. (1977). The effect of tracheostomy on the laryngeal closure reflex. *Laryngoscope, 87*, 1428–1432.

Scatliff, J. (1963). Cinefluorographic evaluation of the soft tissues of the neck. *New York Journal of Medicine, 63*, 1174–1180.

Schultz, A., Niemtzow, P., Jacobs, S., & Naso, F. (1979). Dysphagia associated with cricopharyngeal dysfunction. *Archives of Physical Medicine and Rehabilitation, 60*, 381–386.

Shanahan, T. K., Logemann, J. A., Rademaker, A. W., Pauloski, B. R., & Kahrilas, P. J. (1993). Chin down posture effects on aspiration in dysphagic patients. *Archives of Physical Medicine and Rehabilitation, 74*, 736–739.

Shin, T., Maeyama, T., Morikawa, I., & Umezaki, T. (1988). Laryngeal reflex mechanism during deglutition—Observing of subglottal pressure and afferent discharge. *Otolaryngology—Head and Neck Surgery, 99*, 465–471.

Sloan, R. (1977). Cinefluorographic study of cerebral palsy deglutition. *Journal of the Osaka Dental University, 11*, 58–73.

Splaingard, M. L., Hutchins, B., Sulton, L. D., & Chauhuri, G. (1988). Aspiration in rehabilitation patients: Videofluoroscopy vs. bedside clinical assessment. *Archives of Physical Medical Rehabilitation, 69*, 637–640.

Taniguchi, M. H., & Moyer, R. S. (1994). Assessment of risk factors for pneumonia in dysphagic children: Significance of videofluoroscopic swallowing evaluation. *Developmental Medicine and Child Neurology, 36*, 495–502.

Thompson-Henry, S., & Braddock, B. (1995). The modified Evan's blue dye procedure fails to detect aspiration in the tracheostomized patients: Five case reports. *Dysphagia, 10*(3), 172–174.

Tippett, D. C., & Siebens, A. A. (1995). Reconsidering the value of the modified Evan's blue dye test: A comment on Thompson-Henry and Braddock (1995) [Letter to editor]. *Dysphagia, 11*, 78–79.

Tuch, B. E., & Neilsen, J. M. (1941). Apraxia of swallowing. *Bulletin of Los Angeles Neurologic Society, 6*, 52–54.

Weathers, R., Becker, M., & Genieser, N. (1974). Improved technique for study of swallowing function in infants. *Radiologic Technology, 46*, 98–100.

Welch, M. V., Logemann, J. A., Rademaker, A. W., & Kahrilas, P. J. (1993). Changes in pharyngeal dimensions effected by chin tuck. *Archives of Physical Medicine and Rehabilitation, 74*, 178–181.

Ylvisaker, M., & Logemann, J. A. (1986). Therapy for feeding and swallowing following head injury. In M. Ylvisaker (Ed.), *Management of head injured patients*. San Diego: College-Hill.

Zenner, P. M., Losinski, D. S., & Mills, R. H. (1995). Using cervical auscultation in the clinical dysphagia examination in long-term care. *Dysphagia, 10*(1), 27–31.

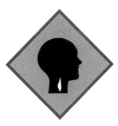

MANAGEMENT OF THE PATIENT WITH OROPHARYNGEAL SWALLOWING DISORDERS

The following three questions need to be answered after evaluation of the patient with an oropharyngeal swallowing problem: First, what type of nutritional management is necessary? Second, should therapy be initiated and what type (compensatory or exercises, direct or indirect)? Third, what specific therapy strategies should be used? The continuous goal of any treatment program is the reestablishment of oral feeding while constantly maintaining adequate hydration and nutrition and safe swallowing (Aguilar, Olson, & Shedd, 1979; American Dietetic Association, 1980). Another question to be answered as therapy progresses is, Does the patient require a maintenance program to maintain the gains in therapy or slow deterioration? This chapter provides clinicians with the types of information needed to answer these questions, including descriptions of the types of management available and a discussion of therapy strategies appropriate for each anatomic or physiologic disorder (Kasprisin, Clumeck, & Nino-Murcia, 1989; Larsen, 1972; Logemann, 1983; Newman, Dodaro, & Welch, 1980).

Treatment Planning

A therapy regimen involves progressive exercise programs or sensory stimulation activities designed to improve oropharyngeal swallow physiology. During and after each therapy session, the patient's performance should be evaluated in terms of quantitative measures, such as extent or coordination of structural movement, pattern of structural movement, strength and frequency of cough in a set of delineated exercises, and so on. A decision to provide therapy for a patient with dysphagia should be based on the patient's potential for improvement or recovery of swallowing ability or longer maintenance of oral intake because of exercise. If the patient has the potential to recover full or partial oral intake with a course of therapy or has the potential to maintain oral intake for a longer period of time, then an intervention program is appropriate.

The clinician should consider a number of patient characteristics when deciding whether to initiate swallowing therapy with a dysphagic patient and what type of therapy to provide. These include the following:

- **Diagnosis**—Knowledge of the speed and potential for recovery of the patient's swallowing disorder should be a primary factor in deciding whether to initiate therapy. If a patient is likely to recover his or her swallow quickly (e.g., within a week or two, as is often seen in a stroke patient who has suffered a first-time infarct uncomplicated by other medical problems) and is otherwise healthy and has no medical complications. Only compensatory strategies may be needed to allow oral intake as the patient's swallow recovers. An active exercise program may or may not be appropriate. If the patient has motor neuron disease, any therapy that requires active muscle exercise, such as range-of-motion exercises or effortful swallow maneuvers, is inappropriate because it creates fatigue. If the patient has dementia, any therapy requiring direction following may be inappropriate.

- **Prognosis**—The patient's prognosis should be considered when determining whether to initiate a therapy program. Recovery of full or partial oral intake is possible if the patient has suffered sudden-onset neurologic damage, such as stroke, head injury, or spinal cord injury, or structural damage, such as from surgical or radiation therapy for head and neck cancer, gunshot wounds, or other trauma. In these patients, swallowing therapy is quite appropriate. In patients with a degenerative process, such as Parkinson's disease, motor neuron disease, myasthenia gravis, multiple sclerosis, various types of muscular dystrophy, and Alzheimer's disease, a course of swallowing therapy may be appropriate, depending upon its goals. However, with these disease processes, there may come a time in the patient's disease process when swallowing therapy is no longer effective because the patient has lost enough neuromotor control that therapy cannot effect change, or the patient is presenting with cognitive deficits that significantly affect his or her ability to follow directions and even apply some or any of the compensatory strategies.

- **Reaction to Compensatory Strategies**—If compensatory strategies successfully eliminate the symptoms of the patient's dysphagia (i.e., aspiration and/or residual food) such that full oral intake is safe and adequately efficient to maintain hydration and nutrition, swallowing therapy may not be warranted, if spontaneous recovery is also likely to take place. Use of compensatory strategies with a reevaluation of the patient's swallowing function after 3 to 4 weeks (or more) may be more appropriate than initiating an active exercise program.

- **Severity of the Patient's Dysphagia**—If the patient's dysphagia is severe and cannot be ameliorated with compensatory strategies during the radiographic study, it is likely that indirect therapy consisting of a variety of exercises to improve the range and coordination of oral and oropharyngeal movements will be necessary without giving any food or liquid. Certainly, the patient's saliva could be used if some swallow attempts are desired.

- **Ability To Follow Directions**—Some of the swallowing therapy strategies require that the patient be able to follow simple or more complex directions. Swallow maneuvers require particularly complex direction following. In contrast, compensatory strategies involve little if any need to follow directions. Compensatory strategies are also largely under the control of the caregiver.

- **Respiratory Function**—Normal swallowing requires airway closure for a brief period of time (i.e., 0.3 to 0.6 seconds for liquids, 3 to 5 seconds or more during continuous cup drinking). If the patient's respiratory function is poor, he or she may not be able to tolerate even the normal brief duration of airway closure. Some swallowing therapy procedures require modifying airway closure duration (supraglottic swallow, super-supraglottic swallow) or affect the duration of airway closure as a side effect of the procedure (the effortful swallow and the Mendelsohn maneuver). If respiratory function is severely affected, some types of swallowing therapy may need to be postponed until respiration improves.

- **Availability of Caregiver Support**—For some patients, reliable caregiver support must be available to ensure regular practice of therapy procedures. For patients with mild memory deficits, this support can be critical to attaining therapy goals. Often, regular reminders to practice exercises are all that is needed.

- **Patient Motivation and Interest**—To be successful in therapy, a patient should be motivated to work to regain swallowing function. Most dysphagic patients are extremely motivated to return to oral intake. However, occasionally, a patient will find nonoral feeding easier than the continued efforts required to reestablish the neuromuscular control needed for adequate and safe oral intake.

Oral Versus Nonoral Feeding

An important decision is whether the patient should continue to be fed orally, or be placed on a nasogastric tube or given some type of gastrostomy or jejunostomy.

At this time, there are no absolute guidelines the clinician can use to make this decision. The results of several studies may be helpful, however. In 1980, Logemann, Sisson, and Wheeler examined the relationship between speed of swallowing and diet choices. Patients studied were those with oral cancer who had been treated surgically, and who were provided with an oral prosthesis to assist in eating and talking. Patients were studied over a 6-month period, and careful records were kept regarding diet choices, amount of food eaten, and speed of eating. Measures of oral and pharyngeal transit time taken at 1-, 2-, 3-, and 6-month intervals were compared with the food consistencies actually included in the patient's diet. These data are shown in Figure 6.1. Examination of these data reveals that patients do not include a particular food consistency in their diet unless the combined oral and pharyngeal transit time for swallow of that mate-

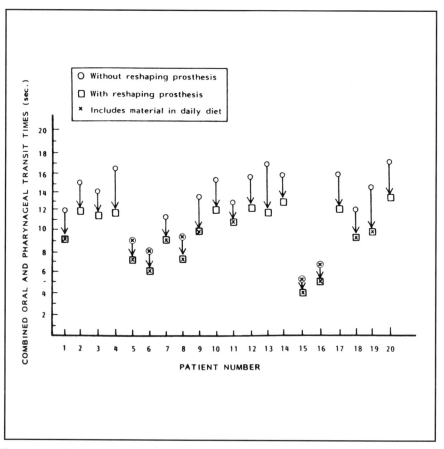

Figure 6.1. Combined oral and pharyngeal transit times for surgically treated oral cancer patients for paste consistency foods and notation of whether patients included paste consistency foods in their daily diet.

rial is approximately 10 seconds or less. These data corroborate earlier patient reports. When it takes a long time to eat a particular food consistency (i.e., more than 10 seconds), most patients will discontinue eating that consistency of food or will not get a sufficient amount of food down to maintain their weight.

Thus, *time* taken to swallow a single bolus of a particular consistency of food appears to be an important parameter in nutritional management. If the radiographic study indicates that it takes the patient more than 10 seconds for oral and pharyngeal transit time combined to swallow *every* consistency of food attempted, but there is no aspiration, the patient may feed by mouth but will need a nonoral feeding to supplement oral feedings and to provide adequate nutrition and hydration. If the swallowing therapist indicates that the patient's progress in therapy is slow, and it appears that it will take more than 3 to 4 weeks to improve the patient's swallowing to the point that he or she will not need the supplemental feedings, the managing physician may prefer to give the patient some type of gastrostomy or jejunostomy rather than leave a nasogastric tube in place for that long a period. Some physicians do not like to leave a nasogastric tube in place for more than 3 to 4 weeks. Or, the patient may be taught to place the nasogastric tube at each meal and remove it after feeding. Generally, the swallowing therapist does not make the decision regarding the type of nonoral nutrition appropriate for the patient other than to discourage the use of wide-diameter, semiflexible feeding tubes. Many factors are used to determine the type of nonoral feeding used, including (1) the patient's gastrointestinal history, (2) the cost of feedings and insurance coverage, (3) the patient's behavior, (4) the patient's preference, and (5) the patient's medical diagnosis. The swallowing therapist may not be as aware of all of these factors as the patient's physician. In some cases, if the patient's swallowing function is borderline (i.e., approximately 10 seconds for oral and pharyngeal transit times), the dietitian may provide the patient with diet supplements to increase the caloric content of the foods eaten orally.

A second parameter of swallowing function that Logemann et al. (1980) examined in relation to diet choices was *aspiration*. The gross approximation of amount of material aspirated was correlated with selection of diet choices by the patient. All of these patients were cognitively intact and aware of their aspiration and coughed in response. These data are shown in Figure 6.2. If patients aspirate any more than 10% of each bolus, and they are aware of that aspiration, they will eliminate that food consistency from their diet. These data indicate that if a patient is unable to swallow any food consistency with less than 10% aspiration, he or she will stop eating because of the discomfort of frequent coughing. However, those patients who are unaware of having a swallowing disorder or who do not cough when they aspirate, particularly those with neurologic disorders, will persevere in attempting to feed by mouth despite aspiration of excessive amounts.

After the radiographic examination is completed, the swallowing therapist

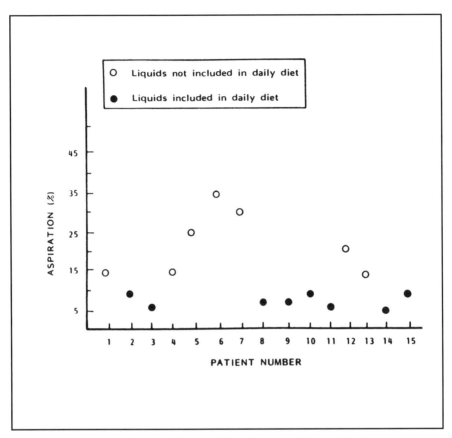

Figure 6.2. Percent aspiration on liquid swallows for surgically treated oral cancer patients and notation of whether patients included liquids in their daily diet.

should inform the patient's managing physician about the gross percentage of each bolus consistency that is aspirated, despite all therapy attempts (e.g., posture change, sensory enhancement, voluntarily protecting the airway). The managing physician should then make the decision regarding oral feeding. In general, however, a patient who is aspirating more than 10% of every bolus, regardless of consistency of food, should not be feeding orally.

Compensatory Treatment Procedures

Compensatory treatment procedures are usually introduced first in the diagnostic procedure. Compensatory treatment procedures are those that control the flow of food and eliminate the patient's symptoms, such as aspiration, but do not necessarily change the physiology of the patient's swallow. These procedures are largely under the control of the caregiver or clinician and can, therefore, be used with patients of all ages and cognitive levels. Compensatory procedures gener-ally involve less muscle effort or work for the patient and thus do not fatigue the patient as quickly as some swallow exercises. Compensatory strategies include (1) postural changes, which potentially change the dimensions of the pharynx and the direction of food flow without increasing the patient's work or effort; (2) increasing sensory input; (3) modifying volume and speed of food presenta-tion; (4) changing food consistency or viscosity; and (5) introducing intraoral prosthetics.

Postural Techniques

Posture changes are suggested as therapy techniques for a number of types of dys-phagic patients. Although some authors recommend a single posture for opti-mum swallowing, generally with the head tilted forward at a 45° angle (Buckley, Addicks, & Maniglia, 1976; Gaffney & Campbell, 1974; Larsen, 1973), no single posture improves swallowing in all patients. Rather, a variety of postural changes will improve specific swallowing disorders. The swallowing therapist must first correctly diagnose the physiologic or anatomic disorder in the patient's degluti-tion and then identify the posture that will facilitate most normal swallowing.

Changing the patient's head or body posture can be effective in eliminating aspiration on liquids in 75% to 80% of dysphagic patients, including infants and children and some patients with cognitive or language impairments (Drake, O'Donoghue, Bartram, Lindsay, & Greenwood, 1997; Horner, Massey, Riski, Lathrop, & Chase, 1988; Larnert & Ekberg, 1995; Logemann, 1989, 1993a; Logemann, Kahrilas, Kobara, & Vakil, 1989; Logemann, Rademaker, Pauloski, & Kahrilas, 1994; Rasley et al., 1993; Shanahan, Logemann, Rademaker, Pauloski, & Kahrilas, 1993; Welch, Logemann, Rademaker, & Kahrilas, 1993). However, some patients are unable to use postural strategies because of head sta-bilization devices or cognitive or other physical constraints.

Postural techniques redirect food flow and change pharyngeal dimensions in systematic ways. Table 6.1 presents the postures currently used therapeuti-cally and their effects on specific swallowing disorders and pharyngeal dimen-sions. In general, postural techniques work equally well with patients having neurological impairments, in patients who have experienced head and neck can-cer resections or other structural damage, and in patients of all ages (Logemann, 1993a; Rasley et al., 1993).

During the diagnostic radiographic procedure, the clinician cannot intro-duce all of the postures to assess their individual effects. Rather, the clinician must select a postural technique to fit the patient's physiologic or anatomic swal-lowing disorders identified in the earlier portion of the radiographic study (Loge-mann, 1993b). Then, the patient is asked to use the postural technique dur-ing swallows of the same type as those that previously exhibited aspiration or

Table 6.1
Postural Techniques Successful in Eliminating Aspiration or
Residue Resulting from Various Swallowing Disorders
and the Rationale for Their Effectiveness

Disorder Observed on Fluoroscopy	Posture Applied	Rationale
Inefficient oral transit (Reduced posterior propulsion of bolus by tongue)	Head back	Utilizes gravity to clear oral cavity
Delay in triggering the pharyngeal swallow (Bolus past ramus of mandible, but pharyngeal swallow not triggered)	Chin down	Widens valleculae to prevent bolus entering airway; narrows airway entrance; pushes epiglottis posteriorly
Reduced posterior motion of tongue base (Residue in valleculae)	Chin down	Pushes tongue base backward toward pharyngeal wall
Unilateral laryngeal dysfunction (Aspiration during swallow)	Head rotated to damaged side; chin down	Places extrinsic pressure on thyroid cartilage, increasing adduction
Reduced laryngeal closure (Aspiration during swallow)	Chin down; head rotated to damaged side	Puts epiglottis in more protective position; narrows laryngeal entrance; increases vocal fold closure by applying extrinsic pressure
Reduced pharyngeal contraction (Residue spread throughout pharynx)	Lying down on one side	Eliminates gravitational effect on pharyngeal residue
Unilateral pharyngeal paresis (Residue on one side of pharynx)	Head rotated to damaged side	Eliminates damaged side from bolus path
Unilateral oral and pharyngeal weakness on the same side (Residue in mouth and pharynx on same side)	Head tilt to stronger side	Directs bolus down stronger side
Cricopharyngeal dysfunction (Residue in pyriform sinuses)	Head rotated	Pulls cricoid cartilage away from posterior pharyngeal wall, reducing resting pressure in cricopharyngeal sphincter

significant residue. In this way, the effectiveness of the posture in eliminating the aspiration or reducing the residue can be defined (Logemann, 1993b).

Postural techniques are usually used temporarily until the patient's swallow recovers or direct therapy procedures to improve oropharyngeal motor function take effect. Occasionally, patients with severe neurologic or structural damage must use postural techniques permanently to eliminate aspiration and facilitate swallow efficiency.

The Chin-Down Posture

The chin-down posture involves touching the chin to the neck. This pushes the anterior pharyngeal wall posteriorly (Welch et al., 1993). With the chin down, the tongue base and epiglottis are pushed closer to the posterior pharyngeal wall. The airway entrance (i.e., the space between the epiglottic base and the arytenoid cartilage) is narrowed. In many patients, the vallecular space is also widened. Thus, the chin-down posture is helpful if patients have a delay in triggering the pharyngeal swallow, reduced tongue base retraction, and/or reduced airway entrance closure.

The Chin-Up Posture

The chin-up posture is used to drain food from the oral cavity using gravity. It is helpful to patients with reduced tongue control. If the clinician is concerned about airway protection when the patient's head is tilted back, the patient may be taught the supraglottic swallow, a swallowing maneuver described later, to close the vocal folds before and during the swallow voluntarily.

Head Rotation

Head rotation to the damaged side twists the pharynx and closes the damaged side of the pharynx so that food flows down the more normal side (Logemann, Kahrilas, Kobara, & Vakil, 1989). This posture is used when there is a unilateral pharyngeal wall impairment or a unilateral vocal fold weakness. In the latter disorder, head rotation pushes the damaged side toward midline, thus improving adduction.

Chin Down and Head Rotation

Chin-down and head rotation positions may be combined to achieve the best airway protection in some patients.

Head Tilt

Head tilting is used when a patient has both a unilateral oral impairment and a unilateral pharyngeal impairment on the same side. The head is always tilted to the better or stronger side, thus using gravity to drain food down the stronger side, where there is better control.

Lying Down

If the patient has bilateral reduction in pharyngeal wall contraction or reduced laryngeal elevation, resulting in residue in the pharynx that is aspirated after the swallow, lying down may eliminate the aspiration (Drake et al., 1997; Rasley et al., 1993). By lying down, the effect of gravity on the residual food will change. While sitting up, gravity will drop residual food down the airway. When lying down, gravity holds the bolus on the pharyngeal walls. Before advising the patient to eat when lying down, the patient's straw drinking should be observed radiographically to be sure the patient is creating suction in the mouth rather than using inhalation to draw material from the straw. When lying down, straw drinking is the only way to take liquids efficiently. Patients who exhibit a buildup of residue in the pharynx with successive swallows are not good candidates for this posture. Also, patients with gastroesophageal reflux may need to have the upper body elevated 15° to 30° to prevent reflux but still eliminate aspiration. All of these issues should be observed as part of the radiographic study before recommending that the patient begin eating lying down. At the end of the meal taken while lying down, the patient should cough to clear any last residue before sitting up.

When postural techniques are successful and the patient is able to eat using them, the patient may or may not be given additional swallowing therapy. The patient may be scheduled for a return in 3 to 4 weeks and allowed to eat using the posture as the major exercise. Because swallowing involves greater muscle contraction and generates greater pressures than speech, it has often been concluded that the best exercise for swallowing is swallowing when it can be done safely and efficiently (McCulloch, Perlman, Palmer, & Van Daele, 1996; Perlman, Luschei, & DuMond, 1989). Thus, although the patient is not necessarily doing other exercises, the use of the mechanism in swallowing food may in fact result in best muscle function. When the patient returns for reevaluation after several weeks, the clinician should begin the reassessment with the patient in a normal upright eating position to assess recovery at that time. If the patient still has a significant swallowing impairment, then reassessment should be done with the patient in the posture of choice. Generally within 1 to 2 months after using a posture, the patient can return to oral intake without using the postural strategy. However, some patients do not recover and need to use the postural strategy permanently.

Patients and families should be warned that the postural strategy will become quite easy to do and they may believe patients' swallowing has improved and want to stop using the posture before reassessment. They should be counseled if this occurs, to call the clinician in order to receive a reevaluation early rather than stopping the postural strategy when they actually may need it.

Techniques To Improve Oral Sensory Awareness

Techniques to improve oral sensory awareness prior to a swallow are generally utilized in patients with swallow apraxia, tactile agnosia for food, delayed onset of the oral swallow, reduced oral sensation, or delayed triggering of the pharyngeal swallow (Logemann, 1993b). In some ways, procedures to enhance pre-swallow sensory input are both compensatory and therapy techniques. They are compensatory because they are under the control of the caregiver and do not change the motor control of the swallow, but therapeutic because they change the timing of the swallow by reducing both oral onset time and pharyngeal delay time. These procedures all involve providing a preliminary sensory stimulus prior to the initiation of the patient's swallow attempt and, we hypothesize, alert the central nervous system, resulting in lowering the threshold of the swallowing centers (Fujiu, Toleikis, Logemann, & Larson, 1994). Sensory enhancement techniques include (1) increasing downward pressure of the spoon against the tongue when presenting food in the mouth; (2) presenting a sour bolus (50% lemon juice, 50% barium); (3) presenting a cold bolus; (4) presenting a bolus requiring chewing; (5) presenting a larger volume bolus (3 ml or more); and (6) thermal–tactile stimulation (Helfrich-Miller, Rector, & Straka, 1986; Lazarus, Logemann, Rademaker, et al., 1993; Lazzara, Lazarus, & Logemann, 1986; Logemann, Pauloski, et al., 1995; Tippett, Palmer, & Linden, 1987; Ylvisaker & Logemann, 1986). In some patients with swallow apraxia, oral onset and oral transit of the swallow may be facilitated by increasing oral sensation with a preliminary stimulus, such as the downward pressure of a spoon; the presentation of a bolus with increased volume, taste, or temperature characteristics; or thermal–tactile stimulation. These techniques, which enhance sensory input, such as bolus taste, temperature, volume, and viscosity, may also result in reduced pharyngeal delay times in some patients (Lazzara et al., 1986). The clinician will have tested the patient's oral reaction to bolus taste, temperature, and texture in the bedside assessment using cloth and various flavored liquids, as described earlier.

Thermal–tactile stimulation and suck–swallow are most commonly used to improve triggering of the pharyngeal swallow. *Thermal–tactile stimulation* involves vertically rubbing the anterior faucial arch firmly, four or five times, with a size 00 laryngeal mirror (which has been held in crushed ice for several seconds) in advance of the presentation of a bolus and the patient's attempt to swallow. This technique is designed to heighten oral awareness and provide an alerting sensory stimulus to the cortex and brainstem such that, when the patient initiates the oral stage of swallow, the pharyngeal swallow will trigger more rapidly. This technique has been demonstrated to facilitate faster trigger-ing of the pharyngeal swallow after the stimulation and reducing the delay for several swallows thereafter (Lazzara et al., 1986).

An exaggerated *suck–swallow*, using increased vertical tongue–jaw sucking movements with the lips closed, facilitates triggering of the pharyngeal swallow. This technique also draws saliva to the back of the mouth, which is helpful for patients with poor saliva control.

Measures of the effectiveness of these sensory enhancement procedures in increasing oral sensory input include (1) duration of time from command to swal-low until initiation of the oral stage of swallow, (2) oral transit time, and (3) pha-ryngeal delay time (Logemann, 1993b). These can be roughly observed and approximated with fingers *lightly* contacting the submandibular area and ante-rior neck at the bedside or measured from videofluoroscopy. In some patients, pharyngeal delay time can be measured from videoendoscopy. However, if a patient exhibits premature spillage of a bolus because of oral abnormalities, videoendoscopy will not be capable of distinguishing premature spillage from the onset of pharyngeal delay time with the same accuracy as videofluoroscopy, because the oral stage of swallow cannot be visualized with videoendoscopy.

Modifying Volume and Speed of Food Presentation

For some patients, a particular volume of food per swallow elicits the fastest pha-ryngeal swallow. In some patients with a delay in pharyngeal triggering, a larger bolus may facilitate triggering. In patients with a weakened pharyngeal swallow that requires two to three swallows per bolus, taking too much food too rapidly can result in a severe collection of food in the pharynx and aspiration. Simply taking smaller boluses at a slower rate may eliminate any risk of aspiration in these patients.

Food Consistency (Diet) Changes

Generally, elimination of certain food consistencies from the diet should be the last compensatory strategy examined (Logemann, 1993b). Eliminating consis-tencies, such as thin liquids, from the diet can be difficult for the patient. This should be done only if other compensatory or therapy strategies are not fea-sible, as in a patient who has a movement disorder and whose posture changes continuously or who cannot follow directions and use swallow maneuvers, or a patient for whom oral sensory procedures are inappropriate. Table 5.3 in Chap-ter 5 presents the food consistencies that are easiest and those that should be avoided for each swallowing disorder. Unfortunately, there are no uniform national viscosity categories or available lists of foods falling into various viscos-

Table 6.2
Bolus Consistencies and the Swallow Problems
for Which They Are Most Appropriate

Food Consistencies	Disorders for Which These Foods Are Most Appropriate
Thin liquids	Oral tongue dysfunction[a] Reduced tongue base retraction Reduced pharyngeal wall contraction Reduced laryngeal elevation Reduced cricopharyngeal opening
Thickened liquids	Oral tongue dysfunction[a] Delayed pharyngeal swallow[b]
Purees and thick foods, including thickened liquids	Delayed pharyngeal swallow Reduced laryngeal closure at the entrance Reduced laryngeal closure throughout

[a] Initially thickened liquids are easier for a patient with oral tongue dysfunction to manage since thin liquids may splash from the mouth quickly, entering the pharynx and open airway. When the clinician understands the patient's pharyngeal swallow and if there is good triggering of the pharyngeal swallow and ability to voluntarily protect the airway, then liquids will be easier. The patient will be able to use the dump and swallow technique to take in a large volume of liquid.

[b] The level of thickness needed may vary from patient to patient. Some patients with a pharyngeal delay will need pureed viscosity in order to prevent aspiration, whereas others may do well with nectar or honey-thickened liquids. Both viscosities should be introduced during the modified barium swallow to determine which is effective with each patient.

ity categories. Swallowing therapists must work with facility dietitians to define specific foods prepared that fit into each category (see Table 6.2).

Intraoral Prosthetics

Intraoral prosthetics can be an important compensatory procedure to improve swallowing in oral cancer patients with significant loss of oral tongue tissue (25% or more) or tongue movement, and in neurologic patients with bilateral hypoglossal paralysis, and in both patient groups with velopharyngeal deficits.

A *palatal lift prosthesis* lifts the soft palate into an elevated (closed) position in patients with velar paralysis. A *palatal obturator* can be used in oral cancer patients with significant resection of the soft palate. A *palatal augmentation or reshaping prosthesis* can be extremely effective in patients with significant tongue resections or bilateral tongue paralysis (J. W. Davis, Lazarus, Logemann, & Hurst, 1987; Logemann, Kahrilas, Hurst, et al., 1989). The *palatal reshaping prosthesis* recontours the hard palate to interact with the remaining tongue, filling in the areas of the hard palate where the patient's tongue cannot make contact postoperatively and enabling the patient to control and propel the bolus more efficiently (see Figure 6.3). After resection of part of the tongue, patients often indicate that it feels as if their tongue "fits their mouth again" with the prosthesis in place. Without the prosthesis, the patient has a large oral cavity and a very small tongue that is incapable of controlling food in the mouth for chewing or swallowing.

These intraoral prosthetics are usually constructed by a maxillofacial prosthodontist in cooperation with the swallowing therapist. Construction should begin within the first 4 to 6 weeks postoperatively to prevent the patient's development of poor habits for swallowing that will need to be dishabituated when he or she receives the prosthesis.

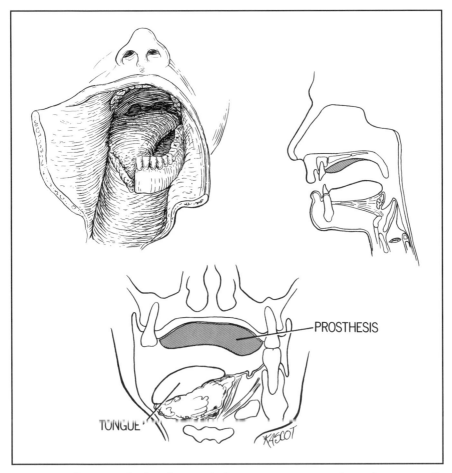

Figure 6.3. Diagrams of palate lowering/palate augmentation prostheses for a surgically treated oral cancer patient.

Therapy Procedures by Category

Therapy procedures are designed to *change* swallow physiology, in contrast to compensatory strategies, which are designed to eliminate symptoms. Therapy procedures are generally designed to improve range of motion of oral or pharyngeal structures, to improve sensory input prior to the swallow, or to take voluntary control over the timing or coordination of selected oropharyngeal movements during swallow (Logemann, 1983). Therapy procedures generally, but not always, require the patient to follow directions and practice independently of the clinician to get best effect. This section on therapy procedures describes procedures by category. Later in the chapter, procedures are discussed according to specific swallowing disorders.

Direct Versus Indirect Therapy

One of the important decisions in management of the patient with disordered feeding, as introduced in the first paragraph of this chapter, is whether to work directly on swallowing—that is, to introduce food into the mouth and attempt to reinforce the appropriate behaviors and motor control during the swallow—or to work indirectly on swallowing, using exercises to improve those neuromotor controls that are prerequisites for normal swallowing or to practice swallowing on saliva only. In general, this decision is made on the basis of information on aspiration gained from the radiographic study. Any of the therapy procedures described here can be done indirectly or directly.

Indirect therapy involves exercise programs or swallows of saliva, but no food or liquid is given. Indirect therapy is used in patients who aspirate on all food viscosities and volumes such that they are unsafe for any oral intake (Logemann, 1983; Neumann, 1993). Even swallow maneuvers can be practiced with saliva only. Typically, information on aspiration should be provided to the patient's physician and he or she should decide whether the patient can tolerate aspiration of the designated amount. In general, if the patient is aspirating more than 10% of each bolus swallowed, and therapeutic techniques applied at the time are unable to reduce this aspiration, the patient will function better if therapy focuses on improving the control of muscles required for swallowing rather than working directly on swallowing by using food or liquid (Griffin, 1974). It is of no help to place the patient in a situation where he or she is continuously aspirating with no hope of deterring material from entering the airway during the swallowing regimen.

Only the radiographic study can provide the data necessary to make these decisions. Aspiration can be clearly observed during the radiographic study, sometimes during videoendoscopy. The clinician working on swallowing without benefit of data from a radiographic study is likely to make a number of erroneous management decisions relative to swallowing physiology.

Direct therapy involves presenting food or liquid to the patient and asking him or her to swallow it while following specified instructions. In some cases, these exercises involve simply positioning the head or body in a particular way so aspiration is eliminated. In other cases, the sequence of instructions may include as many as seven steps and may improve his or her swallowing only a moderate amount. In all instances, the patient should be given written instructions describing the appropriate steps to follow. The rationale for the procedures should be discussed with the patient and the patient should be given ample time to practice the sequence of instructions on dry swallows before proceeding to swallows of liquid or food (Buckley et al., 1976; Griffin, 1974).

Whenever liquid or food is provided for practice swallows, only small amounts should be given (Buckley et al., 1976). The amount to be swallowed should be shown to the patient as reassurance that the food or liquid cannot obliterate the airway. The patient should also be encouraged to cough whenever needed to clear the airway. Patients should never be allowed to feel that coughing should be restrained because it is a sign of failure to swallow correctly. Instead, they should be positively reinforced for coughing as needed (Dobie, 1978).

Types of Therapy Techniques

Another decision in management of the patient with swallowing disorder(s), as introduced in the first paragraph of this chapter, involves selecting the type of therapy to be used and the specific exercises to be provided. This section presents the types of therapy procedures currently suggested. These include oral motor control and range-of-motion exercises, procedures to heighten sensory input, and swallow maneuvers. Then, specific therapy recommendations for various swallowing disorders are presented. The exercises discussed are not meant to be prescriptions or the only options. Rather, they are methods that have been found to improve swallowing in a number of patients with each disorder.

Oral Control and Oral and Pharyngeal Range-of-Motion Exercises

Range-of-motion exercises can be used to improve the extent of movement of the lips, jaw, oral tongue, tongue base, larynx, and vocal folds (adduction exercises) (Logemann, 1983; Logemann, Pauloski, Rademaker, & Colangelo, 1997). Bolus control and chewing exercises can be used to improve fine motor control of the tongue.

Oral Motor Control Exercises. Most frequently, patients have difficulty with the following aspects of tongue control during swallowing: lateralization of the tongue during chewing, elevation of the tongue to the hard palate, cupping of the tongue around the bolus to hold it in a cohesive manner with the sides of the tongue sealed to the lateral alveolar ridge, and anterior–posterior movement of the midline of the tongue in the initiation of the voluntary or oral stage of the swallow. The exercises described below target each of these goals. In all cases, directions for exercise regimens should be written down for the patient, family, or other caregiver so the exercises can be completed without the therapist present.

Range-of-Motion Tongue Exercises. Exercises to increase range of tongue motion, including tongue elevation and lateralization, should improve oral transit. The patient should be asked to open his or her mouth as wide as possible and elevate the tongue as high as possible in the front, hold it there for 1 second, and release it. Then the patient should elevate the back of the tongue as far as possible, hold it there for 1 second, and release it. This procedure should continue with the patient stretching the tongue to each side as far as possible in the mouth, as if cleaning the lateral sulcus, and extending the tongue straight out of his or her mouth as far as possible, and pulling it back as far as possible, holding for 1 second in each direction. The latter is a tongue base range-of-motion exercise. This entire series of range-of-motion exercises should be repeated 5 to 10 times in one session so the exercise lasts approximately 4 to 5 minutes. The entire set of exercises should be repeated 5 to 10 times a day. Range-of-motion exercises have been found to improve both speech understandability and oropharyngeal swallow efficiency in oral cancer patients (Logemann et al., 1997).

Resistance Exercises. Pushing the tongue against a tongue blade, popsicle, sucker, or the clinician's finger will improve both range of motion and strength (Jordan, 1979). The patient can be asked to push his or her tongue up against the tongue blade, to the side against the vertically positioned tongue blade, or thrust forward against it with the tongue blade pushing back against the tongue tip. In each case the patient should hold the pressure against the tongue blade for 1 second.

Bolus Control Exercises. A number of exercises can be used to improve lingual control of the bolus without asking the patient to swallow.

EXERCISES TO IMPROVE GROSS MANIPULATION OF MATERIAL. The patient should be given something large to manipulate in the mouth, which can also be controlled by the clinician, such as a rolled 4″ × 4″ gauze pad or a flexible licorice whip. The patient can manipulate one end of the gauze or the licorice with the tongue while the clinician holds the other end, thereby preventing patient loss of control and choking. At first, the patient is asked simply to grasp the gauze or licorice whip between the tongue and palate, to move it from one side to the other and to slide it forward and backward. After each attempt, the patient should be asked to judge the success of the attempt and to identify where the material is in the mouth. When the patient is able to move the gauze or licorice in a gross way, he or she should be asked to move it in a circular fashion from the middle of the mouth to the teeth on one side, back to the middle of the mouth and back to the teeth on the same side, in the way that the tongue manipulates food during chewing. When the patient is able to make these movements with some speed (approximately three directions in 1 second), he or she should be asked to repeat the same motions with a Lifesaver candy tied to a thread held by the clinician, and then with a thin cloth tape soaked in a small amount of orange or cranberry juice (only if aspiration is minimal). This last provides the patient with some taste, a very small amount of liquid to swallow, and a smaller object (still controlled by the clinician) to manipulate in the mouth. When control improves, the patient can be given chewing gum that must be manipulated without the clinician's control (Ford, Grotz, Pomerantz, Bruno, & Flannery, 1974).

EXERCISES TO HOLD A COHESIVE BOLUS. In addition to manipulating material from side to side in the mouth without losing control of it, the patient needs to be able to hold both a liquid and paste bolus in a cohesive fashion. Exercises to help the patient hold a cohesive bolus should be started only when the patient has demonstrated the ability to manipulate material grossly in the mouth, as described in the previous exercise. It is usually easiest to begin with a paste-consistency bolus, approximately ⅓ teaspoon. The bolus is placed on the patient's tongue and he or she is asked to move the bolus around the mouth, without losing the material or allowing it to spread out around the mouth. This requires that the patient cup the tongue around the bolus. When the patient is finished, the bolus can be expectorated rather than swallowed, and the clinician can examine the patient's mouth for any residue. When the patient is successful at this task, the paste bolus can be varied in size, repeating the same procedure.

Then a liquid bolus can be used. Liquid, ⅓ teaspoon, can be placed in the patient's mouth, and the patient asked to keep the liquid together and to move it about the mouth without losing it or swallowing it. When finished, the patient can spit out the material.

Bolus Propulsion Exercises. The patient may also need to practice posterior propulsion of the bolus. This can be accomplished using a 4″ long, narrow roll of gauze soaked in cranberry or orange juice. With this placed in the mouth, the patient can be asked to push upward and backward against the gauze with the tongue, squeezing liquid out of the gauze and pushing the liquid backward at the same time. With the clinician holding the front of the gauze, it cannot be swallowed but can give the patient practice in pushing material upward and backward with the tongue. The small amount of liquid can stimulate a swallow. The amount of liquid placed in the gauze will depend on the patient's ability to control liquid once it enters the pharyngeal stage of the swallow. If the patient's vertical tongue range of motion is severely reduced, the roll of gauze can be made larger in diameter by placing two or three 4″ × 4″ gauze pads on top of one another and then rolling them. When the end of the gauze roll is dipped into some small amount of liquid, it will fill the space between the patient's tongue and the hard palate and enable the patient to practice the patterning of up and backward tongue pressure on the palate during swallowing. Effectively, the gauze acts as a pseudopalate for the patient to push against. As range of tongue motion improves, the thickness of the gauze roll can be reduced.

Range-of-Motion Exercises for Pharyngeal Structures

AIRWAY ENTRANCE. If laryngeal incompetence during swallowing cannot be managed quickly by postural assists or by teaching the patient to voluntarily close the airway at the vocal folds (the supraglottic swallow) or at the entrance to the airway (the super-supraglottic swallow), a sequence of range-of-motion exercises for airway entrance closure should be initiated. The patient is asked to complete the series 5 to 10 times daily for 5 minutes each time. Initially, the patient should be seated and told to hold his or her breath and to bear down for a second, then to let go. The patient may do this while pushing down or pulling up on the chair with both hands for several seconds. This exercise should not be done with a patient who has a problem with uncontrolled blood pressure as bearing down can increase blood pressure. For such a patient, rapid repeated glottal attack on a vowel may produce the same result, as described below.

VOCAL FOLD ADDUCTION EXERCISES. If the patient has poor vocal fold adduction, the following exercises should be done. The patient is asked to bear down against a chair with only one hand (rather than two) and to produce clear voice simultaneously. After repeating this exercise 5 times, the patient is asked to repeat "ah" 5 times with hard glottal attack on each vowel. These two exercises are repeated 3 times in a sequence, 5 to 10 times a day. It should be carefully explained that the patient can monitor improvements in laryngeal function by listening to the clarity of voice quality. It should also be explained that the exercises involving lifting, pushing, and vocalization are directly applicable to swallowing as these increase muscle activity in the larynx and are basic to good laryngeal closure during swallowing. The patient should continue to practice this series of exercises for about 1 week. After 1 week of these exercises, if swallowing reevaluation does not reveal sufficient improvement, with the larynx providing good airway protection during swallowing, the exercises should be changed. This is to prevent monotony for the patient more than to provide a hierarchy of difficulty.

The second set of exercises involves lifting or pushing with simultaneous voicing, such as sitting and pulling up on the seat of the chair with both hands while prolonging phonation. The repeated glottal attack exercise may be made more difficult by asking the patient to begin phonation on "ah" with a hard attack and to sustain the phonation with clear, smooth vocal quality for 5 to 10 seconds. Finally, the patient should be asked to practice a "pseudo" supraglottic swallow or super-supraglottic swallow—that is to take a breath, hold it, and cough as strongly as possible. In this way the patient practices the adduction and expectoration steps of the super-supraglottic swallow. These movements may be incorporated into the practice of the entire supraglottic or super-supraglottic swallow sequence without giving the patient any material to be swallowed. The entire sequence involves taking a breath, holding the breath while swallowing, and releasing the breath into a cough to expectorate any residual material, as described further later in this chapter.

In most cases, these exercises will effect improvement within 2 to 3 weeks. Occasionally, however, a patient may require 6 to 8 months to attain adequate airway protection. Most often these are the patients who have undergone an extended supraglottic laryngectomy or had other extensive laryngeal damage.

TONGUE BASE EXERCISES. Several exercises help to improve the tongue base range of motion. For the first exercise, the patient can be asked to pull the tongue straight back in the mouth as far as possible and to hold it for 1 second. A second exercise is to pretend to gargle, which pulls the tongue base back. The patient should pull back and pretend to gargle as hard as possible and then release. A third exercise involves pretending to yawn, which also pulls the tongue base back. The patient can be asked to do all three of these during their modified barium swallow procedure so the clinician can determine which of the three exercises results in best tongue base retraction. In my experience, the gargle exercise produces the best tongue base retraction. The effortful swallow, as described later in the section on swallow maneuvers, also improves tongue base retraction. In a supraglottic laryngectomy, the super-supraglottic swallow also pulls the tongue base back, as does the initial part of the super-supraglottic swallow, i.e., maintain the effortful breath-hold for several seconds and release.

LARYNGEAL ELEVATION EXERCISE—THE FALSETTO EXERCISE. In the falsetto exercise, the patient is asked to slide up the pitch scale as high as possible to a high squeaky voice. When the patient reaches the top of the scale, he or she should hold the high note for several seconds with as much effort as possible. During the production of falsetto, the larynx elevates almost as much as it does during swallow. The patient may take a hand and gently pull up on the larynx to assist laryngeal elevation during this procedure. This manual assist should not be done during swallow attempts as the hand may actually get in the way of the swallow.

Sensory-Motor Integration Procedures:
Heightening Sensory Awareness Before the Swallow Attempt

Another set of treatment strategies involves increasing oral sensory stimulation prior to the patient's swallow attempt. These techniques can be considered compensatory or can be therapeutic. In some cases they are compensatory and need to be used as part of a maintenance program by the caregiver or the patient. This is true in patients who have motor neuron disease and in those who have Alzheimer's disease and other degenerative processes. In patients who have suffered stroke, head injury, head and neck cancer treatment, and other procedures from which some recovery is anticipated, the procedures are therapeutic and are designed to regularly improve and maintain an improved onset of the oral swallow and the triggering of the pharyngeal swallow.

Generally, this set of strategies is appropriate for a patient with reduced recognition of food in the mouth or very slowed oral transit because of an apraxic component or a delay in triggering the pharyngeal swallow. This increased sensory stimulation may take a number of forms, as described previously in this chapter, including (1) increasing the downward pressure of the spoon against the tongue as the bolus is delivered into the mouth; (2) introducing a bolus with increased sensory characteristics, such as a cold bolus or a textured bolus (e.g., rice pudding) or a bolus with a strong flavor; (3) providing a bolus requiring chewing so that the mastication provides preliminary oral stimulation; (4) thermal–tactile stimulation to the anterior faucial arches prior to the swallow; and (5) providing a larger volume bolus. Some patients respond to one or more of these techniques by producing a more normal swallow, particularly at the sensorimotor integration points (i.e., onset and speed of the oral stage) and in the triggering of the pharyngeal swallow.

For some patients, the sensorimotor act of swallowing begins with the arm-and-hand action of the feeding act itself. These patients do best when they are given the spoon containing the desired bolus and are allowed to place the food in the mouth themselves. When food is placed in the mouth for these patients, there may be no oral tongue motion or other response, but when they place food in their own mouth, there is normal onset of tongue movement for the oral stage of swallow and speed of the oral stage of swallow. For patients who are unable to use an arm or hand for self-feeding, the caregiver placing the food in the mouth may lift the patient's hand toward the mouth as the food is being placed in the mouth. This may provide the patient with additional preliminary sensory input, alerting the cortex and brainstem that something is coming to the mouth. Techniques to increase sensory input do not fatigue the patient and are relatively easy to implement in a wide variety of patients because they are largely under the control of the caregiver.

Thermal–tactile stimulation is designed to improve the speed of triggering of the pharyngeal swallow in patients who have been identified from assessment of previous swallows as having a delay in triggering the pharyngeal swallow (Lazzara et al., 1986; Rosenbek, Roecker, Wood, & Robbins, 1996). Thermal–tactile stimulation should be done only when a delay in triggering the pharyngeal swallow has been defined radiographically on at least *two* consecutive swallows. Some patients with neurologic impairments, such as those with cerebrovascular accidents, exhibit a "warm-up" period when eating, so that triggering of the pharyngeal swallow may be most delayed on the first swallow and may improve somewhat on the second swallow. Thus, the second swallow may be more representative of the patient's usual functional pattern than the first swallow.

To perform thermal–tactile stimulation, the patient is asked to open his or her mouth while the clinician places a cold, size 00 laryngeal mirror at the base of the anterior faucial arch (Figure 6.4). Complete contact of the back side of the laryngeal mirror to the faucial arch is maintained while rubbing up and down vertically five times. The stimulation is repeated on the opposite side of the oral cavity, if both sides are equally sensitive. In the case of patients with damage to one side of the oral cavity, as in oral surgical patients or trauma patients, the contact is always made on the normal side of the oral cavity. If the patient has a bite reflex and may bite on the mirror, injury to the patient can be prevented by coating the mirror and handle with Teflon™ so that the metal back side of the mirror used for the stimulation is left uncoated (K. R. Helfrich-Miller, personal communication, 1984). Upon completion of the stimulation, the patient

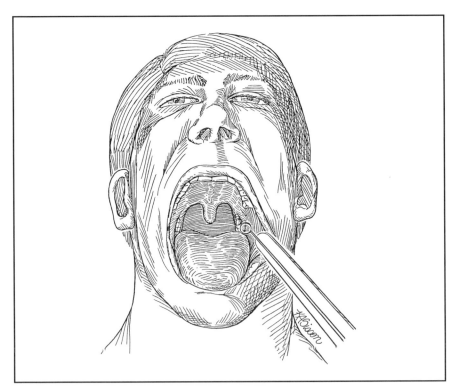

Figure 6.4. Front view of the oral cavity showing placement of the size 00 laryngeal mirror at the anterior faucial arch. It is critical for the clinician to distinguish between the anterior faucial arch and the retromolar trigone area, which is immediately behind the last molar.

is immediately given a small amount of iced liquid barium and told to swallow it. Results of a study by Lazzara et al. (1986) indicate that 95% of those patients identified radiographically as having a delay in triggering of the pharyngeal swallow will improve in speed of triggering the pharyngeal swallow after thermal–tactile stimulation. This 1986 study does not address the role of thermal–tactile stimulation in recovery of functional swallow, but documents the immediate effects of the procedure.

If the procedure is introduced during the radiographic study, the clinician can then use the videotaped example of the immediate effects of thermal–tactile stimulation in education of the patient's family, other caregivers, physician, and other health care professionals regarding the rationale for the procedure. It is important to note that thermal–tactile stimulation does not trigger the pharyngeal swallow at the time of the stimulation. Rather, the purpose of the stimulation is to *heighten the sensitivity* for the swallow in the central nervous system and to alert the central nervous system so that when the patient voluntarily attempts to swallow, he or she will trigger a pharyngeal swallow more rapidly (Fujiu et al., 1994; Logemann, 1983).

With a patient whose physician has ordered no oral feeding, the clinician can ask the patient to swallow saliva after the stimulation without presenting any liquid. Even if the patient cannot follow directions, the stimulation will "tickle" and make the patient want to swallow. Then the clinician should carefully observe the swallowing mechanism by placing outstretched fingers lightly on the patient's neck, with the forefinger under the tip of the mandible on the soft tissue, second finger on the hyoid bone, and third and fourth fingers on the thyroid cartilage and cricoid cartilages respectively, as discussed in Chapter 5. With the index finger on the soft tissue under the tip of the mandible and the second finger on the hyoid, the first lingual movement at the initiation of the posterior propulsion of the bolus (which defines the beginning of the oral transit time) can be felt. When the pharyngeal swallow is initiated, the larynx elevates and the hyoid bone moves upward and backward. Triggering the pharyngeal swallow marks the end of the oral stage of the swallow. Therefore, oral transit time and pharyngeal delay time can be measured by the time interval between the initiation of lingual movement and the elevation of the larynx, indicating that the pharyngeal swallow has triggered. If oral transit plus delay is greater than 2 seconds, it is abnormal.

If the patient can tolerate small amounts of material, the clinician may introduce a small amount of liquid as follows and ask the patient to swallow. After rubbing vertically up and down with the laryngeal mirror against the faucial arches, a straw can be effectively used as a pipette, filling it with approximately ¼ inch of ice water. The pipette is then placed with its fluid-filled end at the anterior faucial arch, where contact of the laryngeal mirror was made during stimulation. The patient is then instructed to attempt to swallow when the clinician releases the liquid and gives the command, "Now." For added stimulation, iced ginger ale or other carbonated beverage may be used rather than ice water. To assure that any liquids swallowed can be detected if expectorated orally or through a tracheostomy site after the swallow, food coloring can be added to the liquid.

In severely impaired patients, it is likely that no pharyngeal swallow will be triggered with attempts to swallow (with or without liquid) during the early sessions of stimulation. In such patients stimulation will need to be repeated three or four times daily for 5 to 10 minutes each time for several weeks to a month.

Once the pharyngeal swallow begins to trigger, therapy may be expanded by (1) increasing, in very small steps, the amount of material presented to the patient in a single swallow (still in the pipette at the base of the faucial arches) and (2) changing the consistency of the food presented at the faucial arches (increasing thickness). The progression of therapy in these patients is often slow, with restoration of oral feeding often taking a number of months. During this time, these patients need nonoral feeding to maintain nutrition. There is evidence that some types of severely involved patients, such as those with cerebral palsy and developmental delay, and those with severe head injury, will require this procedure to be done as a part of a feeding maintenance program (Helfrich-Miller et al., 1986).

Swallow Maneuvers

Swallow maneuvers are designed to place specific aspects of pharyngeal swallow physiology under voluntary control. Four swallow maneuvers have been developed to date: (1) the supraglottic swallow, designed to close the airway at the level of the true vocal folds before and during the swallow (Logemann, 1983, 1993b; Martin, Logemann, Shaker, & Dodds, 1993); (2) the super-supraglottic swallow, designed to close the airway entrance before and during the swallow (Logemann, 1993a, 1993b; Martin et al., 1993; Ohmae, Logemann, Kaiser, Hanson, & Kahrilas, 1996); (3) the effortful swallow, designed to increase posterior motion of the tongue base during the pharyngeal swallow and thus improve bolus clearance from the valleculae (Kahrilas, Lin, Logemann, Ergun, & Facchini, 1993; Logemann, 1993b; Pouderoux & Kahrilas, 1995); and (4) the Mendelsohn maneuver, designed to increase the extent and duration of laryngeal elevation and thereby increase the duration and width of cricopharyngeal opening (Bartolome & Neumann, 1993; Bryant, 1991; Kahrilas, Logemann, Krugler, & Flanagan, 1991; Lazarus, Logemann, & Gibbons, 1993; Logemann & Kahrilas, 1990; Neumann, 1993). This latter maneuver can also improve the overall coordination of the swallow (Lazarus, Logemann, & Gibbons, 1993). These maneuvers are summarized in Table 6.3.

These maneuvers, however, require the ability to follow directions carefully

Table 6.3
Swallow Maneuvers, the Swallowing Disorders for Which
They Are Appropriate, and Their Rationale

Swallow Maneuvers	Problem for Which Maneuver Was Designed	Rationale
Supraglottic swallow	Reduced or late vocal fold closure	Voluntary breath hold usually closes vocal folds before and during swallow (Martin et al., 1993)
	Delayed pharyngeal swallow	Closes vocal folds before and during delay
Super-supraglottic swallow	Reduced closure of airway entrance	Effortful breath hold tilts arytenoid forward, closing airway entrance before and during swallow (Martin et al., 1993)
Effortful swallow	Reduced posterior movement of the tongue base	Effort increases posterior tongue base movement (Pouderoux & Kahrilas, 1995)
Mendelsohn maneuver	Reduced laryngeal movement	Laryngeal movement opens the upper esophageal sphincter (UES); prolonging laryngeal elevation prolongs UES opening (Cook et al., 1989; Jacob et al., 1989)
	Discoordinated swallow	Normalizes timing of pharyngeal swallow events (Lazarus, Logemann, & Gibbons, 1993)

and are not feasible in patients who have cognitive or significant language impairment. These maneuvers also require increased muscular effort and are not appropriate in patients who fatigue easily. However, some patients can swallow safely and efficiently only using a voluntary maneuver (Kahrilas, Logemann, & Gibbons, 1992; Lazarus, Logemann, & Gibbons, 1993; Logemann & Kahrilas, 1990; Robbins & Levine, 1993). Usually, voluntary maneuvers are used temporarily as the patient's swallow recovers, and are then discarded as the patient's swallow physiology returns to normal.

Each swallow maneuver has a specific goal to change a selected aspect of pharyngeal swallow physiology (Logemann, 1993a). Changes in these target components of the oropharyngeal swallow can be observed or measured. In general, the effects of swallow maneuvers are best observed and measured using videofluoroscopy. The effects of these maneuvers on swallowing safety (aspiration) and efficiency (residue) may be observed at times using videoendoscopy; however, videoendoscopy does not allow visualization of these maneuvers *during* the swallow, a significant limitation.

All of these maneuvers can be practiced by giving the patient slow, step-by-step instructions and asking him or her to swallow saliva. Food is not needed to teach the patient these maneuvers.

Supraglottic Swallow. The goal of the supraglottic swallow is to close the vocal folds before and during the swallow, thus protecting the trachea from aspiration (Logemann, 1983), as illustrated in Figure 6.5. The supraglottic swallow, or the voluntary airway closure technique, can be attempted with a patient for the first time during the videofluoroscopic study or at bedside. The patient must be alert, relatively relaxed, and able to follow simple directions without becoming upset or confused. The patient can be directed through the procedure step by step by the clinician during the radiographic study. To do this, the patient is given material to swallow and told to keep it in his or her mouth while directions are given. The directions should be as follows:

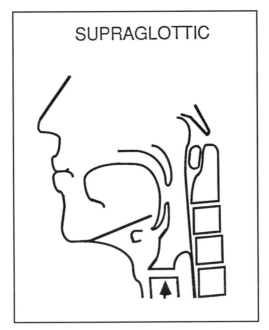

Figure 6.5. Lateral drawing of the head and neck showing the focus of the supraglottic swallow as the closure of the true vocal folds.

1. Take a deep breath and hold your breath.

2. Keep holding your breath and lightly cover your tracheostomy tube (if a tracheostomy is present).

3. Keep holding your breath while you swallow.

4. Immediately after you swallow, cough.

These steps should be practiced with the patient on saliva swallows prior to giving him or her the actual food to swallow. However, the patient cannot take a great deal of time to practice while in radiology. If the patient is able to follow the directions correctly several times without food, then the procedure may be tried under fluoroscopy with some expectation of success. At all times, the clinician should continue to provide verbal directions for each step.

If the patient becomes confused or cannot follow directions easily, this technique should not be tried initially during the modified barium swallow. Instead, the clinician should work with the patient later until the technique has been learned. When the supraglottic procedure has been mastered, the patient can be rescheduled for another fluorographic study and the success of this technique in improving airway closure can be assessed. If the patient has a large gap in glottic closure, such as may be seen following extended partial laryngectomy or in bilateral adductor paralysis, the supraglottic swallow procedure alone will not be sufficient to achieve airway protection. The patient will also need adduction exercises, which must be practiced for a week or more, before improvement in vocal cord adduction can be expected (Logemann, 1983).

In some patients, the direction to "Take a deep breath and hold your breath" does not result in vocal fold closure (Martin et al., 1993). Instead, some patients hold their breath by stopping chest wall movement. These patients appear to be performing the supraglottic swallow procedure correctly, but fluorographic examination of swallow reveals an open airway. For these patients, a change in instructions is needed. The clinician can instruct the patient to "Inhale and then exhale slightly; hold the breath and swallow while holding the breath." Because the vocal folds move toward each other slightly during exhalation, holding the breath on exhalation may result in vocal fold closure. Or, the clinician may ask the patient to "Inhale and then say 'ah'; stop voicing and hold the breath." Usually, one of these techniques will elicit vocal fold closure on the breath hold.

Some patients with severe reductions in tongue mobility or severely reduced tongue bulk because of oral cancer surgical procedures essentially have little or no oral transit. They need to take a sufficient volume of liquid to drop the bolus by gravity from the mouth to the pharynx with chin elevation (head extension). During the radiographic study, these patients should be taught the extended supraglottic swallow or "dump and swallow" technique. First, these patients should be given very small amounts (1 or 3 ml) of liquid on a spoon. These small volume swallows should be observed as the patient tosses his or her head back and dumps the liquid into the pharynx to determine whether (1) the pharyngeal swallow triggers on time and (2) airway closure is sufficient to protect the airway. If both triggering of the pharyngeal swallow and airway closure are normal, the patient can be given 5 to 10 ml of liquid in a cup and taught the following sequence:

1. Hold the breath tightly.

2. Put the entire 5 to 10 ml of liquid in the mouth.

3. Continue to hold the breath and toss the head back, thus dumping the liquid into the pharynx as a whole.

4. Swallow two to three times or as many times as needed to clear the majority of the liquid *while continuing to hold the breath*.

5. Cough to clear any residue from the pharynx.

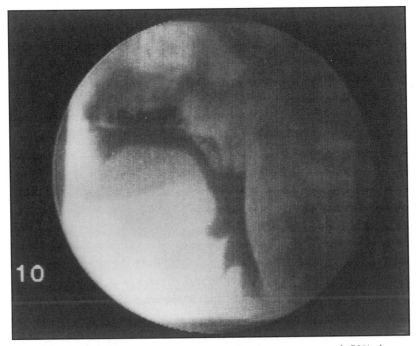

Figure 6.6. Lateral videoprint of a radiographic study as a patient with 70% glossectomy uses the extended supraglottic swallow. One third of a cup of liquid barium has been dumped into the oral cavity and pharynx and will be cleared by repeated swallows.

This process is much like a normal swallow when taking consecutive swallows of liquid from a cup. A normal swallower usually holds the breath throughout all of the consecutive swallows.

As the patient's confidence and efficiency with the procedure increase, up to 20 ml may be taken at one time, using five to six repeated swallows while holding the airway closed. Figure 6.6 illustrates this technique. At the end of the sequence of swallows, the patient should cough to clear any residual food from the pharynx. This technique enables the patient with severe lingual impairment to take a significant amount of calories in a short period of time.

Super-Supraglottic Swallow. The super-supraglottic swallow is designed to close the *entrance* to the airway voluntarily by tilting the arytenoid cartilage anteriorly to the base of the epiglottis before and during the swallow and closing the false cords tightly, as illustrated in Figure 6.7. This is the normal mechanism for closure of the entrance to the airway, and is facilitated during normal swallow by the elevation of the larynx. Laryngeal elevation brings the arytenoid cartilage closer to the posterior surface of the epiglottis, so that the arytenoid does not have to move as far anteriorly. The effort involved in the super-supraglottic swallow increases the anterior tilt of the arytenoid and the false vocal cord closure to close the entrance to the airway early, before and during the swallow.

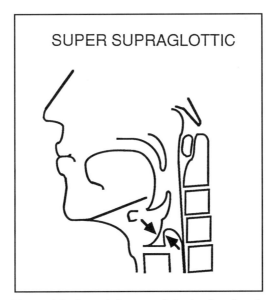

Figure 6.7. Lateral diagram of the head and neck showing the focus of the super-supraglottic maneuver as the closure of the airway entrance at the arytenoid cartilage and base of epiglottis, as well as closure of the false vocal folds.

The patient is given the following *instructions:* "Inhale and hold your breath very tightly, bearing down. Keep holding your breath and bearing down as you swallow. Cough when you are finished."

The bearing down helps to tilt the arytenoid forward, close the false vocal folds, and close the entrance to the airway. This strategy is used in patients with reduced closure of the airway entrance, particularly those who have undergone a supraglottic laryngectomy (Logemann, Gibbons, et al., 1994). During supra-glottic laryngectomy, the epiglottis is removed so that the laryngeal entrance comprises the tongue base and arytenoid cartilage. These differences in anatomy of the airway entrance or vestibule are illustrated in Figure 6.8. In the case of the supraglottic laryngectomy, the arytenoid cartilage tilts forward to contact the tongue base, rather than the base of the epiglottis. In the supraglottic laryngec-tomy, the super-supraglottic swallow improves tongue base retraction as well as anterior tilt of the arytenoid and adduction of the false vocal folds.

The *super-supraglottic swallow* also improves the rate of laryngeal elevation at the beginning of the swallow and is particularly helpful in the patient who has undergone a full course of radiotherapy to the neck (Logemann, Pauloski, Rademaker, & Colangelo, in press). The super-supraglottic swallow can also be

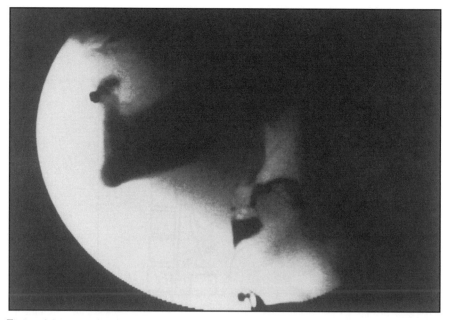

Figure 6.8. Lateral radiographic view of the laryngeal entrance in a supraglottic laryngec-tomee showing the absence of the vallecula, epiglottis, hyoid bone, and false vocal folds with the base of tongue and arytenoid cartilage coated with barium, the remainder of which is sit-ting on the top surface of the vocal folds.

used as an exercise to improve tongue base retraction in patients with normal anatomy.

Effortful Swallow. The effortful swallow is designed to increase posterior motion of the tongue base during the pharyngeal swallow (as shown in Figure 6.9) and thus improve bolus clearance from the valleculae (Kahrilas et al., 1993; Kahrilas, Logemann, Lin, & Ergun, 1992; Logemann, 1993a). The clinician should provide the following *instructions* for the effortful swallow: "As you swallow, squeeze hard with all of your muscles." This will improve the pressure exerted by the oral tongue at all points along the palate and at the tongue base (Pouderoux & Kahrilas, 1995) and will increase tongue base movement.

Mendelsohn Maneuver The Mendelsohn maneuver is designed to increase the extent and duration of laryngeal elevation and thereby increase the duration and width of cricopharyngeal opening (Bartolome & Neumann, 1993; Bryant, 1991; Kahrilas et al., 1991; Lazarus, Logemann, & Gibbons, 1993; Logemann & Kahrilas, 1990; Neumann, 1993; Robbins & Levine, 1993). (See Figure 6.10.) This maneuver can also improve the overall coordination of the swallow (Lazarus, Logemann, & Gibbons, 1993). The clinician should provide the patient with the following *instructions* for the Mendelsohn maneuver: "Swallow your saliva several times and pay attention to your neck as you swallow. Tell me if you can feel that something (your Adam's apple or voice box) lifts and lowers

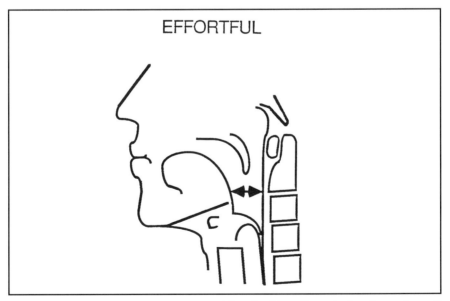

Figure 6.9. A lateral diagram of the effects of the effortful swallow, which is designed to pull the tongue base more posteriorly and improve pharyngeal pressure during swallowing.

as you swallow. Now, this time, when you swallow and you feel something lift as you swallow, don't let your Adam's apple drop. Hold it up with your muscles for several seconds."

Alternative instructions are as follows: "As you swallow, can you feel that everything squeezes together in the middle of the swallow? When you can feel this, swallow and hold the squeeze." "Holding the squeeze" translates to prolonging the moment when the larynx is most elevated, the tongue base is most retracted and in contact with the pharyngeal wall and the airway is closed.

Therapy and Management for Specific Swallowing Disorders

Disorders Affecting the Oral Preparatory Phase of the Swallow

During the oral preparatory phase of the swallow, the patient must be able to manipulate food in the mouth while maintaining complete closure of the lips and while controlling the bolus so that nothing spills into the pharynx. The

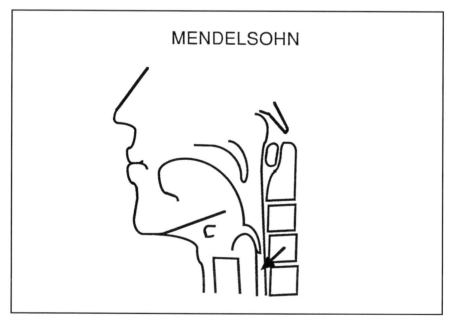

Figure 6.10. A lateral diagram of the focus for the Mendelsohn maneuver, which is the improvement in laryngeal elevation with prolonged and expanded cricopharyngeal opening during the swallow.

clinician should be sure that the patient can maintain comfortable nasal breathing while maintaining lip closure from the time that food is placed in the mouth until the pharyngeal swallow is completed.

Reduced Labial Closure

To improve labial closure, range-of-motion lip exercises may be necessary first. These exercises include (1) stretching the lips in the /i/ position as far as possible and holding in extreme extension for 1 second; (2) puckering the lips as tightly as possible and holding for 1 second; and (3) bringing the lips together and holding tightly for 1 second. If lip closure is not possible on the third exercise, the patient can close his or her lips against a pile of tongue blades, a spoon, or other object. As strength and range of motion improve, the size of the object can be reduced until it is only the thickness of a single tongue blade, and closure can be obtained. Once the patient is able to obtain lip closure, but has not habituated it, a graduated increase in the time required to maintain closure should be used. The patient may be asked to hold lip closure for 1 minute. This should be repeated 10 times a day. The next day the patient should maintain lip closure for 2 minutes, 10 times a day. The schedule should be increased by 1 minute each day or two, or more as needed, until the patient reaches 10 minutes of closure 10 times per day. After 2 weeks of following the regimen regularly, the patient should have habituated normal lip closure. Mitchell (1967) described a buccinator apparatus to remind the patient to keep the mouth closed until closure can be accomplished automatically. The device consisted of flat-shaped, 16-gauge indoor–outdoor wire, cut to the length that encircles the patient's lips. The overlapped ends are wrapped with tape and positioned on the outside of the lower lip at the base of the lower teeth. Mitchell wrote, "By contouring the wire around the buccinator muscle and by applying pressure at the base of the nose and at the base of the lower teeth, the device pulls the lips in and holds the teeth together" (p. 1135).

Closing the lips against resistance both laterally and anteriorly may help to improve lip closure. Using a tongue blade, the patient can be asked to close the lips tightly around the tongue blade and hold it with the lips while the patient or the clinician attempts to extract it. This exercise will also increase lip strength.

Another exercise involves maintaining lip closure while the patient or the clinician tries to manually part the lips.

Reduced Range of Tongue Movement Laterally During Mastication

Mastication is critical to a normal diet. As a temporary measure, the patient with difficulty chewing may restrict his or her diet to liquids and soft foods while working on mastication.

Exercises to improve range of lateral tongue movement have been described earlier in the section on indirect swallowing therapy procedures. As a temporary measure, the patient whose tongue elevation is normal may be taught to mash food by pressing the tongue against the roof of the mouth. Alternatively, the patient may position food on the most mobile side of the tongue (Buckley et al., 1976) and tilt the head slightly to that side to keep food on the side of better control.

Reduced Buccal Tension or Buccal Scarring

To improve buccal tension, the patient may be given facial exercises. These include rounding the lips tightly for "oh" and stretching the lips broadly for "ee." Rapidly alternating these two postures may increase buccal tension. Also, smiling broadly and spreading the lips tightly across the teeth may also improve cheek tension, as will pulling the lips as far as possible to one side, holding in extension for 1 second, and then to the other, holding in extension for 1 second.

In the interim, the patient may be taught to place external pressure on the affected cheek and thus close the sulcus between the cheek and the lower alveolus. Gently resting one hand against the affected cheek should provide sufficient pressure.

Placing food on the unaffected side and tilting the head toward the unaffected side may also be helpful, as it will keep food on the stronger side (Buckley et al., 1976).

Reduced Range of Mandibular Movement Laterally

The patient may be given mandibular range-of-motion exercises to improve lateral movement range. These exercises involve opening the jaw as widely as possible and holding the maximum opening for 1 second; opening and moving the jaw to each side as far as possible and holding the extended position in each direction for 1 second; and moving the jaw around in a circle as far as possible in each direction. Occasionally, the clinician may assist the patient's attempts at jaw movement by placing gentle external pressure on the mandible in the desired direction of movement. The patient should always be instructed to move the jaw as far as possible in each direction, feeling a strong pull but no pain. If any pain occurs, the exercise should be discontinued until the patient can talk with the swallowing therapist or the doctor. This kind of exercise is particularly important for postoperative oral cancer patients and for patients undergoing oral radiotherapy, as they may experience some scarring/fibrosis of the muscles of mastication. The exercises should be continued through radiotherapy and for at least 6 to 8 weeks after radiation therapy, as radiotherapy may increase fibrosis in the muscles of mastication, narrow the mouth opening, and restrict mandibular movement.

If the patient is completely unable to lateralize the mandible and thus get normal occlusion, the individual may be taught to mash food with the tongue against the palate in order to broaden diet options.

In some cases a guide plane prosthesis is helpful. Such a prosthesis involves a vertical bar attached to a lower denture or partial plate. When the patient closes his or her mouth, the vertical bar guides the mandible into proper alignment, and thus proper occlusion.

Reduced Range of Tongue Movement Vertically

Exercises for improving vertical tongue range of movement were described previously in the section on indirect therapy for swallowing. If, however, the patient has not achieved tongue–palate contact after several months of repeating these exercises daily at regular intervals, a palate reshaping prosthesis may be given (Logemann, Sisson, & Wheeler, 1980; Trible, 1967; Wheeler, Logemann, & Rosen, 1980). If such a prosthesis is made and the patient's tongue elevation continues to improve, the palate can be reshaped with some of the bulk removed to allow for this improved tongue movement.

The speech–language pathologist and maxillofacial prosthodontist work together to construct the prosthesis, which is designed to lower the palatal vault to complement tongue function. Several prostheses are illustrated in Figure 6.11 A–D. If a patient has generalized reduction in tongue elevation both anteriorly and posteriorly, the palate would be lowered uniformly. If the patient exhibits a hemiparesis or has lost one longitudinal half of the tongue in ablative surgery, the prosthesis would contain more material on the affected side.

The ultimate design of the prosthesis depends on speech needs as well as swallowing patterns, so the final configuration may be a compromise between the optimum shape for the two functions. The prosthesis may contain no teeth and be designed to clasp to the patient's existing dentition; or it may have several teeth to replace missing dental units; or it may be constructed as a full upper denture.

Other types of prostheses, such as mandibular tongue prostheses to improve the patient's oral manipulation of food and speed of oral transit, may also be considered (Leonard & Gillis, 1982).

Reduced Tongue Movement To Form the Bolus

Exercises to improve tongue movement in formation of the bolus are discussed in the section on indirect swallowing procedures. However, as an interim measure, the clinician may suggest that the patient tilt his or her head slightly forward to keep the bolus in the anterior part of the mouth until the patient is ready to initiate the swallow, thus preventing him or her from losing the bolus in one of the lateral sulci. With the start of the swallow, the patient may then change head posture as appropriate.

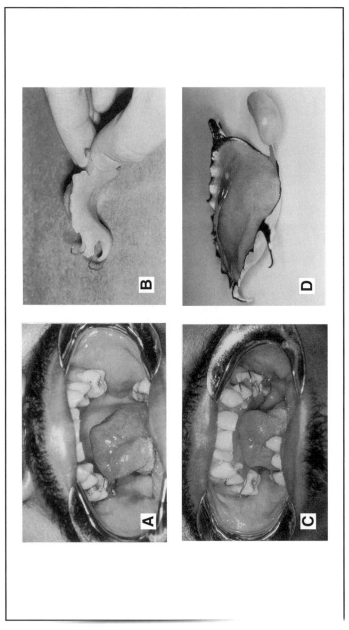

Figure 6.11. (A) Postsurgical anatomy of a patient who has had a lateral resection of the tongue reconstructed by tongue flap. He is unable to make contact with his tongue to the hard palate. (B) The same patient's prosthetic device, which clasps around his teeth and fills in the hard palatal area where his tongue could not make contact. (C) The same patient with the prosthesis in place, clasping around his teeth and enabling his tongue to contact the prosthetic palate. (D) An intraoral tongue reshaping/palate augmentation prosthesis containing not only the reshaped palate with clasps to hold it in place around the teeth but also a palatal lift extension to lift the patient's soft palate into an elevated position. This prosthesis is designed for a patient with neurologic tongue and palatal involvement.

226

Reduced Range and Coordination of Tongue Movement To Hold the Bolus

Exercises for range and coordination of tongue movement in controlling the bolus are discussed in the section on indirect therapy techniques for swallowing. As an interim measure, the clinician may suggest that the patient not attempt to manipulate the bolus once it is in the mouth but to hold the material securely against the front of the roof of the mouth and to initiate the swallow immediately.

In addition, the patient may hold his or her head slightly downward to keep the bolus in the more anterior position and then lift the head or tilt backward to initiate the swallow.

Reduced Ability To Hold the Bolus in Normal Position

The patient may be given a bolus of thick paste consistency (approximately ⅓ teaspoon) and asked to hold it consciously against the anterior to mid-portion of the palate with the tongue. This exercise requires that the tongue tip and the lateral margins of the tongue be contacting the alveolar ridge immediately posterior to the teeth. Then, the bolus can be made thinner and thinner in consistency, which makes the task more difficult.

Reduced Oral Sensitivity

The patient with reduced oral sensitivity should position food on the more sensitive side of his or her oral cavity. In addition, the use of cold material may help the individual to localize the material in the mouth. The use of mild spices or tastes to which the patient is sensitive may also improve his or her localization of material in the mouth.

Disorders Affecting the Oral Phase of the Swallow

A number of techniques may be employed to improve the oral phase of the swallow. Some of these are compensatory in nature—that is, they are not designed to improve function, but are designed to allow the patient to compensate for his or her problem. Others are rehabilitative in nature—that is, designed to help the patient reclaim normal movement patterns.

Tongue Thrust

In tongue thrust, the patient pushes the tongue anteriorly against the central incisors to initiate the swallow. This text does not address the problem of developmental tongue thrust, which is a complicated one, requiring more attention than is given here. The emphasis is on the patient with neurologic impairment who acquires a tongue thrust as a result of a neurologic lesion. In these patients, heightening their awareness of the thrust pattern and asking them to consciously position their tongue on the alveolar ridge and begin the swallow with an upward–backward push often reduces the thrusting. Applying downward pressure to the middle of the tongue may also reduce the thrust. This should be done during feeding.

As a compensatory measure, the patient may be taught to position food posteriorly on the tongue and thus avoid the thrusting pattern. In some instances, the tongue thrust is severe enough to actually throw material from the mouth. Tilting the head slightly backward may also assist in keeping food in the mouth. Tilting the patient's body backward 60° may be helpful if the individual is in a wheelchair.

Reduced Tongue Elevation

Exercises to improve tongue elevation have been discussed in the section on indirect exercises to improve swallowing. As an interim measure, the patient may be taught to position food posteriorly in the oral cavity or to syringe 5 to 10 ml of liquid into the oral pharynx and bypass the necessity of tongue elevation (Buckley et al., 1976; Trible, 1967). This should be done only when the clinician knows that the patient triggers the pharyngeal swallow in a timely fashion and has good airway protection. If the patient is able to suck, positioning a straw far posteriorly in the oral cavity, almost at the level of the faucial arches, may facilitate liquid swallows.

The patient also may be taught to tilt the head backward to allow gravity to assist in propelling food from the oral cavity into the pharynx (Trible, 1967). This technique does not increase the patient's chances of aspiration if the patient has normal pharyngeal swallow triggering and normal laryngeal control. If the clinician is concerned that the patient may aspirate because of the rapidity with which food is thrust into the pharynx, the clinician may teach the patient to voluntarily protect his or her airway using the supraglottic swallow technique. In this technique, the patient is taught to take a breath and hold it during the swallow (Larsen, 1973). In the case of the individual with reduced tongue elevation, the patient's swallowing sequence may be as follows: First, take a breath and hold it; second, place the food in the mouth; third, tilt the head backward and swallow; and fourth, cough after the swallow to rid the pharynx of any residue of material. In this sequence, voluntarily closing the airway prevents any aspiration that may occur before the pharyngeal swallow is triggered.

Reduced Anterior–Posterior Tongue Movement

Exercises to improve range of anterior–posterior tongue movement are discussed in the section on techniques for indirectly working on swallowing. The same compensatory postures and positions of food in the oral cavity described in the previous section on exercises to improve tongue elevation also may be used for patients with reduced anterior–posterior tongue movement. Frequently, the same patients experience reduced tongue range of motion in both elevation and anterior–posterior movement.

Disorganized Patterns of Anterior–Posterior Tongue Movement

Some types of patients exhibit specific patterns of tongue movement that are severely disorganized and result in long delays in oral transit. Patients with Parkinson's disease are such a group. They exhibit a rapidly repeating tongue pumping action that keeps food in the oral cavity for long periods of time. One way to reduce this activity is to alert the patient to the pumping, and ask him or her to consciously hold the bolus against the palate with the tongue and to initiate the swallow with a single strong backward movement of the tongue. This will normally eliminate or reduce the disorganized tongue pattern as long as the patient can remain aware of his or her swallowing pattern.

Reduced Tongue Strength

Reduced tongue strength can be improved with resistance exercises, which have been discussed earlier in this chapter. These exercises involve either a tongue blade or other flat object to push vertically down on the tongue, asking the patient to resist against the tongue blade, if possible. Then, the tongue blade can be turned vertically and pushed laterally against one side of the tongue with the patient resisting, and then moved to the other side of the tongue with a similar patient response. Then the tongue blade can be put down vertically in the front of the mouth and used to push back against the tongue tip, with the patient again applying resistance. The Iowa Oral Pressure Instrument (IOPI) (Breakthrough, 131 Technology Innovation Center, Oakdale, IA) can also be used to help the patient gauge the amount of pressure applied vertically against the IOPI, which rests between the tongue and the palate.

Swallowing Apraxia

Swallowing apraxia usually manifests itself with searching motions or lack of any response to placement of food in the mouth. Generally, techniques to improve sensory input work best for apraxic patients. These include changing the bolus characteristics to heighten the patient's awareness and thermal–tactile stimulation. All have been described earlier in the section on indirect management.

Scarred Tongue Contour

A scarred tongue contour cannot be improved with exercises. It may be compensated for by teaching the patient to position food posterior to this scarring, and to tilt the head backward to use gravity to assist in oral transit. Actual treatment for the scarring involves surgical release of the scar, and the patient should be referred to a head and neck surgeon for corrective measures. In many cases, it is necessary to show the patient's fluoroscopic study, which has been recorded on videotape, to the head and neck surgeon in order for the physician to appreciate the seriousness of the disorder as it impacts on swallowing. The effect of scarring is usually not seen except in the dynamics of movement. If the head and neck surgeon simply examines the patient's oral cavity at rest, the scar may seem rather small and insignificant. However, during tongue movement for swallowing, when the anterior and posterior tongue segments elevate and the scar tissue does not, a large depression is created into which most or all of the bolus of food collects. The patient is thus unable to move food posteriorly.

Delayed or Absent Triggering of the Pharyngeal Swallow

Treatment for a delayed or absent triggering of the pharyngeal swallow involves thermal–tactile stimulation, suck–swallow, or using a bolus with a particular sensory characteristic, such as sour or cold, or a particular volume, as described earlier in this chapter under indirect techniques. Thermal–tactile stimulation usually needs to be repeated three to four times a day for 5 to 10 minutes each time. The patient or a family member or other caregiver may be taught to do this stimulation when the patient leaves the hospital.

One technique to compensate for delayed triggering of the pharyngeal swallow is to ask the patient to tilt the head forward when swallowing. Tilting the head forward protects the airway more and in some people widens the vallecular space and increases the chance that the bolus will hesitate in the valleculae during the delay, rather than falling into the open airway. Patients with delayed or absent pharyngeal swallow should also limit the amount of each bolus so the bolus can be held in the pharyngeal recesses and the volume is not so large that it will overflow into the open airway.

The speed at which the patient swallows is also an important factor. Once the radiographic study has determined the duration of the delay in the pharyngeal triggering, the patient and his or her caregiver should be warned that the patient needs this amount of time between swallows to ensure that each bolus has cleared the pharynx before a new swallow is initiated. Otherwise, the patient will overflow his or her pharyngeal recesses and aspirate significantly.

Heimlich and O'Connor (1979a, 1979b) described an unusual technique employed with three patients who had "forgotten" how to swallow. The procedure involved four sequential steps. First, the patient placed one gloved index finger in the instructor's mouth and the other hand against the upper throat and chin of the instructor so the patient could experience the sensation of the instructor sucking the finger while feeling the swallowing movements in the therapist's neck. Second, the patient put a finger into his or her own mouth, trying to imitate the sucking sensation, and placed the other hand on his or her own upper neck to attempt to duplicate the swallowing process. Third, a specially designed plastic tube was placed in the cervical esophagus with its flared end above the cricopharyngeus, allowing free access of saliva into the upper esophagus, and the patient repeated the sucking and swallowing process. Fourth, when the ability to swallow liquids was mastered with the tube, the tube was removed and instruction continued until a normal diet was resumed. Care was taken not to perforate the esophagus with the tube and not to allow displacement of the prosthesis upward or downward. This technique has not been broadly used.

Disorders Affecting the Pharyngeal Stage of the Swallow

Techniques used to improve disorders affecting the pharyngeal stage of swallow also can be compensatory or rehabilitative.

Bilateral Reduction in Pharyngeal Contraction

No direct therapy technique improves pharyngeal contraction at all levels. The tongue holding, or Masako, maneuver is designed to exercise the portion of the superior constrictor known as the glossopharyngeus muscle. These inferior fibers of the superior constrictor come from the median raphe of the pharyngeal wall around into the tongue base on each side. This muscle is believed to be responsible for retraction of the tongue base and anterior bulging of the posterior pharyngeal wall at the level of the tongue base. The maneuver involves holding the tongue between the teeth with the tip of the tongue extended out approximately ¾ inch. This stabilizes the anterior attachment of the muscle in the tongue base and effectively directs all of the effect of muscle contraction on the posterior attachment. The result of the maneuver is to pull the pharyngeal wall more forward during the swallow while doing the tongue holding (Fujiu & Logemann, 1996; Fujiu, Logemann, & Pauloski, 1995). The maneuver can be difficult to do if the patient has a delay in the pharyngeal swallow since holding the tongue changes tongue motion and usually introduces a slight increase in pharyngeal delay, even in normal subjects. The patient should feel a strong pulling on the back of the throat when doing the maneuver.

Compensatory techniques include (1) alternating liquid and semisolid or solid swallows so the liquid washes the material of thicker consistency through the pharynx; (2) limiting the diet to liquids or thin paste materials requiring less pressure to clear the pharynx; and (3) following each swallow of food or liquid with several repetitive dry swallows to clear the pharynx of any residual material. The effectiveness of these techniques should be examined radiographically.

In some cases, teaching the patient a supraglottic swallow or voluntary airway protection may be helpful. The patient's expectoration may clear residual material from the pharynx.

Unilateral Pharyngeal Paralysis

No exercise improves pharyngeal paralysis; however, a number of compensatory techniques can be used.

The patient may be taught to *turn* his or her head toward the *affected* side, thus closing the pyriform sinus on the affected side and directing material down the more normal side (Kirchner, 1967; Logemann, Kahrilas, Kobara, & Vakil, 1989).

If the patient has a unilateral paralysis in lingual function as well as the pharynx, the patient may function better by *tilting* the head toward the *stronger* side, thus keeping material on the stronger side in the oral cavity as well as through the pharynx.

Additionally, the patient may be taught the supraglottic swallow in order to expectorate any residual material that remains in the pharynx. Or the patient may alternate liquid and solid swallows in order to wash away thicker food that remains in the pharynx after the swallow.

Scarred Pharyngeal Wall

The same techniques that improve or compensate for unilateral pharyngeal paralysis may be used for a scarred pharyngeal wall. The indentation in the area of the scarring often collects material, which will remain at the scar site after the swallow. The supraglottic swallow sequence may help to eliminate this residue.

Cervical Osteophyte

A cervical osteophyte, or boney overgrowth of one of the cervical vertebra, may be surgically reduced, or the patient may acclimate to it by thinning out the consistency of material swallowed. Foods of a thicker consistency will be more difficult. Changing head posture, particularly rotating to one side or the other, may also be helpful. (See Chapter 11 for medical management of osteophytes.)

Pseudoepiglottis at the Base of the Tongue in Total Laryngectomees

Many total laryngectomees whose surgical wound was closed with vertical closure will develop a fold of tissue coming from the side of the pharynx which, on lateral radiography, appears to be an epiglottis (Bremner et al., 1993; R. Davis, Vincent, Shapshay, & Strong, 1982). When the patient attempts to swallow, this tissue fold widens with the pull of the pharyngeal constrictors and acts as a side pocket in the pharynx. This fold of tissue can be surgically removed, or the patient can adjust to it by swallowing only liquids and thin paste consistencies. Sometimes head rotation will keep the fold out of the bolus path.

Cricopharyngeal Dysfunction

Cricopharyngeal dysfunction may result from (1) failure of the cricopharyngeal muscular portion of the cricopharyngeal or upper esophageal sphincter to relax adequately, thereby keeping the larynx from lifting and moving forward; (2) reduced laryngeal motion up and forward; and/or (3) poor pressure to drive the bolus through the sphincter and widen the opening. Before defining therapy for the disorder, the clinician must determine which of these factors is impaired in each patient. If the problem is truly spasm in the cricopharyngeal muscle strong enough to prevent the larynx from moving up and forward, then a cricopharyngeal myotomy should be considered after the patient has adequate time to recover spontaneously (5 to 6 months). If the problem is poor laryngeal motion up and forward, the Mendelsohn maneuver may be very helpful. Most patients with this swallowing disorder are capable of doing the Mendelsohn maneuver, as long as they can follow directions. Patients with this disorder include those who have suffered a cervical spinal cord injury and had cervical fusion from the anterior or posterior approach, those who have had a brainstem stroke, and those who have had radiation therapy or surgery to the pharynx affecting laryngeal elevation. The Mendelsohn maneuver is described in the earlier section on swallowing maneuvers. The maneuver may be used as a therapy procedure to improve laryngeal motion or as a strategy to enable the patient to eat (Logemann & Kahrilas, 1990; Lazarus, Logemann, & Gibbons, 1993). If pharyngeal pressure is found to be inadequate during the swallow, exercises to improve tongue base action may be appropriate. Generally, dilatation is not helpful unless there is scar tissue that is restricting laryngeal motion up and forward; this can occur after radiotherapy to the neck or after surgical procedures. In my experience, the problem has most frequently been caused by reduced laryngeal movement with a unilateral pharyngeal weakness. The combination of the Mendelsohn maneuver and head rotation to the weaker side may be most helpful.

Reduced Laryngeal Elevation

The Mendelsohn maneuver is a specific swallowing maneuver designed to improve laryngeal elevation. This technique is explained earlier in the section on swallowing maneuvers. A technique to compensate for reduced laryngeal elevation involves teaching the patient the supraglottic swallow. This technique is helpful because the patient will expectorate the residual material left above the larynx after the swallow. Thus, aspiration after the swallow is minimized. In some cases, the patient does not need to learn the entire supraglottic sequence, but instead can be taught to simply clear the throat immediately after the swallow and thus expectorate any residue. The super-supraglottic swallow may be helpful as it speeds the onset of laryngeal elevation. The falsetto exercise may also be used as a range-of-motion exercise for laryngeal elevation.

Such techniques as light pressure upward on the thyroid cartilage to assist in laryngeal elevation are of questionable impact except as an assist to the falsetto exercise.

Reduced Laryngeal Closure at the Airway Entrance

Therapy for reduced closure of the airway entrance involves the super-supraglottic swallow. The entire swallow maneuver does not need to be done. The patient can simply take a breath, hold the breath, and bear down. This is a range-of-motion exercise for the anterior tilting of the arytenoid and false vocal fold closure. The super-supraglottic swallow can also be used to allow the patient to swallow some food or liquid. However, the effort involved may be more than the patient can sustain over a full meal.

Reduced Laryngeal Closure at the Vocal Folds

Exercises to improve laryngeal adduction during swallowing have been outlined in the section on indirect procedures for working on swallowing. The supraglottic swallow, or voluntary airway closure, is often sufficient to increase closure in many patients. In this technique the patient is taught to hold his or her breath and swallow simultaneously and to release the air into a cough after the swallow. It is a useful technique because the patient may be directed by the clinician as the individual performs the procedure. The clinician can essentially "cheerlead" by giving step-by-step directions as the patient holds his or her breath and continues to hold it while swallowing. A reminder to cough immediately after the swallow is important. It is difficult for patients to remember to continue to hold their breath and to release the air into a cough rather than inhaling first. Obviously, if they inhale first, they will aspirate the material instead of clearing it from their airway. The supraglottic sequence is a technique that can be practiced using dry swallows without giving the patient any actual food or liquid to swallow. When the clinician is satisfied that the patient has mastered the sequence, food or liquid can be given. The patient with reduced laryngeal closure may do best with a thicker consistency. However, if the reduced laryngeal closure is combined with a reduction in pharyngeal contraction, thinner material will be easier because thicker consistencies will have a greater tendency to remain in the pharynx after the swallow and be aspirated at that time.

Some patients benefit from a forward, chin-down head posture during swallowing, which widens the vallecular space, narrows the airway entrance, puts the epiglottis in a more posterior position, and pushes the tongue base posteriorly. The hemilaryngectomee who has swallowing disorders because of slightly reduced airway closure may exhibit normal swallowing without aspiration with the head tilted forward. However, the patient must have an epiglottis for this procedure to be successful. Therefore, it will not work well for a supraglottic laryngectomee whose epiglottis has been included in the resection.

Turning the patient's head to the nonfunctional side or placing pressure on the thyroid cartilage on the nonfunctional side may improve laryngeal closure (Buckley et al., 1976). However, placement of downward pressure on the head or manipulation of the larynx from side to side or up and down will have little effect on laryngeal closure and may, in fact, inhibit laryngeal elevation and closure during the swallow. Best airway closure may be obtained by a combination of head rotation and chin-down postures.

Disorders Affecting the Esophageal Phase of the Swallow

Disorders affecting the esophageal phase of deglutition are normally handled with medication or surgery. They may be diagnosed in the radiographic study completed by the swallowing therapist and the radiologist, but are not normally treated by the swallowing therapist.

Other Issues in Swallowing Therapy

Combining Postures and Swallow Maneuvers

In some cases, patients require use of both a swallow maneuver and a postural technique to attain a safe and efficient swallow. For example, in patients with severe problems with airway entrance closure, head rotation to the damaged side and chin down while using a super-supraglottic swallow may result in optimal airway protection. In patients with poor tongue base motion, a combination of the chin-down posture, which pushes the tongue base posteriorly, and the effortful swallow may be needed. In patients with poor cricopharyngeal opening because of both a reduction in laryngeal elevation and a unilateral pharyngeal wall weakness, a combination of head rotation to the damaged side and the Mendelsohn maneuver may be optimal. In most instances, the effectiveness of the posture and the maneuver should be examined separately during the modified barium swallow and then the combination of the two assessed.

Biofeedback as an Assist to Swallowing Therapy

Some of the instrumental procedures described in Chapter 3 can be used to provide biofeedback to patients who are undergoing swallowing therapy.

Surface Electromyography

Surface electromyography, with the surface electrodes placed on the lips, can be used to provide biofeedback regarding amount of effort utilized in attempts at lip closure. With the surface electrodes under the chin on the submandibular muscles—that is, on the neck above the larynx on the laryngeal elevators—the patient can be provided with additional information on the degree of muscle effort used during the effortful swallow maneuver or the Mendelsohn maneuver. In the case of the Mendelsohn maneuver, the electrode above the larynx would provide information on electrical activity in the laryngeal elevators during the maneuver. The patient could look at both the amplitude and the duration of the signal, trying to increase both muscle effort (amplitude) and duration of muscle effort while doing the maneuver.

Ultrasound

Ultrasound can be used to provide biofeedback regarding tongue movement patterns during swallowing. After the patient is taught how to interpret the ultrasound image, he or she could then observe tongue motion over time while practicing the upward and backward movement of the tongue to propel the bolus through the oral cavity.

Videoendoscopy

Videoendoscopy could be used to provide biofeedback regarding closure of the true vocal folds before a swallow attempt or closure of the airway entrance before a swallow attempt. If the patient was having difficulty in attaining vocal fold or airway entrance closure, the patient could observe the movement of these structures during various breath hold maneuvers (Martin et al., 1993; Ohmae et al., 1996).

Videofluorography

Videofluorography also can be used as a biofeedback tool if the patient is allowed to observe his or her pharyngeal swallow movements during the X-ray study (Logemann & Kahrilas, 1990). Sometimes patients ask to see the X-ray study as it is ongoing in order to better understand the goal(s) of therapy. The clinician can point out the various elements of the swallow and identify those that are defective and need increased range of motion. The patient can then observe his or her swallowing videofluorographically while attempting to improve range of motion.

When To Begin Swallowing Therapy

As soon as an inpatient is medically stable and identified as dysphagic, a videofluorographic assessment of his or her swallow function should be accomplished by the swallow therapist and radiologist. From this assessment, an appropriate therapy plan should be initiated, with the patient seen daily in the hospital and weekly thereafter. For surgically treated head and neck cancer patients, assessment and treatment of swallow dysfunction should begin as soon as healing has progressed enough to allow them to try to swallow (usually 7 to 14 days postoperatively, with no healing complications). If a patient is undergoing radiation therapy and begins complaining of swallowing problems, assessment and treatment should begin at that time (Lazarus, 1993). For stroke patients, assessment should take place when they are awake and alert, usually 2 to 3 days postictus.

Outpatients who are dysphagic should receive the same careful videofluorographic assessment and therapy as inpatients. Even if patients have been dysphagic for some time, they should receive the same type of assessment and intensive therapy (Perlman, 1993; Sonies, 1993). Patients who receive therapy months or years after the onset of their problem are still capable of achieving oral intake (Lazarus, Logemann, & Gibbons, 1993; Lazarus, Logemann, Rademaker, et al., 1993; Logemann & Kahrilas, 1990). Therapy is usually provided daily for inpatients and weekly for outpatients.

In general, tracheostomy tubes and nonoral feeding tubes are left in place during swallowing assessment and therapy, as there have not been any studies that indicate that these tubes significantly deter swallowing rehabilitation. However, the cuff of the tracheostomy tube should be deflated if medically feasible during the assessment and therapy. An inflated cuff can restrict laryngeal elevation and cricopharyngeal opening during the swallow as discussed earlier. An inflated tracheostomy cuff can also cause tracheal irritation by rubbing on the tracheal walls as the larynx elevates during each swallow. Therefore, it is inappropriate to feed a patient with a tracheostomy cuff inflated. If the patient is aspirating, he or she should not be fed orally. On occasion it may be absolutely necessary to leave the cuff inflated, such as when the patient is ventilator dependent, because many ventilators require cuff inflation. If the patient is terminal, and wishes to attempt to take food orally, leaving a tracheostomy cuff inflated will have negligible effect.

Maintenance Program

As mentioned in the opening paragraph of this chapter, another critical question that the clinician needs to answer while doing therapy is whether the dysphagic patient requires a maintenance program. Maintenance programs are the applications of therapy strategies in a continuous way with patients in order to assist them in maintaining their function for a period of time. In general, maintenance programs most often involve compensatory strategies, such as postural changes or diet changes, and repeated use of particular swallow therapy techniques to maintain the mechanism's coordination for swallowing such as thermal–tactile stimulation. Typically, maintenance programs are needed in patients who are unable to monitor their own performance (i.e., those with cognitive deficits or dementia) or those whose diagnosis involves deterioration and the maintenance program is designed to maintain compensatory function as long as possible (e.g., those with amyotrophic lateral sclerosis, Parkinson's disease, or Alzheimer's disease). Some patients in the latter category are able to monitor their own performance and therefore are on a maintenance set of exercises or strategies for eating but do not need the active involvement of a speech–language pathologist or swallowing therapist for the long term. They generally need to be reevaluated at intervals of perhaps 6 months or 1 year to define needed changes in their maintenance program, but the therapist does not need to be present at meals.

Patients with cognitive and language deficits, however, generally need to be monitored when in a maintenance program. Typically, the swallowing therapist would design the maintenance program that enables the patient to eat safely and then transfer the monitoring operation to the caregiver after teaching the caregiver the appropriate strategies for use with the patient during feeding. Most third-party payers define maintenance programs as a caregiver's responsibility once they have been designed and taught to the caregiver by the swallowing therapist. This typically means that the therapist will not be reimbursed once the plan has been designed and the caregiver trained to implement it reliably. Some evidence in the literature indicates that patients with severe neurologic damage, such as those with head injury or cerebral palsy, require chronic maintenance therapy in order to maintain their gains (Helfrich-Miller et al., 1986). These patients often need chronic use of thermal–tactile stimulation to maintain the gains they achieved in therapy. This likewise means that the caregiver is providing the thermal–tactile stimulation after being taught how to do so correctly by the swallowing therapist.

Incorporating Swallowing Therapy into Eating

In general, swallowing therapy should be done at a time separate from mealtime. The swallowing therapist's first goal with a dysphagic patient should be to identify the safest way for the patient to eat and the most efficient and quickest way for the person to swallow. Typically, this means using compensatory strategies in the beginning, if compensatory strategies that eliminate aspiration on all foods or at least a selected group of foods can be identified. If such a combination of strategies or a single strategy cannot be identified, then the patient should remain nonoral and be provided swallowing therapy. If the patient can use a compensatory strategy to eat and the clinician believes that therapy is needed to improve the function so that the patient does not need to use the compensatory strategy forever, then swallowing therapy should be initiated but at a time separate from eating, or if the patient cannot use a compensatory strategy and the clinician believes swallowing therapy is appropriate, then therapy should be initiated, again at a time separate from any oral or nonoral intake. Most people consider eating to be a pleasurable activity; if a patient is required to do too much exercise and work while eating, he or she is likely to find eating unpleasant and withdraw from the task to some extent.

Swallowing therapy is not feeding. Once the patient has attained the ability to eat safely under whatever circumstances, this task of monitoring eating is turned over to a caregiver as a maintenance task, as described earlier. Occasionally, patients can swallow only when incorporating some swallow therapy procedures, particularly swallowing maneuvers such as the Mendelsohn maneuver or the supraglottic swallow. In this case, the patients may be provided with short-term therapy during mealtime to learn these procedures and to incorporate them in their eating. However, this is, in general, a small number of patients.

Group Therapy

Group therapy may be appropriate if several patients are in the facility at the same time who are working on the same therapy procedures. In this case, the patients may be brought together to reinforce each others' use of particular procedures or exercise programs. Patients often gain support from each other and learn by observation of each other. If group therapy is done, the therapy cost should be divided by the number of individuals being provided with concurrent treatment. Group therapy is not monitoring patients while they eat to assure that they use their feeding strategies. Maintenance programs can be done in groups with a caregiver, such as a nursing aide, monitoring more than one patient at the same time. Again, this maintenance task should be turned over very quickly to the caregiver. The swallowing therapist may spend a few sessions teaching the caregiver how to monitor each patient's eating but, as described earlier, after a few sessions, maintenance becomes the responsibility of a caregiver.

Cultural Differences in Dysphagia Management

The dysphagia therapist should talk with the patient, family, and significant others regarding the patient's food preferences and any issues surrounding mealtime. In most cultures, meals are social events where a great deal of communication takes place. What is the patient's role in the family structure? What have been the patient's usual communication patterns during meals? What are the patient's most and least favorite foods? Are there any cultural preferences for foods, spices, and so on? Are there any cultural preferences or aversions for certain foods when someone is ill (e.g., cold foods should be avoided when a person is ill, chicken soup is a good remedy, etc.)? Whenever possible, these issues should be identified and honored in therapy.

Mealtime Management

Mealtimes generally place the aerodigestive tract under stress because rapid switching occurs between respiration, swallowing, and talking. Mealtimes should be as pleasant as possible. Patients should be given the foods that are easiest for them to swallow and that taste best to them. Cultural preferences should be respected as much as possible. Swallowing therapy should not be conducted at mealtime unless absolutely necessary. In general, once a safe strategy or set of strategies for oral intake have been identified, the patient should use these with or without caregiver supervision as appropriate.

The swallowing therapist's role is to identify the safe swallowing strategies, including optimal diet; to teach these to the caregiver; to monitor the caregiver's performance as needed; and to provide therapy to improve or compensate for the patient's abnormal neuromuscular control for swallowing at a time different from mealtime. The therapist also should (1) warn the family or significant others not to encourage talking immediately after the patient takes a bite of food or immediately after swallowing as this increases the risk of aspiration, and (2) encourage them to include the dysphagic patient at mealtime by providing the kinds of foods the patient can swallow easily, even if it is only one food or food viscosity. The importance of socialization at meals should not be underestimated.

Medications To Improve Swallowing Disorders

Few studies have been done of the therapeutic benefits of medications on oropharyngeal swallowing disorders. The use of atropine to reduce drooling (Dworkin & Nadal, 1991) has been documented; however, no other medications to improve specific oropharyngeal swallowing disorders have been identified.

Patients with progressive neurologic disease (e.g., Parkinson's disease, multiple sclerosis, and myasthenia gravis) sometimes experience improvement in oropharyngeal swallowing when placed on medications for their disease process. Unfortunately, detailed studies of the effects of specific medications on the oropharyngeal function of these patients have not been completed.

Surgical Interventions

Generally surgical interventions to improve oropharyngeal swallowing should not be attempted until swallowing therapy has had at least a 6-month trial. The oropharyngeal swallow mechanism is a sensitive one in which any surgical intervention may create more damage through scar tissue than benefit accrued. Any surgical intervention should be carefully planned based on the patient's oropharyngeal anatomy and swallow physiology and be as noninvasive as possible. Surgical management strategies are described further in Chapter 11.

Issues in the Management of Dysphagia in Various Settings

The setting in which dysphagia management is given can present particular challenges to the swallowing therapist. Various issues should be kept in mind in each setting.

Acute Care Hospitals

With the decreasing length of stay for dysphagic patients of almost any etiology in the acute care hospital, the pressure is on the speech–language pathologist or swallowing therapist to identify dysphagic patients, define their swallow physiology, and outline a treatment plan as quickly as possible. Before the patient is discharged, the swallowing therapist should complete the necessary assessments and have a clear idea of the patient's swallow symptomatology and anatomic or physiologic disorders. There may be time to begin management to return the patient to oral intake or to maintain oral intake, or there may be only enough time to develop a thorough assessment and therapy plan that should be passed along to the swallowing therapist in the rehabilitation facility or nursing home. It is critical, however, that when the patient leaves acute care, the swallowing therapist has completed the physiologic and anatomic assessment of the patient's swallowing disorders and identified those treatment strategies most likely to be successful. If at all possible, the patient's management or therapy for swallowing disorders should begin in acute care. The communication between the swallowing therapist in the acute care facility and the swallowing therapist in the next facility where the patient will receive care is most important to a successful outcome of the patient's dysphagia.

Schools

Speech–language pathologists or swallowing therapists in the schools are under the same limitations as those in nursing facilities and home care; that is, they do not have regular on-site access to diagnostic procedures to define the exact nature of a child's swallowing disorder. Therefore, it is essential that the swallowing therapist complete a thorough screening and clinical assessment. Indirect therapy—that is, treatment without food—can be initiated until a physiologic or diagnostic study can be obtained. If the child shows any of the symptoms of significant pharyngeal dysphagia or aspiration resulting from oropharyngeal dysphagia, a radiographic study is necessary for adequate diagnosis and management. Liability in this situation is a significant factor. Clinicians always seek the highest level of safety for the children and themselves. If there is any question about a child's aspirating during feeding experiences in school, it is suggested that the caregivers in the school refrain from further oral feeding of the child until the diagnostic studies are completed. If parents insist that the child be fed, it is suggested that the school offer the parents the opportunity to come and feed the child themselves, thereby accepting their own liability for any medical complications resulting from eating.

Nursing Home Settings

Dysphagic patients in the nursing home setting may offer great challenges to the swallowing therapist, both because of some restrictions in the types of assessment procedures readily available and because of the nature of the populations served. The swallowing therapist in the nursing home often finds it a challenge to obtain the necessary radiographic studies for evaluation. With the advent of mobile videofluoroscopic units, the availability of radiographic studies within the nursing home is increasing significantly. Swallowing therapy for suspected pharyngeal disorders without a radiographic diagnostic study or other physiologic diagnostic procedure that enables assessment of interventions will not allow the clinician to focus therapy efforts appropriately and may potentially waste time and money.

Unfortunately, the use of videoendoscopy does not provide the same physiologic information as videofluoroscopy and often serves only as a screening procedure to identify patients who aspirate. Screening information (i.e., symptoms) does not enable the clinician to develop a workable and effective treatment plan for the patient's swallowing dysfunction. Also, should the patient have an adverse reaction either to the anesthetic used in the nose or to the stimulation of the pharynx with the endoscopic tube, use of endoscopic procedures without a physician available may be risky for the patient and the clinician (Kidder, Langmore, & Martin, 1994).

In addition to the issue of achieving an appropriate physiologic assessment of the patient's oropharyngeal swallowing function in the nursing home setting, it is important for the clinician to keep the general philosophy of rehabilitation and therapy in mind in selecting patients for treatment: The patient should have reasonable chance of improving function with whatever type of therapy is provided. In the case of dysphagia, the clinician should feel that the management provided to the patient will, in fact, improve his or her functional abilities to eat orally while keeping the patient medically healthy. Feeding a patient without understanding his or her swallow physiology can cause aspiration and is not facilitating the patient's health, but rather is increasing risk of illness. Therefore, the swallowing therapist must be sure to have the most accurate physiologic evaluation of swallowing possible before feeding a dysphagic patient in therapy or before recommending oral feeding for nutrition and hydration.

It is critical to incorporate assessment of feeding into the patient's bedside assessment, if appropriate and low risk, and to incorporate observation of the patient's oral intake at one or two meals to define any behavioral characteristics that interfere with eating a meal. The act of eating combines behavioral controls with the physiology of swallowing. Damage of any significance to either behavior control, cognition, or swallow physiology can make getting adequate oral intake significantly more difficult. In the case of patients with dementia, the clinician should be sure to observe the patients' reactions to their surroundings, including the specific other residents with whom they appear to have a good relationship and whose behavior they may mimic; the kinds of foods they tend to enjoy the most; their reactions to auditory and visual distractions; and their general ability to manipulate eating utensils and to self-feed. If the patient is being fed by a caregiver rather than self-feeding, the clinician should observe the way in which food is placed in front of the patient, the positioning of food in the patient's mouth, the patient's reaction to the foods being presented, the length of time it takes to place one serving of food into the patient's mouth, and the time it takes from oral placement of the food until the food is swallowed, as determined by movement of the larynx in the neck. The patient's general neuromuscular fatigue level, attention span, general attentiveness to the feeding situation, awareness of food as it is placed in the mouth, and typical oral manipulative abilities with the foods should all be examined.

The swallowing therapist's interactions with feeding staff in the nursing facility are also important. Feeding staff should follow the directions of the swallowing therapist in terms of the type of foods to be fed to the patient, the timing and length of feedings, the way in which food is placed in the mouth, and the observations to be made with each patient prior to placing another food serving into the patient's mouth. The feeder should focus on the patient and not on the television set or other auditory or visual distractions. The feeding staff should also concentrate on the patient's behavior and reaction to the placement of food in the mouth. Any changes in the patient's respiratory rate, voice quality, or general alertness throughout a meal should be noted. The feeding staff should report immediately to the swallowing therapist any changes in the patient's function during a meal and discontinue feeding until the swallowing therapist has assessed the situation. The feeding staff should also be aware of the patient's general posture and be sure that the patient is in his or her optimal feeding posture before oral feeding begins. The feeding staff should also examine the food tray to be sure that inappropriate foods are not included and that the placement of food on the tray is appropriate for the patient's visual field. The feeding staff should provide additional tactile and/or olfactory stimulation if necessary prior to starting or during feeding. The swallowing therapist should supervise the feeding staff and provide them with any cues to change their behavior in feeding various patients.

If the speech–language pathologist is having difficulty obtaining adequate physiologic assessments of his or her dysphagic patients in a nursing facility, the clinician should work with the administration of the nursing facility to require radiographic or other physiologic studies of swallowing prior to admission to the nursing home of any patients with nonoral feeding in place or a history of dysphagia. This policy will save money for the health care system by eliminating the need to transport the patient to an acute care hospital to get the radiographic study after the patient has been admitted to the nursing facility. Although the availability of mobile videofluoroscopic units has eased the difficulty in obtaining this kind of study in the nursing home population, not every nursing home resident is appropriate for a radiographic study. Some patients are simply too advanced in their dementia or other medical diagnosis to be able to obtain benefit from any swallowing therapy. The clinician should determine whether the patient has potential to improve swallowing ability through compensatory techniques and ability to manipulate posture and other feeding variables before referring the patient for radiographic study. If there is no potential for use of any strategies and the family has said that they will not approve use of any nonoral feeding, even if the patient is aspirating, it is recommended that the swallowing therapist not proceed with intervention as no improvement can be anticipated.

In-service education of staff regarding swallowing and feeding is critical in the skilled nursing facility. Staff members need to understand that swallowing is a complex neuromuscular activity and that watching someone eat does not constitute an adequate swallowing assessment. They also need to be taught that simply feeding a resident with swallowing problems will not necessarily be helpful or supportive and that feeding can endanger the patient. The need to be nurturing to patients can often mislead other health care professionals into thinking that any feeding, whether safe or not, is helpful to the patient. The swallowing therapist needs to maintain a continual educational program regarding swallowing management for the staff.

Once the swallowing therapist has defined the nature of the patient's anatomic or physiologic swallowing problems and defined the optimal way for the patient to eat, this must be taught to the feeding staff and left to them to implement. Implementation of the feeding program is a maintenance function after caregivers have been trained to feed each patient appropriately and is not reimbursable as a professional service. In general, swallowing therapy should not be incorporated into mealtime but should be conducted at a separate time unless the patient is being taught to use certain strategies during mealtime swallowing.

Home

As in the nursing facility, the patient who is receiving home care presents a number of challenges to the swallowing therapist. Because the availability of physiologic studies of swallow, such as radiographic evaluations, becomes more difficult in the home, if the patient has a nonoral feeding in place, the home health agency should request that the patient receive the needed physiologic studies of swallowing prior to being discharged from the acute care hospital, acute rehabilitation facility, or nursing facility. In this way, the studies can be provided in a more cost-effective way. As in other care locations, the swallowing therapist must understand the patient's swallowing anatomy and physiology in order to provide appropriate, efficient, and cost-effective treatment.

In home care, the family can be engaged in providing the appropriate feeding after training by the swallowing therapist and can, in fact, continue home practice with the patient between the swallowing therapist's visits. In a randomized study of follow-up in dysphagic patients who had suffered strokes, DePippo, Holas, Reding, Mandel, and Lesser (1994) found that family reinforcement can be as effective as reinforcement by any other caregiver or professional. In this study, all patients first received the professional swallowing therapist's intervention through the radiographic study, during which the optimal posture and diet for each patient were identified. Then, patients were randomized to one of three follow-up strategies: (1) the swallowing therapist provided reminders during meals to follow the designated diet and posture, (2) the family member provided that type of monitoring and reminder, or (3) the patient provided self-monitoring. Outcome measures after 6 months were rate of pneumonia, rate of death, and several other physiologic measures. Not surprisingly, the three groups had no significant differences in the outcome measures. This is not surprising because all patients received the same professional intervention, that is, the X-ray study that identified the optimal posture and diet for each patient. The follow-up was simply a nonprofessional task of reminding the patient to follow the instructions.

This study indicates that caregivers are capable of following and observing the patient's behavior and assuring good compliance with professional recommendations. In home care, it is critical that the swallowing therapist provide the patient and family with the tools needed to practice exercises correctly. For example, if the patient is to receive thermal–tactile stimulation, the swallowing therapist should provide the caregiver with a size 00 laryngeal mirror with which to provide the therapy. As in other settings, if the patient requires a repeat videofluoroscopy to assure that his or her progress is adequate to return to oral intake, this can be scheduled on an outpatient basis at most acute care hospitals or through a mobile videofluoroscopic unit.

Summary

Research has shown that swallowing rehabilitation, including compensatory procedures and direct and indirect therapy, can be successful in returning over 80% of oropharyngeal dysphagic patients to oral intake (Rademaker et al., 1993). It can eliminate aspiration and reduce the risk of pneumonia and other pulmonary complications, as well as improve nutritional status (Rademaker et al., 1993; Silverman & Elfant, 1979; Strandberg, 1982). Usually, the swallowing therapist is a speech–language pathologist. In some instances, another professional plays this role. The swallowing therapist participates actively in the radiographic assessment and other diagnostic procedures, as well as in designing and implementing the swallowing rehabilitation program in cooperation with the patient's attending physician, other health care professionals, the patient, and his or her family or other caregivers.

References

Aguilar, N., Olson, M., & Shedd, D. (1979). Rehabilitation of deglutition problems in patients with head and neck cancer. *American Journal of Surgery, 138*, 501–507.

American Dietetic Association. (1980). *Study guide: Dysphagia—The dietitian's role in patient care* [Audiocassette series]. Chicago: Author.

Bartolome, G., & Neumann, S. (1993). Swallowing therapy in patients with neurological disorders causing cricopharyngeal dysfunction. *Dysphagia, 8*, 146–149.

Bremner, R. M., Hoeft, S. F., Costantini, M., Crookes, P. F., Bremner, C. G., & DeMeester, T. R. (1993). Pharyngeal swallowing: The major factor in clearance of esophageal reflux episodes. *Annals of Surgery, 218*, 364–370.

Bryant, M. (1991). Biofeedback in the treatment of a selected dysphagic patient. *Dysphagia, 6*, 140–144.

Buckley, J., Addicks, C., & Maniglia, J. (1976). Feeding patients with dysphagia. *Nursing Forum, 15*, 69–85.

Cook, I. J., Dodds, W. J., Dantas, R. O., Massey, B., Kern, M. K., Lang, I. M., Brasseur, J. G., & Hogan, W. J. (1989). Opening mechanisms of the human upper esophageal sphincter. *American Journal of Physiology, 257*, G748–G759.

Davis, J. W., Lazarus, C., Logemann, J. A., & Hurst, P. (1987). Effect of a maxillary glossectomy prosthesis on articulation and swallowing. *Journal of Prosthetic Dentistry, 57*(6), 715–719.

Davis, R., Vincent, M., Shapshay, S., & Strong, M. (1982). The anatomy and complications of "T" versus vertical closure of the hypopharynx after laryngectomy. *Laryngoscope, 92*, 16–22.

DePippo, K. L., Holas, M. A., Reding, M. J., Mandel, F. S., & Lesser, M. L. (1994). Dysphagia therapy following stroke: A controlled trial. *Neurology, 64*, 1665–1669.

Dobie, R. (1978). Rehabilitation of swallowing disorders. *American Family Physician, 17*, 84–95.

Drake, W., O'Donoghue, S., Bartram, C., Lindsay, J., & Greenwood, R. (1997). Eating in side-lying facilitates rehabilitation in neurogenic dysphagia. *Brain Injury, 11*, 137–142.

Dworkin, J. P., & Nadal, J. C. (1991). Nonsurgical treatment of drooling in a patient with closed head injury and severe dysarthria. *Dysphagia, 6,* 40–49.

Ford, M., Grotz, R., Pomerantz, P., Bruno, R., & Flannery, E. (1974). Dysphagia therapy. *Archives of Physical Medicine and Rehabilitation, 55,* 571.

Fujiu, M., & Logemann, J. A. (1996). Effect of a tongue holding maneuver on posterior pharyngeal wall movement during deglutition. *American Journal of Speech-Language Pathology, 5,* 23–30.

Fujiu, M., Logemann, J. A., & Pauloski, B. R. (1995). Increased postoperative posterior pharyngeal wall movement in patients with anterior oral cancer: Preliminary findings and possible implications for treatment. *American Journal of Speech-Language Pathology, 4,* 24–30.

Fujiu, M., Toleikis, J. R., Logemann, J. A., & Larson, C. R. (1994). Glossopharyngeal evoked potentials in normal subjects following mechanical stimulation of the anterior faucial pillar. *Electroencephalography and Clinical Neurophysiology, 92,* 183–195.

Gaffney, T., & Campbell, R. (1974). Feeding techniques for dysphagic patients. *American Journal of Nursing, 74,* 2194–2195.

Griffin, K. (1974). Swallowing training for dysphagic patients. *Archives of Physical Medicine and Rehabilitation, 55,* 467–470.

Heimlich, H., & O'Connor, T. (1979a). Patients relearn swallowing process. *Journal of the American Medical Association, 241,* 2355–2360.

Heimlich, H., & O'Connor, T. (1979b). Relearning the swallowing process. *Annals of Otology, Rhinology and Laryngology, 88,* 794–797.

Helfrich-Miller, K. R., Rector, K. L., & Straka, J. A. (1986). Dysphagia: Its treatment in the profoundly retarded patient with cerebral palsy. *Archives of Physical Medicine and Rehabilitation, 67,* 520–525.

Horner, J., Massey, E. W., Riski, J. E., Lathrop, D., & Chase, K. N. (1988). Aspiration following stroke: Clinical correlates and outcomes. *Neurology, 38,* 1359–1362.

Jacob, P., Kahrilas, P. J., Logemann, J. A., Shah, V., & Ha, T. (1989). Upper esophageal sphincter opening and modulation during swallowing. *Gastroenterology, 97,* 1469–1478.

Jordan, K. (1979). Rehabilitation of the patients with dysphagia. *Ear, Nose and Throat Journal, 58,* 86–87.

Kahrilas, P. J., Lin, S., Logemann, J. A., Ergun, G. A., & Facchini, F. (1993). Deglutitive tongue action: Volume accommodation and bolus propulsion. *Gastroenterology, 104,* 152–162.

Kahrilas, P. J., Logemann, J. A., Krugler, C., & Flanagan, E. (1991). Volitional augmentation of upper esophageal sphincter opening during swallowing. *American Journal of Physiology, 260,* G450–G456.

Kahrilas, P. J., Logemann, J. A., Lin, S., & Ergun, G. A. (1992). Pharyngeal clearance during swallow: A combined manometric and videofluoroscopic study. *Gastroenterology, 103,* 128–136.

Kasprisin, A. T., Clumeck, A., & Nino-Murcia, M. (1989). The efficacy of rehabilitative management of dysphagia. *Dysphagia, 4,* 48–52.

Kidder, T. M., Langmore, S. E., & Martin, B. J. W. (1994). Indications and techniques of endoscopy in evaluation of cervical dysphagia: Comparison with radiographic techniques. *Dysphagia, 9,* 256–261.

Kirchner, J. (1967). Pharyngeal and esophageal dysfunction: The diagnosis. *Minnesota Medicine, 50,* 921–924.

Larnert, G., & Ekberg, O. (1995). Positioning improves the oral and pharyngeal swallowing function in children with cerebral palsy. *Acta Pædiatrica, 84,* 689–692.

Larsen, G. (1972). Rehabilitation for dysphagia paralytica. *Journal of Speech and Hearing Disorders*, *37*, 187–193.

Larsen, G. (1973). Conservative management for incomplete dysphagia paralytica. *Archives of Physical Medicine and Rehabilitation*, *54*, 180–185.

Lazarus, C. L. (1993). Effects of radiation therapy and voluntary maneuvers on swallow functioning in head and neck cancer patients. *Clinics in Communication Disorders*, *3*, 11–20.

Lazarus, C., Logemann, J. A., & Gibbons, P. (1993). Effects of maneuvers on swallowing function in a dysphagic oral cancer patient. *Head & Neck*, *15*, 419–424.

Lazarus, C. L., Logemann, J. A., Rademaker, A. W., Kahrilas, P. J., Pajak, T., Lazar, R., & Halper, A. (1993). Effects of bolus volume, viscosity and repeated swallows in nonstroke subjects and stroke patients. *Archives of Physical Medicine and Rehabilitation*, *74*, 1066–1070.

Lazzara, G., Lazarus, C., & Logemann, J. A. (1986). Impact of thermal stimulation on the triggering of the swallowing reflex. *Dysphagia*, *1*, 73–77.

Leonard, R., & Gillis, R. (1982). Effects of a prosthetic tongue on vowel intelligibility and food management in a patient with total glossectomy. *Journal of Speech and Hearing Disorders*, *47*, 25–30.

Logemann, J. A. (1983). *Evaluation and treatment of swallowing disorders*. Austin, TX: PRO-ED.

Logemann, J. A. (Ed.). (1989). Swallowing disorders and rehabilitation. *Journal Head Trauma Rehabilitation*, *4*.

Logemann, J. A. (1993a). The dysphagia diagnostic procedure as a treatment efficacy trial. *Clinics in Communication Disorders*, *3*(4), 1–10.

Logemann, J. A. (1993b). *Manual for the videofluoroscopic study of swallowing* (2nd ed.). Austin, TX: PRO-ED.

Logemann, J. A., Gibbons, P., Rademaker, A. W., Pauloski, B. R., Kahrilas, P. J., Bacon, M., Bowman, J., & McCracken, E. (1994). Mechanisms of recovery of swallow after supraglottic laryngectomy. *Journal of Speech and Hearing Research*, *37*, 965–974.

Logemann, J. A., & Kahrilas, P. J. (1990). Relearning to swallow post CVA: Application of maneuvers and indirect biofeedback: A case study. *Neurology*, *40*, 1136–1138.

Logemann, J. A., Kahrilas, P. J., Cheng, J., Pauloski, B. R., Gibbons, P. J., Rademaker, A. W., & Lin, S. (1992). Closure mechanisms of the laryngeal vestibule during swallowing. *American Journal of Physiology*, *262*, G338–G344.

Logemann, J. A., Kahrilas, P., Hurst, P., Davis, J., & Krugler, C. (1989). Effects of intraoral prosthetics on swallowing in oral cancer patients. *Dysphagia*, *4*, 118–120.

Logemann, J., Kahrilas, P., Kobara, M., & Vakil, N. (1989). The benefit of head rotation on pharyngoesophageal dysphagia. *Archives of Physical and Medical Rehabilitation*, *70*, 767–771.

Logemann, J. A., Pauloski, B. R., Colangelo, L., Lazarus, C., Fujiu, M., & Kahrilas, P. J. (1995). The effects of a sour bolus on oropharyngeal swallowing measures in patients with neurogenic dysphagia. *Journal of Speech and Hearing Research*, *38*, 556–563.

Logemann, J. A., Pauloski, B. R., Rademaker, A. W., & Colangelo, L. (1997). Speech and swallowing rehabilitation in head and neck cancer patients. *Oncology*, *11*(5), 651–659.

Logemann, J. A., Pauloski, B. R., Rademaker, A. W., & Colangelo, L. (in press). Super-supraglottic swallow in irradiated head and neck cancer patients. *Head & Neck*.

Logemann, J. A., Rademaker, A. W., Pauloski, B. R., & Kahrilas, P. J. (1994). Effects of postural change on aspiration in head and neck surgical patients. *Otolaryngology—Head and Neck Surgery*, *110*, 222–227.

Logemann, J., Sisson, G., & Wheeler, R. (1980). The team approach to rehabilitation of surgically treated oral cancer patients. *Proceedings of the National Forum on Comprehensive Cancer Rehabilitation and its Vocational Implications* (pp. 222–227).

Martin, B. J. W., Logemann, J. A., Shaker, R., & Dodds, W. J. (1993). Normal laryngeal valving patterns during three breath-hold maneuvers: A pilot investigation. *Dysphagia, 8*, 11–20.

McCulloch, T. M., Perlman, A. L., Palmer, P. M., & Van Daele, D. J. (1996). Laryngeal activity during swallow, phonation, and the Valsalva maneuver: An electromyographic analysis. *Laryngoscope, 106*, 1351–1358.

Mitchell, P. (1967). Buccinator apparatus to improve swallowing. *Physical Therapy, 47*, 1135.

Neumann, S. (1993). Swallowing therapy with neurologic patients: Results of direct and indirect therapy methods in 66 patients suffering from neurological disorders. *Dysphagia, 8*, 150–153.

Newman, L., Dodaro, R., & Welch, M. (1980, May). *A comprehensive program for dysphagia rehabilitation.* Workshop conducted at Mercy Hospital and Medical Center, Chicago.

Ohmae, Y., Logemann, J. A., Kaiser, P., Hanson, D. G., & Kahrilas, P. J. (1996). Effects of two breath-holding maneuvers on oropharyngeal swallow. *Annals of Otology, Rhinology and Laryngology, 105*, 123–131.

Perlman, A. L. (1993). Successful treatment of challenging cases. *Clinics in Communication Disorders, 3*(4), 37–44.

Perlman, A. L., Luschei, E. S., & DuMond, C. E. (1989). Electrical activity from the superior pharyngeal constrictor during reflexive and nonreflexive tasks. *Journal of Speech and Hearing Research, 32*, 749–754.

Pouderoux, P., & Kahrilas, P. J. (1995). Deglutitive tongue force modulation by volition, volume, and viscosity in humans. *Gastroenterology, 108*, 1418–1426.

Pouderoux, P., Logemann, J. A., & Kahrilas, P. J. (1996). Pharyngeal swallowing elicited by fluid infusion: Role of volition and vallecular containment. *American Journal of Physiology, 270*, G347–G354.

Rademaker, A. W., Logemann, J. A., Pauloski, B. R., Bowman, J., Lazarus, C., Sisson, G., Milianti, F., Graner, D., Cook, B., Collins, S., Stein, D., Beery, Q., Johnson, J., & Baker, T. (1993). Recovery of postoperative swallowing in patients undergoing partial laryngectomy. *Head & Neck, 15*, 325–334.

Rasley, A., Logemann, J. A., Kahrilas, P. J., Rademaker, A. W., Pauloski, B. R., & Dodds, W. J. (1993). Prevention of barium aspiration during videofluoroscopic swallowing studies: Value of change in posture. *American Journal of Roentgenology, 160*, 1005–1009.

Robbins, J. A., & Levine, R. (1993). Swallowing after lateral medullary syndrome plus. *Clinics in Communication Disorders, 3*(4), 37–44.

Rosenbek, J. C., Roecker, E. B., Wood, M. L., & Robbins, J. A. (1996). Thermal application reduces the duration of stage transition in dysphagia after stroke. *Dysphagia, 11*, 225–233.

Shanahan, T. K., Logemann, J. A., Rademaker, A. W., Pauloski, B. R., & Kahrilas, P. J. (1993). Chin down posture effects on aspiration in dysphagic patients. *Archives of Physical Medicine and Rehabilitation, 74*, 736–739.

Silverman, E., & Elfant, L. (1979). Dysphagia: An evaluation and treatment program for the adult. *The American Journal of Occupational Therapy, 33*, 382–392.

Sonies, B. C. (1993). Remediation challenges in treating dysphagia post head/neck cancer— A problem oriented approach. *Clinics in Communication Disorders, 3*(4), 21–26.

Strandberg, T., (1982, January). *Establishment of a swallowing rehabilitation program.* Lecture presented at workshop on swallowing rehabilitation, Sarah Bush Lincoln Health Center, Mattoon, IL.

Tippett, D. C., Palmer, J., & Linden, P. (1987). Management of dysphagia in a patient with closed head injury: A case report. *Dysphagia, 1,* 221–226.

Trible, W. (1967). The rehabilitation of deglutition following head and neck surgery. *Laryngoscope, 77,* 518–523.

Welch, M. V., Logemann, J. A., Rademaker, A. W., & Kahrilas, P. J. (1993). Changes in pharyngeal dimensions effected by chin tuck. *Archives of Physical Medicine and Rehabilitation, 74,* 178–181.

Wheeler, R., Logemann, J., & Rosen, M. (1980). Maxillary reshaping prostheses: Effectiveness in improving speech and swallowing of post-surgical oral cancer patients. *Journal of Prosthetic Dentistry, 43,* 313–319.

Ylvisaker, M., & Logemann, J. A. (1986). Therapy for feeding and swallowing following head injury. In M. Ylvisaker (Ed.), *Management of head injured patients.* San Diego: College-Hill.

SWALLOWING DISORDERS
AFTER TREATMENT FOR ORAL
AND OROPHARYNGEAL CANCER

Malignant tumors of the oral cavity can be managed by one of two primary treatment modalities, surgical resection or radiotherapy with or without chemotherapy, in addition to a combination of the two treatment procedures with adjuvant chemotherapy (U.S. Department of Health, Education, and Welfare, 1979). Each type of treatment may affect deglutition. Selection of the treatment modality or combination generally depends on the exact site and extent of the tumor. Smaller tumors are frequently treated with radiotherapy alone or surgery alone. Radiation therapy in the oral cavity may be by implant into the gross tumor, external beam methods, or both. Chemotherapy may be given in a variety of protocols, concurrent with and/or following radiotherapy.

Larger tumors positioned more posteriorly in the oral cavity may be treated with combined modalities—that is, surgical resection and radiotherapy or by radiotherapy plus or minus chemotherapy in what are known as organ preservation protocols. These protocols are designed in an attempt to reduce morbidity (i.e., the functional impact of the tumor treatment) by preserving the patient's oropharyngeal structures and, hopefully, their function.

At this time, chemotherapy for head and neck cancer patients is an adjuvant experimental treatment designed to attempt to control regional and metastatic disease, rather than a primary treatment designed to eradicate the tumor itself. Although many patients have tumor shrinkage during or immediately after a course of chemotherapy, this is often of short duration. In the case of larger tumors, when both surgery and radiation are used, radiation therapy is considered the adjuvant treatment, designed to control disease within the region of the tumor, whereas surgery is the treatment designed to eradicate the tumor itself. When surgery is used to control tumors in the *oral cavity*, the general rule is that the malignant tumor must be resected along with a margin of at least 1.5 to 2 cm of normal tissue. Therefore, it is easy to see why very small lesions result in large ablative surgeries. Often these surgeries require removal of more than one structure or parts of more than one structure, such as the mandible, floor of the mouth, and tongue. When only one structure is resected, the surgery is known as a simple resection. When more than one structure or parts of more than one structure are included in the resection, it is known as a composite resection. Usually a composite resection in the oral cavity includes some part of the floor of the mouth and perhaps the mandible. There is one major rule of cancer surgery: No ablative surgical procedure should be compromised because of the desire to maintain the patient's function. Rehabilitation and reconstruction cannot be considered until the cancer is removed with normal margins.

Once the tumor and the required margin of normal tissue have been resected, the surgeon can attend to the problem of reconstruction to maximize functional capacity. In some cases, where sufficient tissue remains or where tissue can be borrowed from another site, options are available to the surgeon in the way the defect can be reconstructed. These options, as discussed later in this chapter, often determine how the patient functions for speech and swallowing after surgery. In other cases, when the resection has been very large and little tissue remains to reconstruct the surgical defect, the surgeon has fewer choices in the way the patient's oral cavity defect can be reconstructed.

Currently, when radiotherapy is scheduled as an adjunct to surgery, it is usually given postoperatively. This is because radiotherapy tends to devascularize tissue and make healing after surgery more difficult. The full course lasts for 5 to 6 weeks to a dose of 6,000 to 7,000 cGy. The exposed field usually includes all of the regional lymph nodes. When postoperative radiotherapy is used, the patient is operated and the surgical wound is allowed to heal. Radiotherapy is then initiated approximately 4 to 6 weeks after surgery, assuming that there are no problems with healing. This is considered the optimal time to initiate radiotherapy, because malignant cells that may have been released during surgery will be at their weakest.

Pretreatment Dental Assessment

When the radiotherapy field includes the oral cavity, careful dental evaluations should be performed prior to initiating radiotherapy treatments. Radiotherapy can have devastating effects on salivary flow, causing an increase in the rate of dental disease (caries). If patients enter radiotherapy with poor oral hygiene and rampant dental disease, the caries can rapidly worsen after radiotherapy because of reduced salivary flow. In addition, any teeth that are infected should be removed prior to radiotherapy, as any extractions after a full course of radiotherapy can put the patient at risk for osteoradionecrosis of the mandible. This is a condition in which portions of the mandible become infected and gradually break from the main body of the mandible to extrude or protrude through the soft tissue, necessitating removal of the infected portions. This is an extremely difficult condition to manage once it has begun and should be avoided at all costs by preventive dental evaluation before radiotherapy.

Tumor Staging

Tumors in the oral cavity are staged according to size and location (American Joint Committee on Cancer, 1992). Tumor staging is generally conducted by the attending physician and permits comparisons of the results of various treatments across patients with the same tumor. The staging procedure creates a standard for comparison of tumor reaction to treatment. Staging for the oral cavity is divided into eight sites, each staged according to the tumor size (T), nodal status (N), and presence or absence of metastasis (M), otherwise called the TNM system. The tumor size is assigned a number from 1 to 4, with T1 being the smallest and T4 the largest lesion. Metastasis to the nodes in the head and neck is noted by recording an N followed by a number representing the number of nodes thought to be involved with the tumor. The location of nodes in the head and neck region is shown in Figure 7.1. The M in the TNM staging refers to the

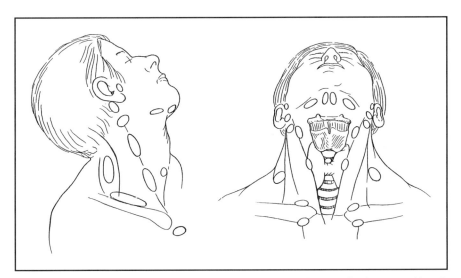

Figure 7.1. Frontal and lateral views of the head and neck showing the location of lymph nodes in the head and neck.

Table 7.1
Stage Group for All Head and Neck Sites (Except Salivary Glands
and Thyroid Gland) According to the International Union Against Cancer
and the American Joint Committee on Cancer

Stage	TNM System
I	T1 N0 M0
II	T2 N0 M0
III	T3 N0 M0
	T1 or T2 or T3 N1 M0
IV	T4 N0 or N1 M0
	any T N2 or N3 M0
	any T any N M1

Note. T = tumor size; N = number of nodes thought to be involved in the tumor; M = number of distant metastases. From "Evaluation and Staging of the Patient with Head and Neck Cancer," by G. Snow, 1989, in E. N. Meyer and J. Y. Suen (Eds.), Cancer of the Head and Neck (2nd ed., p. 33). New York: Churchill Livingston.

presence of metastasis or seeding of the tumor outside of the region. The M is also followed by a number, indicating the number of distant metastases. An M1 would indicate that the patient had one metastasis in an area other than the head and neck, often in the lung or brain. In summary, then, each tumor is staged prior to treatment using the TNM system, with each initial followed by a number and the stage assigned accordingly, as shown in Table 7.1. In general, the larger the tumor, the more aggressive the treatment, with T3 and T4 lesions more frequently treated by combined therapies (Givens, Johns, & Cantrell, 1981). At this time, combined treatment usually includes surgery followed by radiotherapy, with chemotherapy also provided, sometimes preoperatively and continuing for some time postoperatively. The nature and schedule of radiation and chemotherapy depends on the particular protocol (study).

Typical Tumor Locations and Resections in the Oral Cavity

Tumors in the oral cavity most frequently occur in the six locations shown in Figure 7.2: the anterior floor of the mouth or the lower alveolar ridge in the anterior floor of the mouth, the tongue (either anteriorly or laterally), the lateral floor of the mouth or lateral alveolar ridge, the tonsil (between the pillars of

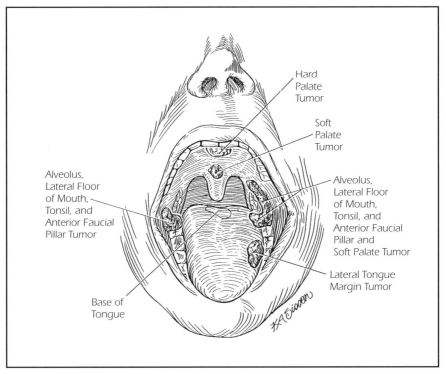

Figure 7.2. Frontal view of the oral cavity showing six typical locations of tumors in the oral cavity and oropharynx.

fauces), the base of the tongue area, the hard palate, and the soft palate. A small tumor located on the anterior floor of the mouth under the tongue, as shown in Figure 7.3, or on the alveolar ridge in the anterior floor of the mouth can frequently be treated by a small resection including only tissues of the floor of the mouth or the rim of the mandible, as shown in Figure 7.4 (Som & Nussbaum, 1971). Larger tumors in this region often require a composite resection; removal of parts of more than one structure, including the floor of the mouth, a portion of the mandible, and often a portion of the tongue; and a radical neck dissection on the side of the tumor (Kremen, 1951), as shown in Figure 7.5. This tissue is removed *en bloc* so that tissues that may contain cancerous cells are taken in continuity, and the cancer is not spread by the surgical procedure itself. Resection of the anterior floor of the mouth and a full section of the anterior mandible frequently results in an "Andy Gump" appearance (i.e., with the mandible smaller and retracted in relation to the maxilla).

Small tumors on the lateral margin or anterior portion of the tongue, as shown in Figure 7.6, often can be removed by resecting only tongue tissue. Larger

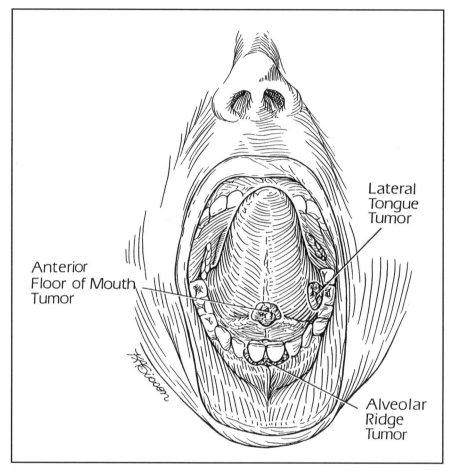

Lateral
Tongue
Tumor

Anterior
Floor of Mouth
Tumor

Alveolar
Ridge
Tumor

Figure 7.3. Frontal view of the oral cavity with the tongue elevated so that a tumor of the anterior floor of the mouth is clearly visible as are tumors on the anterior alveolar ridge and lateral tongue.

tumors of the tongue may also be treated with a simple resection of part or all of the tongue (total glossectomy). If the tumors are close to or involve adjacent tissues, such as the alveolar ridge of the mandible or the floor of the mouth, a composite resection may be necessary, including not only the tongue but also the alveolar ridge or a larger portion of the mandible and the floor of the mouth. Often, a radical neck dissection is also included in the resection on the side of the tumor. A radical neck dissection removes the submandibular lymph nodes, the lymph nodes in the neck, and the sternocleidomastoid and omohyoid muscles. The spinal accessory nerve (C11) often must be sacrificed. A modified

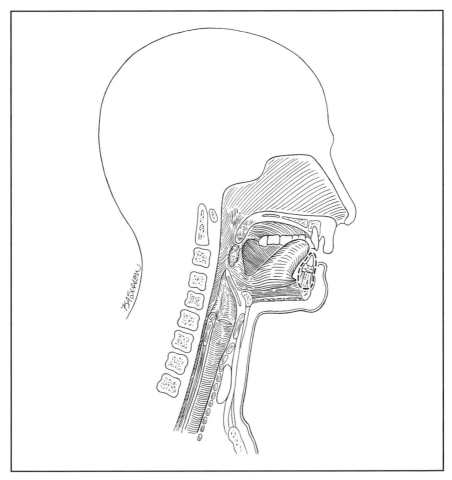

Figure 7.4. Lateral view of the oral cavity with the dotted line indicating the extent of resection for tumor involving the anterior alveolar ridge.

radical neck dissection generally spares the spinal accessory nerve (Suen, 1989).

A tumor occurring on the lateral floor of the mouth, if small, may be treated with wide local excision, including only tissues of the floor of the mouth. However, as is more likely, a larger tumor may require removal of not only part of the floor of the mouth, but also the portion of the lateral mandible adjacent to the tumor and a part of the tongue, as well as a radical neck dissection on the side of the tumor, as shown in Figure 7.7. If the mandible is not invaded by tumor, it may be spared from resection, and simply split vertically, swung out of the way to facilitate the resection, and wired back in place.

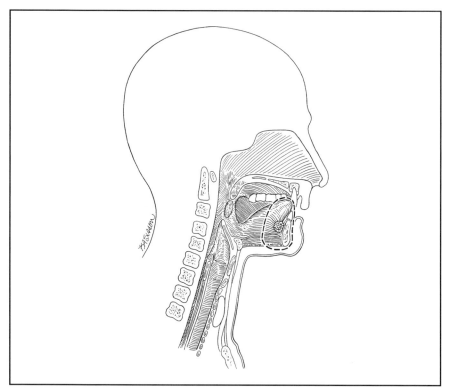

Figure 7.5. Lateral view of the oral cavity with the dotted line indicating the extent of resection for tumor involving the anterior tongue, floor of mouth, and alveolar ridge.

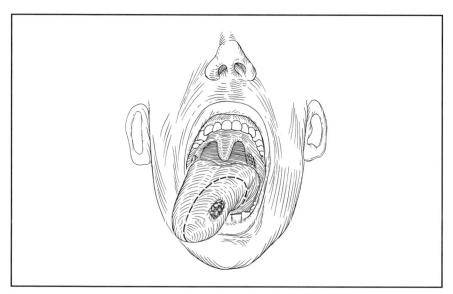

Figure 7.6. Frontal view of the oral cavity and tongue with the dotted line indicating the extent of resection of tumor on the tongue.

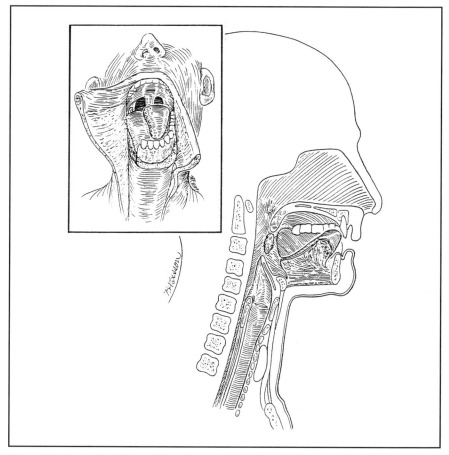

Figure 7.7. Lateral and frontal (inset) view of the oral cavity resection for a lateral floor of mouth tumor, including a portion of the lateral mandible, tongue, floor of mouth, and possibly a radical neck dissection.

A tumor in the tonsil or base of tongue area is usually classified as in the oropharyngeal region (i.e., the region between the oral and the pharyngeal areas). Such tumors often require a composite resection, including removal of the tonsilar area, a portion of the base of the tongue, and a portion of the lateral mandible, with a radical neck dissection (Givens et al., 1981). If the tumor spreads up the faucial arches, a portion of the soft palate and pharyngeal wall may also need to be excised.

A small tumor located on the hard palate may require only partial resection of the maxilla; however, total removal of the hard palate may be necessary if the tumor is large. Tumors on the soft palate may likewise require partial or total removal of the soft palate. In general, rehabilitation of the patient who has had total removal of the soft palate is easier than rehabilitation of the patient with partial removal of the velum. The prosthodontist can more easily develop a prosthesis that adequately occludes the velopharyngeal port when no scar tissue is present than when a portion of the soft palate is scarred down and relatively immobile.

Types of Reconstruction Following the Ablative Procedure

If the resection of tissue is relatively small, the wound may be closed with primary closure (i.e., the soft tissues remaining are simply pulled together and sutured). Small lesions of the tongue are often closed primarily because the tongue is composed of viable muscle that can be easily closed upon itself, as shown in Figure 7.8. Similarly, if the removal of tissues from the soft palate is small, the remaining tissues may be pulled together and sutured. More often, the resection of tissues is so large that there is not sufficient tissue remaining to permit primary closure, or, if primary closure were accomplished, the natural tension or pull of the tissue after closure would be sufficient to separate the tissues, create a fistula or reopening of the wound, and prevent healing. Therefore, to be able to close the surgical defect, the surgeon may need to borrow tissue from another area of the body. Most often this is done by means of a flap or a graft (Sisson & Goldstein, 1970; Yousif, Matloub, Sanger, & Campbell, 1994).

A flap is a piece of tissue that has been elevated or raised away from its normal site. One portion is left attached to its donor site to allow the flap to receive a blood supply from its donor site. The connecting bridge of remaining tissue permits a supply of blood to feed the flap until the portion that is sewn into the wound has an opportunity to heal in place.

Flaps are divided into local and distal (i.e., distant) types. A local flap is one that uses tissue in an area close to the surgical defect. For example, if a portion of the anterior floor of the mouth is resected along with a portion of the mandible, a tongue flap may be raised to fill the defect. In this instance, a portion of the tongue is sliced horizontally, with the posterior attachment to the tongue remaining. The anterior portion of the tongue flap is laid down in the surgical defect, as shown in Figure 7.9 (Som & Nussbaum, 1971). In this procedure, a piece of lingual tissue fills the surgical defect but remains attached to the tongue posteriorly. In many cases, this particular flap does not restrict remaining tongue movement but does reduce to some extent the bulk of the tongue anteriorly. A tongue flap used to close an oral cavity defect would be considered a local flap, as it is tissue taken from the immediate region of the surgical defect.

Two other popular flaps are the skin flap and the myocutaneous flap. The

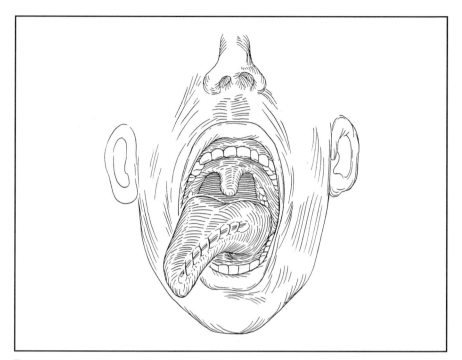

Figure 7.8. Frontal view of the oral cavity and tongue showing primary closure of the tongue after tumor resection.

skin flap consists of skin and subcutaneous tissue that is moved from one part of the body to another, while a pedical or attachment is maintained between it and the body for nourishment. Skin flaps may be taken from the neck, shoulder, or nasolabial fold, for example, to fill a floor of mouth defect. A flap from the shoulder would be considered a distal flap, that is, from a more distant site.

When a large amount of tissue is necessary to close a surgical gap, occasionally myocutaneous distal flaps are used. The myocutaneous flap includes muscle and overlying skin. When added bulk is needed in wound closure, the myocutaneous flap is thought to be more appropriate than a skin flap. The pectoralis major, platysma, and trapizeus are frequently used as myocutaneous flaps in reconstruction of the oral cavity, as shown in Figure 7.10. The myocutaneous flap is usually passed beneath the skin to the reconstruction site, and the donor site is closed at the primary surgery, so that a two-stage approach is not necessary.

Microsurgical techniques are also being used to transplant tissue from far distant parts of the body into the oral cavity, with veins and arteries anastomosed or attached carefully to blood supply at the site to assure viability of the tissue. Often called a microvascular free tissue transfer or graft (Zuker et al.,

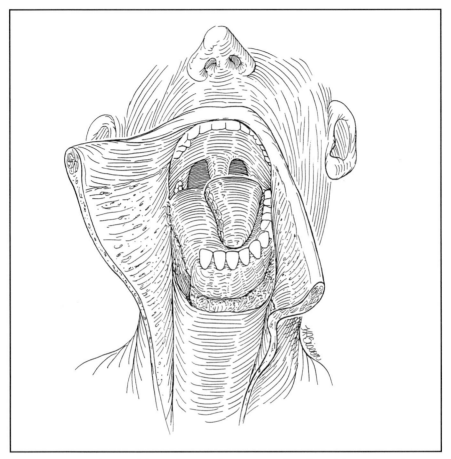

Figure 7.9. Frontal view of the oral cavity after resection for a lateral floor of mouth tumor. The resection included lateral mandible and lateral floor of mouth, which was reconstructed with a tongue flap.

1980), the free flap is a portion of tissue, entirely supplied by a specific artery and drained by a specific vein. It is capable of being revascularized by microvascular techniques at a new site, attaching arteries and veins from the recipient site to the tissue transfer. The donor sites for these flaps are less conspicuous than conventional flaps and can be used when conventional flaps may be difficult to use. However, these surgical techniques are time consuming and are therefore more costly. Also, infection in the oral cavity after microsurgical procedures, with subsequent loss of the graft, can be a complication.

Recently innervated grafts or sensate flaps are being attempted to improve the patient's postoperative function. The concept of these flaps is to bring sensation to the region by including a nerve in the flap or graft and anastomosing a

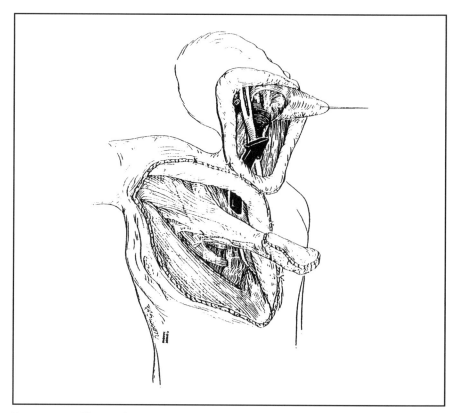

Figure 7.10. Closure of an anterior floor of mouth defect with a myocutaneous flap.

nerve from the site to the nerve in the flap or graft, thereby, hopefully, bringing sensation to the area. Whether the innervated or sensate flaps will, in fact, result in postoperative sensation in the oral cavity that is useful in speech or swallowing function is still open to question.

Rehabilitation Needs and Procedures for the Oral Cancer Patient

Oral cancer patients may experience changes in salivary flow, speech, and swallowing posttreatment, depending on the treatment modalities used for tumor eradication or control. If radiotherapy is used, the patient may experience changes in swallowing, mucositis, and reduced salivary flow. Swallowing disorders may be caused by reduced salivary flow or by intraoral sensory loss. Also, range of motion of the tongue and jaw may be reduced toward the end of the radiation protocol or at some point after completion of the protocol. This reduced range of tongue and jaw motion probably results from fibrosis and can be counteracted with an active range-of-motion exercise program completed morning and night.

If oral cancer patients are treated surgically, the amount of oral tongue or tongue base resected is correlated with the extent of speech and swallowing impairment (McConnel et al., 1994; Skelly, 1973; Zimmerman, 1958). The nature of the surgical reconstruction may also affect the patient's functional ability postoperatively. Although only a few studies have examined the relationship between (1) surgical resection and reconstruction of the oral cavity and (2) speech and swallowing changes postoperatively, results of these studies point toward primary closure as providing optimal function in comparison to distal flaps. Primary closure does not introduce any foreign tissue to the oral cavity and may provide most normal oral sensory input. The specific site of the cancer in the oral cavity also usually contributes to the determination of the particular nature of changes in chewing and swallowing (Logemann et al., 1993; Pauloski et al., 1993).

The typical multimodality pattern of care for more advanced oral cancers involves surgery followed by a full course of postoperative radiotherapy to a total dose of 5,000 to 7,000 cGy. This pattern of care often works against the patient's rehabilitative process. After the surgical procedure, patients are usually provided with swallowing (and speech) therapy to improve their function. They begin to see improvement in their eating and talking. Then, radiation therapy is introduced 4 to 6 weeks postoperatively and continues for a 6-week period. Often, at approximately 4 weeks into radiotherapy, patients experience worsening of their swallowing (and speech) problems. Thus, the patient experiences his or her function slowly improving and then beginning to deteriorate. This is frequently emotionally upsetting to the patient, who may withdraw from the rehabilitation process at 3 to 4 months after surgical treatment and receive no further rehabilitation intervention. Data indicate that at 12 months posttreatment, the oral cancer patient's speech and swallowing function is generally no better than at 3 months posttreatment (Pauloski et al., 1994). It is important that the oral cancer patient receive regular swallowing (and speech) intervention postoperatively and throughout radiotherapy as tolerated and that the patient resume swallowing (and speech) therapy after radiotherapy is completed.

Part of the speech and swallowing intervention may involve development of an intraoral prosthesis, which may obturate any velopharyngeal deficit created in posterior oral cavity resections and/or may recontour the patient's hard palate, lowering it to be able to interact more effectively with the remaining tongue and its reduced range of motion. Generally, patients with 50% or more of the oral tongue resected can benefit from a palatal reshaping (augmentation) prosthesis, as described in Chapter 6 (Davis, Lazarus, Logemann, & Hurst, 1987; Wheeler, Logemann, & Rosen, 1980).

Rehabilitation Needs and Procedures for the Oropharyngeal Cancer Patient

Cancer in the oropharyngeal region often affects the tongue base and/or pharyngeal wall. The base of the tongue is critical in the pharyngeal stage of swallowing, as tongue base and pharyngeal wall motion contributes to the propulsion of the bolus through the pharynx (Kahrilas, Logemann, Lin, & Ergun, 1992). These regions are less critical to speech function unless velopharyngeal closure is affected by the treatment modalities. This can occur when surgery involves the tongue base and lateral pharyngeal walls, which contribute to velopharyngeal closure in some patients. Similarly, muscles extending from the pharyngeal wall to the palate (e.g., the palatopharyngeus muscle), if affected by the resection or included in it, will create some degree of velopharyngeal deficit.

As in the oral cancer patient, swallowing (and speech) intervention should begin early postoperatively and involve exercise programs and possibly intraoral prosthetics. Obturation of the velopharyngeal deficit can significantly improve swallowing if the tongue base is also included in the resection. Exercise programs to improve tongue base motion during swallowing can improve efficiency and safety of the pharyngeal swallow in these patients. Generally, the speech–language pathology postoperative intervention is initiated when the patient's suture lines have healed sufficiently to enable aggressive exercise. In the oral and oropharyngeal cancer patient, this is usually 10 to 14 days after surgery. At this point, the patient is usually out of the hospital and must return for rehabilitation as an outpatient. This can be difficult for patients who are older and have less available transportation to the medical center. However, home health rehabilitation specialists may not be as experienced in care of the head and neck cancer patient as are rehabilitation professionals in the hospital setting.

Optimal Schedule for Rehabilitation

Treatment Selection as the First Line of Rehabilitation

Differing effects on speech and swallowing occur as a result of various extents of surgical resection in the oral cavity and varying surgical reconstruction techniques and radiotherapy for oral carcinoma (Fox, Busch, & Baum, 1987; Herberman, 1958; Logemann & Bytell, 1979; Logemann et al., 1993; Pauloski et al., 1993; Sonies, 1993; Staple & Ogura, 1966). Thus, rehabilitation begins with treatment planning, where the challenge is to identify the optimal treatment strategy for tumor eradication or control while causing least functional impairment in swallowing. Generally, the best decisions are made in a tumor conference where professionals treating the tumor (e.g., radiation oncologist, medical oncologist, surgeons) can discuss possible options for a particular patient and his or her tumor. At the same conference, rehabilitation specialists, including the speech–language pathologist, maxillofacial prosthodontist, and social worker, can contribute their expertise on functional effects of the various treatments in light of the particular patient's history. Patient characteristics and preferences are important in treatment selection. Some patients cannot emotionally tolerate or afford regular daily trips to radiation oncology for treatment. Other patients cannot tolerate surgical intervention because of their medical history. Also, based on their prior knowledge and history, some patients may have a strong preference for a specific treatment modality, particularly when informed of the possible functional sequelae associated with each treatment. Thus, the patient and family or significant other should be critical members of this pretreatment planning team, and consulted in the treatment decision.

Pretreatment Counseling

Patients should receive rehabilitative counseling prior to initiation of their treatment for head and neck cancer. The multidisciplinary rehabilitation team that should be available to the head and neck cancer patient beginning with pretreatment includes the swallowing therapist (usually a speech–language pathologist), social worker, dentist or maxillofacial prosthodontist, and dietitian, in addition to the patient's physicians and nurses.

Preoperative counseling by the swallowing therapist usually includes a swallowing screening, if not a videofluoroscopic assessment, to define any swallowing disorders. A pretreatment dental consultation is critical to identify any dental disease and to ensure preservation of critical teeth that may be needed for prosthetic stabilization after treatment. Indiscriminately pulling a patient's teeth before treatment begins may reduce the patient's rehabilitation alternatives after treatment. Optimal prosthetic devices may not be possible if key dental units needed to stabilize an intraoral prosthesis are missing. A pretreatment psychosocial assessment may identify any preexisting psychosocial problems, as well as enable the social worker or other psychosocial professional to become acquainted with the patient at a time when the patient can typically communicate more easily. The patient and family are often under significant stress pretreatment and can benefit from this psychosocial support.

Sometimes physicians are concerned that pretreatment counseling may scare the patient and cause him or her to refuse treatment. Actually, this counseling is designed to reduce the patient's and family's fears and assure them that rehabilitation professionals will be available to them after treatment to improve their functional status. Generally, the exact details of the functional effects of the patient's treatment cannot be and are not provided to the patient during preoperative counseling, because often these cannot be defined in detail before treatment. Rather, the counseling focuses on informing the patient that there are likely to be changes in swallowing after treatment and that rehabilitation professionals will be available to assist them in their posttreatment rehabilitation. An important concept for the patient to learn during treatment is that he or she is in control and responsible for his or her own rehabilitation. The speech–language pathologist and other professionals involved in the patient's rehabilitation will be providing exercise programs and various intervention strategies to improve the patient's function, but it is the patient's responsibility to practice the specific exercises and to follow through with other rehabilitation strategies on a regular basis. This puts the control back in the patient's hands and facilitates his or her recovery to independence. Prior to treatment, patients often comment that they are not interested in the details of the rehabilitation process but are pleased to know that rehabilitation professionals will be available to them as they recover.

Schedule of Posttreatment Intervention

If the initial treatment is surgical, the rehabilitation team should provide additional counseling to the patient and family beginning 2 to 3 days postoperatively. At that time the patient and family often have many questions about the functional effects of the surgery and more information can be given about swallowing changes. When the patient's healing has progressed sufficiently to enable aggressive exercise (usually 1 to 2 weeks postoperatively, depending on the site and nature of the surgery), the rehabilitation team will reevaluate the patient and begin intensive rehabilitation with daily inpatient therapy and weekly outpatient intervention. If swallowing changes result from treatment, the patient should receive a modified barium swallow to assess oropharyngeal function and evaluate the effectiveness of treatment strategies to improve the patient's swallow as quickly as possible (Dodds, Logemann, & Stewart, 1990; Dodds, Stewart, & Logemann, 1990; Logemann, 1983b, 1993). Dental status is critical, with consideration of the future need for an intraoral prosthesis. Psychosocial support and counseling should be provided. If a radical neck dissection is included in the surgical procedure, a physical therapy assessment should be completed. After completion of these evaluations, all of these professionals can plan and initiate therapy as needed.

Generally, it is optimal if the patient's first postoperative attempt at swallowing is completed during a radiographic assessment (the modified barium swallow), when the exact details of the patient's oropharyngeal anatomy and physiology can be defined and treatment strategies can be introduced and evaluated. During the radiographic study, if the patient aspirates, the aspiration often can be eliminated by introduction of such simple procedures as postural changes, which can change the direction of food flow or the relative position of oropharyngeal structures and dimensions (Logemann, 1983b, 1993; Logemann, Kahrilas, Kobara, & Vakil, 1989; Rasley et al., 1993; Shanahan, Logemann, Rademaker, Pauloski, & Kahrilas, 1993; Welch, Logemann, Rademaker, & Kahrilas, 1993). The videofluoroscopic evaluation of oropharyngeal swallow in head and neck cancer patients (the modified barium swallow) usually facilitates the speed of recovery in these patients (Rasley et al., 1993).

If the patient is undergoing postoperative radiotherapy or if radiotherapy is the primary treatment modality in combination with chemotherapy, the patient may receive rehabilitation interventions throughout the period of radiation treatment and thereafter. If the patient suffers side effects of radiotherapy that prevent regular rehabilitation management, the patient is usually encouraged to try to continue some exercises to preserve range of motion and flexibility of the lips, tongue, jaw, larynx, and pharynx.

Unfortunately, the prospective payment plans currently in place to cover hospital costs often make inpatient rehabilitation more difficult. Because patients are permitted shorter and shorter stays in the hospital after surgical treatment, they are often sent home having minimal contact with members of the rehabilitation team. Because patients are often not as physically strong when discharged, they may not be able to return to the hospital immediately for outpatient rehabilitation. As a result, weeks may go by before outpatient rehabilitation is initiated. Just at the time the patient begins outpatient rehabilitation, he or she may also begin postoperative radiotherapy. At 3 to 4 weeks into radiotherapy, the patient may suffer increasing functional impairment and become depressed as his or her swallowing function deteriorates. Review of data from our prospective study of 186 oral and oropharyngeal cancer patients treated surgically at 10 major medical centers indicated that only 50% of the patients received speech and swallowing therapy and less than 10% received maxillofacial prosthetic intervention. At 3 months posttreatment, 50% of the patients were lost to follow-up. One may hypothesize that these patients became disillusioned with their functional abilities and the lack of active rehabilitation, and stopped trying. Early and active rehabilitation is critical to the successful functioning of head and neck cancer patients. The responsibility for establishing the rehabilitation plan and educating the patient and family regarding its importance falls to the members of the rehabilitation team, including the patient's physician.

Swallowing Disorders Related to Specific Surgical Resections and Reconstruction Techniques

The two most important pieces of information needed by the swallowing therapist to understand the oral cancer patient's swallowing difficulties are (1) the exact nature and extent of the resection that was necessary to totally remove the tumor and (2) the exact nature of the reconstruction of the oral cavity (Logemann, Fisher, & Bytell, 1977; Rappaport, Shramek, & Brummett, 1967; Rappaport, Swirsky, & Chie, 1968; Trible, 1967). In patients who have had less than 50% of their tongue resected in the surgical procedure, the nature of the reconstruction is the major determinant of the pattern of function. In patients with greater than 50% of the tongue resected, the extent of resection and the nature of reconstruction determine the functional abilities of the patient. Thus, the first two pieces of information the swallowing therapist should obtain from the surgeon, before seeing a postsurgical oral cancer patient, are the exact nature of the resection and the reconstruction. It is best for the therapist not to use labels for surgical procedures, such as "anterior floor of mouth" or "lateral composite resection," but to ask the surgeon to define, in terms of the structures involved, the exact extent of the surgical resection and the reconstruction. Surgical labels often cover a wide variety of specific resections and reconstructions and are misleading to the therapist.

Partial Tongue Resection

Patients whose surgical resection is small (less than 50%) and limited to the tongue, with no other tissues involved, and whose reconstruction is by primary closure (pulling the remaining tissues of the tongue together and suturing), have swallowing difficulties of a relatively temporary nature (Conley, 1960). Initially, presumably because of edema or because tongue movement is changed, these patients may have short-term difficulties in triggering the pharyngeal swallow. This may occur even in patients whose resection was not in the tongue adjacent to the faucial arches. Thermal–tactile stimulation of the pharyngeal swallow provided for several days when the patient begins oral feeding can be very helpful. Also, some of these patients experience a sense of clumsiness with their tongue in swallowing. Range-of-motion tongue exercises and exercises to control the bolus in the oral cavity usually improve their control and their confidence within the first 3 to 4 weeks postoperatively.

In those patients whose resection has included 50% or more of the tongue, more severe effects on swallowing can be expected. Obviously, lingual propulsion and control of material in the mouth are severely reduced, as the patient cannot contact the remaining tongue segment to the palate and thus control the movement of food. Usually, a liquid or thinned paste consistency can be managed by tilting the head backward during swallows and allowing gravity to carry material into the pharynx. Some of these patients need to learn to voluntarily protect their airway during the swallow, using the supraglottic swallow as additional defense against aspiration. However, if the resection is limited to the tongue, the pharyngeal and laryngeal aspects of the swallow are usually normal and the patient can tolerate a backward tilted head posture without increasing the chances of aspiration. Again, range-of-motion tongue exercises are necessary to get maximum movement from the remaining tongue remnant. Construction of an intraoral maxillary reshaping prosthesis often improves swallowing to the point where patients can manage all food consistencies except those requiring mastication. Even so, some patients using the prosthesis and fork or spoon can manipulate food over to the teeth and do some chewing of softer foods, such as spaghetti or chopped meat.

Anterior Floor of Mouth Resection

After anterior floor of mouth resection, the oral phase of the swallow is usually impaired but pharyngeal transit is normal unless the floor of mouth muscles have been cut or partially resected (Jacob, Kahrilas, Logemann, Shah, & Ha, 1989; Logemann & Bytell, 1979; Pauloski et al., 1993; Pauloski, Logemann, Fox, & Colangelo, 1995; Shedd, Kirchner, & Scatliff, 1961). The patient who has the upper margin of the mandible and a portion of the floor of the mouth removed, with closure of the defect effected by using a flap of tissue from a site other than the tongue, generally has relatively few functional changes in swallowing after surgery. Because the remaining tongue segment is mobile and the inferior rim of the mandible has been left to maintain the mandibular contour, lingual propulsion of the bolus is good and lingual control of the bolus in the oral cavity is essentially normal (Rappaport et al., 1968). There may be an initial period after surgery when swallowing is best accomplished by positioning the food more posteriorly on the tongue. This will speed oral transit time while edema at the surgical site is most severe. Later, the patient can wear a dental prosthesis or full lower denture.

If, however, the same resection of the margin of the mandible and floor of the mouth is closed by suturing the tongue into the surgical defect (a form of primary closure), as shown in Figure 7.11, the patient will have severe difficulties with lingual control and propulsion of the bolus, and with mastication (Logemann & Bytell, 1979). Because the tongue is sutured down, its anterior range of motion is reduced and the patient's ability to cup and hold material in the anterior mouth in preparation for the swallow is severely affected. Shedd, Scatliff, and Kirchner (1960) wrote that disruption of the mylohyoid support for the tongue contributes significantly to these problems. This can be compensated for by positioning food more posteriorly, but the consistency of the food must be restricted to liquids or pastes. Chewing is impossible because the patient is unable to lateralize the tongue (and thus lateralize the bolus over to the teeth for chewing) and usually cannot wear dentures because there is no alveolus as a foundation. Therefore, unless the tongue is released from this position by subsequent surgery, these patients will be unable to eat any food requiring mastication. If tongue movement is severely reduced, the liquid may have to be syringed

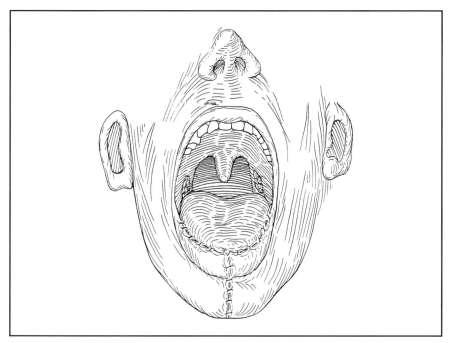

Figure 7.11. Frontal view of the oral cavity showing lingual labial closure (i.e., the tongue sutured to the lower lip).

or "dumped" into the back of the oral cavity. These patients often need to be taught to use the "dump and swallow" or prolonged supraglottic swallow procedure to voluntarily protect the airway during the swallow, not because of reduced laryngeal or pharyngeal control in the swallow but because their oral control is such that they may lose material over the tongue into the airway before they actually initiate a voluntary oral stage swallow.

A composite resection in the area of the anterior floor of the mouth, including a portion of the entire anterior mandible, the anterior floor of the mouth, a portion of the tongue, and a radical neck dissection, may result in a variety of swallowing disorders, from mild to severe, depending on the way the surgical defect is reconstructed, the extent of resection of the tongue, and whether the floor of the mouth muscles are left intact, cut, or resected (Logemann & Bytell, 1979; Pauloski et al., 1995; Pauloski et al., 1993).

Patients who have had the tongue sewn into the surgical defect at the front of the mandible, as described earlier for resection of the rim of the mandible and floor of the mouth, have severe difficulties in swallowing, similar to those already described because of the severe reduction in tongue movement. This is true whether small or larger amounts of tongue have been resected. In contrast, if tissue from a distant site, a local flap, or a tongue flap is used to accomplish closure, mobility of the remaining tongue segment may be good enough to permit functional swallowing. A tongue flap, as described earlier, involves splitting the tongue longitudinally and using one small portion to close the surgical defect while leaving the remaining bulk of tongue to move normally, as shown previously in Figure 7.9.

Figure 7.12 shows the difference in swallowing transit time based on the method of surgical reconstruction in patients after anterior floor of mouth resection. Three groups of patients were studied at Northwestern University, each with only 10% of the tongue resected: (1) five patients who had reconstruction of their surgical defect by tongue flap, as just described; (2) five patients who had their surgical defect reconstructed by lingual labial closure (i.e., sewing the

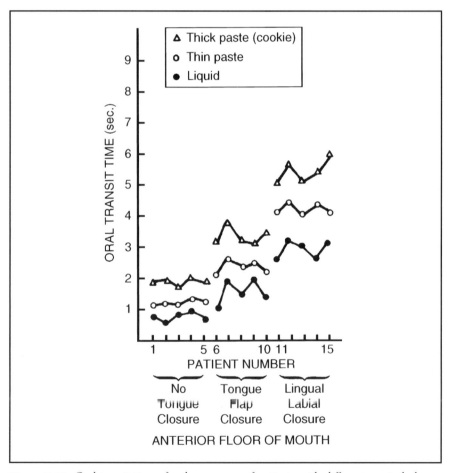

Figure 7.12. Oral transit times for three groups of patients with different surgical closure after anterior floor of mouth resection.

tongue to the lip); and (3) five patients whose closure was accomplished without using any tongue tissue. Those patients with no tongue used in surgical closure functioned most normally, followed by those patients whose reconstruction was completed by tongue flap. Patients whose tongue was sutured into the surgical defect functioned most poorly and, in fact, were not able to handle anything but liquids on a regular basis. Thus, it is clear that surgical reconstruction plays a key role in the functional outcome of the patient.

Patients whose tongue is sewn into the surgical defect anteriorly may be helped by tongue range-of-motion exercises, positioning food more posteriorly in the mouth, tilting the head backward during the swallow, and the introduction of a palatal reshaping prosthesis. However, these patients will always be unable to handle chewing and thicker food consistencies unless the tongue is surgically freed from the floor of the mouth and the floor of the mouth is relined with other tissues such as a skin graft. If the floor of mouth muscles are cut or partially resected, these muscles will at least temporarily lose their ability to pull the hyoid, and thus the larynx, up and forward to open the upper esophageal sphincter. As a result, these patients may have pharyngeal dysphagia with reduced laryngeal movement and food remaining in the pyriform sinuses. The falsetto exercise and the Mendelsohn maneuver should be used to improve laryngeal movement.

Lateral Floor of Mouth/Posterior Composite Resection or Base of Tongue Resection

Patients who have had resection in the lateral floor of the mouth, tonsil, and tongue base area have potential difficulties in both the oral and the pharyngeal stages of the swallow (Logemann & Bytell, 1979; Logemann et al., 1993; Shedd et al., 1961; Shedd et al., 1960). Because the tongue and other oral structures are involved in the resection, the oral stages of the swallow will be affected. However, because the surgical resection is in the area of the faucial arches, where the pharyngeal swallow is normally triggered, and because a portion of the pharynx may be involved in the resection, these patients will often also have problems in triggering the pharyngeal swallow and in the pharyngeal stage of the swallow. As with patients who have had resection of the anterior floor of mouth, the way the surgical closure is accomplished has a definite effect on the patient's swallowing (Logemann, Sisson, & Wheeler, 1980).

The patient who has undergone surgical resection in the tonsil/base of tongue region may have mild to severe disturbances in oral preparation and chewing and in oral transit times, with impaired lingual propulsion of the bolus. Material can collect in the lateral sulcus or on the hard palate, and, because of reduced range of tongue motion, the patient cannot clear this material from the crevices. In addition to these oral problems, the surgical resection is located in the area of the faucial arches, where the pharyngeal swallow is triggered. Thus, these patients may have delayed triggering of the pharyngeal swallow. When the pharyngeal swallow does trigger, patients may have reduced tongue base retraction and reduced pharyngeal wall contraction because the fibers of the glossopharyngeus muscle are cut, causing a residue of material to remain in the valleculae after the swallow. Usually, their laryngeal control in swallowing is normal unless a fistula has developed in healing, causing scar tissue to form in the pharynx that can inhibit laryngeal elevation. A fistula in the pharynx causing scar tissue can also lead to a slight defect, or crevice, that collects material. Therapy to improve oral and tongue base range of motion, improve triggering of the pharyngeal swallow, and promote voluntary protection of the airway during the swallow and clearing of the pharynx after the swallow is often helpful (Logemann, 1983a). Occasionally, following this type of resection, these patients have difficulty with the opening of the cricopharyngeal sphincter because of reduced laryngeal movement. A Mendelsohn maneuver and the falsetto exercise may be helpful.

These patients often benefit from a maxillary reshaping prosthesis. If the patient has teeth, the maxillary prosthesis can be made to clip onto the teeth. If the patient is edentulous, the maxillary prosthesis can be retained by suction. In edentulous patients whose resection included part of the mandible, the purpose of the prosthesis is to speed oral and pharyngeal transit times and to facilitate chewing, if possible. However, many patients with composite resection of the lateral floor of the mouth, tongue, and mandible who have no teeth cannot wear a lower denture because of their altered anatomy postoperatively. Even those patients who have a mobile tongue remnant and who have mandibular reconstruction at some time after their original ablative surgical procedure will usually not have normal function or be able to wear a lower denture without implants for stabilization (Lawson, Balk, Loscalzo, Biller, & Krespi, 1982; Rappaport et al., 1968).

Swallowing Disorders After Radiotherapy to the Oral Cavity and Oropharynx

During a full course of radiotherapy to the oral cavity, patients often experience reduced saliva flow or xerostomia, if some or all of the salivary glands are in the field of radiation, edema, and, occasionally, sores in the mouth (mucositis). The salivary changes are permanent and are the most upsetting to patients as there are no good, effective management strategies. Medications to stimulate saliva and pseudo-saliva products are often only partially effective. Patients frequently become dissatisfied with these and discontinue their use. Xerostomia alone can cause changes in swallowing, including reduced speed of tongue movement causing a delay in oral transit time and a change in pattern of tongue movement probably contributing to a delay in triggering the pharyngeal swallow. These swallowing changes are similar to those experienced by normal swallowers who are asked to quickly and repeatedly dry swallow five or six times in a row (Hughes et al., 1987).

Fibrosis also forms as a result of damage to the small blood vessels in the radiated area. Fibrosis changes muscle fibers to connective tissue in a process that can continue for years. Patients with dentures or prostheses may need to discontinue wearing these during and immediately after radiotherapy, as the contact of the denture or prosthesis against the oral tissues may create irritation and open sores that will have difficulty healing because of the reduced blood supply resulting from radiotherapy. Prior to and during radiotherapy to the oral cavity, patients with some or all of their own teeth should have regular fluoride treatments to prevent caries (Fleming, 1982). Some patients experience delays in triggering of the pharyngeal swallow during or sometimes after radiotherapy. If the pharynx is in the radiation field (e.g., when the back and base of the tongue and tonsil area are the tumor site), there is reduced pharyngeal contraction, tongue base movement, and laryngeal elevation (Lazarus, 1993; Lazarus et al., 1996). These problems result in residue in the pharynx after the swallow, often causing aspiration after the swallow. These patients usually benefit from the super-supraglottic swallow and the Mendelsohn maneuver (Logemann, Rademaker, Colangelo, & Pauloski, 1997; Logemann et al., 1993).

Not all radiotherapy effects occur during or immediately after the series of treatments. It is not uncommon for irradiated patients to develop increasing swallowing problems a year or more after the completion of radiotherapy. Fluoroscopic examination most frequently reveals a delay in triggering the pharyngeal swallow, reduced contraction of the pharyngeal walls, and reduced laryngeal elevation (Lazarus et al., 1996). It is important for patients who will undergo radiotherapy to the oral cavity and/or pharynx to begin range-of-motion exercises for the tongue, jaw, and larynx *before* radiotherapy begins and to continue these at least twice daily through the radiotherapy and for a period of months afterward. Many patients need to continue these exercises forever in order to prevent fibrosis.

General Principles of Swallowing Therapy with Treated Oral Cancer Patients

It is important for the swallowing therapist to counsel the patient before treatment to discuss potential swallowing problems. It is impossible to know the exact extent of the swallowing disorder that will occur after treatment, but it is important to alert the patient that problems may be encountered with swallowing and to provide reassurance that the swallowing therapist will be available to provide any necessary exercise programs. The patient must be informed that he or she has some responsibility for his or her own rehabilitation by cooperating with and carrying through the exercise programs. It is difficult to initiate rehabilitation posttreatment with a patient who has been unprepared for any problems with swallowing. Many patients assume that their swallowing will recover normally without any effort on their part. When it becomes clear several weeks after treatment that swallowing will not improve spontaneously, patients can become quite depressed. Thus, pretreatment discussions of the potential need for therapy to improve swallowing can reduce the patient's emotional reaction to unanticipated problems.

In the surgically treated patient, swallowing therapy, including those preparatory oromotor exercises that are necessary to build muscle control for swallowing, is begun when the surgeon indicates that the patient's healing has progressed to the point where there is no danger to suture lines. In patients without complications, this is usually within 10 to 14 days after surgery. At that time, an aggressive program of tongue and jaw range-of-motion exercises is begun. Jaw range-of-motion exercises are particularly important if the patient will undergo postoperative radiotherapy.

Swallowing therapy is usually begun when the patient has a nasogastric tube or other nonoral feeding in place to maintain nutrition. After the complete assessment of oral functioning and initiation of range-of-motion exercises, a videofluoroscopic examination of swallowing is completed using the three materials: thin liquid of various volumes, paste, and cookie. Thick liquids may be appropriate for some patients. The therapy program is then designed to improve any physiologic dysfunctions noted from fluoroscopy. Most often, patients can begin oral feeding at that time with at least one viscosity of food, usually liquid. As oral function improves, the viscosity of the material can be gradually increased.

Therapy continues until a patient's swallowing has reached a point where the therapist and the patient agree that maximum goals have been attained. This usually involves following the patient weekly for 2 to 3 months on an outpatient basis, and may include developing an intraoral prosthesis with a maxillofacial prosthodontist, as well as working on more difficult tongue exercises to improve control of the bolus (Logemann et al., 1980; Wheeler et al., 1980). Some patients, for example those who have undergone a composite resection including an extensive tongue resection (75% or more) and a partial mandibulectomy, will never be able to chew, so their diet will always be restricted to liquids and soft foods. Often, the ultimate functional outcome cannot be determined until several months postoperatively, and then involves discussions between the various members of the team seeing the patient. If a patient is not referred for swallowing therapy until months after treatment, there is still a good possibility that he or she will be able to return to oral intake with therapy (Lazarus, Logemann, & Gibbons, 1993).

Normally, maximum rehabilitation goals in head and neck cancer patients can be attained only with a team of professionals, including nursing staff, speech–language pathologist or swallowing therapist, social worker, dentist, and maxillofacial prosthodontist (see Chapter 13). Usually the social worker, speech–language pathologist or swallowing therapist, and maxillofacial prosthodontist follow the patient most intensively after hospital discharge, and work to define maximum obtainable functional goals. It is often not possible to know the patient's capabilities until the speech–language pathologist and maxillofacial prosthodontist have had an opportunity to work together to develop optimum prosthetic interventions to assist the patient in his or her rehabilitation.

References

American Joint Committee on Cancer. (1992). *Manual for the staging of cancer* (4th ed.). Philadelphia: Lippincott.

Conley, J. (1960). Swallowing dysfunctions associated with radical surgery of the head and neck. *Archives of Surgery, 80,* 602–612.

Davis, J., Lazarus, C., Logemann, J., & Hurst, P. (1987). Effect of a maxillary glossectomy prosthesis on articulation and swallowing. *Journal of Prosthetic Dentistry, 57,* 715–719.

Dodds, W. J., Logemann, J. A., & Stewart, E. T. (1990). Radiological assessment of abnormal oral and pharyngeal phases of swallowing. *American Journal of Roentgenology, 154,* 965–974.

Dodds, W. J., Stewart, E. T., & Logemann, J. A. (1990). Physiology and radiology of the normal oral and pharyngeal phases of swallowing. *American Journal of Roentgenology, 154,* 953–963.

Fleming, T. (1982). Dental care for cancer patients receiving radiotherapy to the head and neck. *The Cancer Bulletin, 34,* 63–65.

Fox, P. C., Busch, K. A., & Baum, B. J. (1987). Subjective reports of xerostomia and objective measures of salivary gland performance. *Journal of the American Dental Association, 115,* 581–584.

Givens, C., Johns, M., & Cantrell, R. (1981). Carcinoma of the tonsil. *Archives of Otolaryngology, 107,* 730–734.

Herberman, M. (1958). Rehabilitation of patients following glossectomy. *Archives of Otolaryngology, 67,* 182–183.

Hughes, C. V., Baum, B. J., Fox, P. C., Marmary, Y., Yeh, C.-K., & Sonies, B. C. (1987). Oralpharyngeal dysphagia: A common sequellae of salivary gland dysfunction. *Dysphagia, 1,* 173–177.

Jacob, P., Kahrilas, P., Logemann, J., Shah, V., & Ha, T. (1989). Upper esophageal sphincter opening and modulation during swallowing. *Gastroenterology, 97,* 1469–1478.

Kahrilas, P. J., Logemann, J. A., Lin, S., & Ergun, G. A. (1992). Pharyngeal clearance during swallow: A combined manometric and videofluoroscopic study. *Gastroenterology, 103,* 128–136.

Kremen, A. (1951). Cancer of the tongue: A surgical technique for a primary combined enbloc resection of tongue, floor of mouth and cervical lymphatics. *Surgery, 30,* 227–238.

Lawson, W., Balk, S., Loscalzo, L., Biller, H., & Krespi, Y. (1982). Experience with immediate and delayed mandibular reconstruction. *Laryngoscope, 92*, 5–10.

Lazarus, C. L. (1993). Effects of radiation therapy and voluntary maneuvers on swallow functioning in head and neck cancer patients. *Clinics in Communication Disorders, 3*(4), 11–20.

Lazarus, C. L., Logemann, J. A., & Gibbons, P. (1993). Effects of maneuvers on swallowing function in a dysphagic oral cancer patient. *Head & Neck, 15*, 419–424.

Lazarus, C. L., Logemann, J. A., Pauloski, B. R., Colangelo, L. A., Kahrilas, P. J., Mittal, B. B., & Pierce, M. (1996). Swallowing disorders in head and neck cancer patients treated with radiotherapy and adjuvant chemotherapy. *Laryngoscope, 106*, 1157–1166.

Logemann, J. (1983a). Articulation management of the oral pharyngeal impaired patient. In W. H. Perkins (Ed.), *Current therapy for communication disorders.* New York: Thieme and Stratton.

Logemann, J. (1983b). *Evaluation and treatment of swallowing disorders.* Austin, TX: PRO-ED.

Logemann, J. (1993). *Manual for the videofluoroscopic study of swallowing* (2nd ed.). Austin, TX: PRO-ED.

Logemann, J., & Bytell, D. (1979). Swallowing disorders in three types of head and neck surgical patients. *Cancer, 44*, 1075–1105.

Logemann, J., Fisher, H., & Bytell, D. (1977, November). *Functional effects of reconstruction in partially glossectomized patients.* Paper presented at the annual convention of the American Speech and Hearing Association, Chicago.

Logemann, J., Kahrilas, P., Kobara, M., & Vakil, N. (1989). The benefit of head rotation on pharyngoesophageal dysphagia. *Archives of Physical Medicine and Rehabilitation, 70*, 767–771.

Logemann, J. A., Pauloski, B. R., Rademaker, A. W., McConnel, F. M. S., Heiser, M. A., Cardinale, S., Shedd, D., Stein, D., Beery, Q., Johnson, J., & Baker, T. (1993). Speech and swallow function after tonsil/base of tongue resection with primary closure. *Journal of Speech and Hearing Research, 36*, 918–926.

Logemann, J. A., Rademaker, A. W., Colangelo, L., & Pauloski, B. R. (1977). Speech and swallowing rehabilitation in head and neck cancer patients. *Oncology, 11*, 651–659.

Logemann, J., Sisson, G., & Wheeler, R. (1980). The team approach to rehabilitation of surgically treated oral cancer patients. In *Proceedings of the National Forum on Comprehensive Cancer Rehabilitation and Its Vocational Implications* (pp. 222–227).

McConnel, F. M. S., Logemann, J. A., Rademaker, A. W., Pauloski, B. R., Baker, S. R., Lewin, J., Shedd, D., Heiser, M. A., Cardinale, S., Collins, S., Graner, D., Cook, B. S., Milianti, F., & Baker, T. (1994). Surgical variables affecting postoperative swallowing efficiency in oral cancer patients: A pilot study. *Laryngoscope, 104*(1), 87–90.

Pauloski, B. R., Logemann, J. A., Fox, J. C., & Colangelo, L. A. (1995). Biomechanical analysis of the pharyngeal swallow in postsurgical patients with anterior tongue and floor of mouth resection and distal flap reconstruction. *Journal of Speech and Hearing Research, 38*, 110–123.

Pauloski, B. R., Logemann, J. A., Rademaker, A., McConnel, F., Heiser, M. A., Cardinale, S., Shedd, D., Lewin, J., Baker, S., Graner, D., Cook, B., Milianti, F., Collins, S., & Baker, T. (1993). Speech and swallowing function after anterior tongue and floor of mouth resection with distal flap reconstruction. *Journal of Speech Hearing Research, 36*, 267–276.

Pauloski, B. R., Logemann, J. A., Rademaker, A. W., McConnel, F. M. S., Stein, D., Beery, Q., Johnson, J., Heiser, M. A., Cardinale, S., Shedd, D., Graner, D., Cook, B., Milianti, F., Collins, S., & Baker, T. (1994). Speech and swallowing function after oral and oropharyngeal resections: One-year follow-up. *Head & Neck, 16*(4), 313–322.

Rappaport, L., Shramek, J., & Brummett, S. (1967). Functional aspects of cancer of the base of the tongue. *American Journal of Surgery, 114,* 489–492.

Rappaport, L., Swirsky, A., & Chie, S. (1968). Functional considerations after resection of the hyomandibular complex. *American Journal of Surgery, 116,* 581–584.

Rasley, A., Logemann, J. A., Kahrilas, P. J., Rademaker, A. W., Pauloski, B. R., & Dodds, W. J. (1993). Prevention of barium aspiration during videofluoroscopic swallowing studies: Value of change in posture. *American Journal of Roentology, 160,* 1005–1009.

Shanahan, T. K., Logemann, J. A., Rademaker, A. W., Pauloski, B. R., & Kahrilas, P. J. (1993). Chin-down posture effect on aspiration in dysphagic patients. *Archives of Physical Medicine and Rehabilitation, 74,* 736–739.

Shedd, D., Kirchner, J., & Scatliff, J. (1961). Oral and pharyngeal components of deglutition. *Archives of Surgery, 82,* 373–380.

Shedd, D., Scatliff, J., & Kirchner, J. (1960). A cineradiographic study of postresectional alterations in oropharyngeal physiology. *Surgery, Gynecology and Obstetrics, 110,* 69–89.

Sisson, G., & Goldstein, J. (1970). Flaps and grafts in head and neck surgery. *Archives of Otolaryngology, 92,* 599–610.

Skelly, M. (1973). *Glossectomee speech rehabilitation.* Springfield, IL: Thomas.

Snow, G. (1989). Evaluation and staging of the patient with head and neck cancer. In E. N. Meyer & J. Y. Suen (Eds.), *Cancer of the head and neck* (2nd ed., pp. 17–38). New York: Churchill Livingston.

Som, M., & Nussbaum, M. (1971). Marginal resection of the mandible with reconstruction by tongue flap for carcinoma of the floor of the mouth. *American Journal of Surgery, 121,* 679–683.

Sonies, B. C. (1993). Remediation challenges in treating dysphagia post head/neck cancer: A problem-oriented approach. *Clinics in Communication Disorders, 3*(4), 21–26.

Staple, T., & Ogura, J. (1966). Cineradiography of the swallowing mechanism following supraglottic subtotal laryngectomy. *Radiology, 87,* 226–230.

Suen, J. (1989). Cancer of the neck. In E. N. Meyer & J. Y. Suen (Eds.), *Cancer of the head and neck* (2nd ed., pp. 221–254). New York: Churchill Livingston.

Trible, W. (1967). The rehabilitation of deglutition following head and neck surgery. *Laryngoscope, 77,* 518–523.

U.S. Department of Health, Education, and Welfare. (1979). *Management guidelines for head and neck cancer.* Washington, DC: Author.

Welch, M. V., Logemann, J. A., Rademaker, A. W., & Kahrilas, P. J. (1993). Changes in pharyngeal dimensions effected by chin tuck. *Archives of Physical Medicine and Rehabilitation, 74,* 178–181.

Wheeler, R., Logemann, J., & Rosen, M. (1980). Maxillary reshaping prosthesis: Effectiveness in improving speech and swallowing of post-surgical oral cancer patients. *Journal of Prosthetic Dentistry, 43,* 313–319.

Yousif, N. J., Matloub, H. S., Sanger, J. R., & Campbell, B. (1994). Soft tissue reconstruction of the oral cavity. *Clinics in Plastic Surgery, 21*(1), 15–23.

Zimmerman, J. (1958). *Speech production after glossectomy.* Paper presented at the American Speech and Hearing Association Convention, New York.

Zuker, R., Rosen, I., Palmer, J., Sutton, F., McKee, N., & Manktelow, R. (1980). Microvascular free flaps in head and neck reconstruction. *The Canadian Journal of Surgery, 23,* 157–162.

C H A P T E R 8

SWALLOWING DISORDERS AFTER TREATMENT FOR LARYNGEAL CANCER

Over the past 40 years, rehabilitation of the laryngeal cancer patient has been receiving increased emphasis as a component of patient care and has been initiated earlier and earlier relative to diagnosis. In years past, rehabilitation was often considered only long after the patient's treatment was completed, when the patient complained of significant functional impairment. Today, the potential effects of treatment on the patient's swallowing and respiration are frequently considered as a part of treatment planning and selection. These types of considerations began in the 1950s when partial laryngectomy procedures were introduced as an alternative to total laryngectomy in selected patients (Alonso, 1947; Ogura, 1955; Pressman, 1954; Som, 1951). Recently, consideration of potential functional losses prior to treatment selection has driven the development of organ preservation protocols, including high-dose chemotherapy and radiation therapy, as alternatives to total laryngectomy in patients with advanced laryngeal cancer (Pfister et al., 1991; U.S. Department of Veterans Affairs Laryngeal Cancer Study Group, 1991). In an editorial in *Otolaryngology—Head and Neck Surgery*, Weiss (1993) stated quite eloquently the importance of considering the patient's functional status when planning treatment:

> I know that the larynx preservation protocol is extremely hard on the patient, may not culminate in larynx preservation after all the effort, and indeed may not be equally efficacious with respect to survival when compared with standard treatment for tongue and hypopharynx primaries. I also know that many

laryngectomees are rehabilitated well and cope beautifully. I share this knowledge with the patient, but it rarely deters him or her from choosing the larynx
preservation option. The patient's perception of the quality of life governs the
entire decision. . . .

   We all heartily endorse the goal of preserving the patient's life, and when
the choice is a stark one—between aggressive therapy on the one hand and
certain death on the other—then the choice is clear for the physician. But the
choice is rarely so stark. Quality of life counts for a great deal in the patients'
minds. It should matter just as much to us. (p. 311)

The newest combined high-dose chemotherapy and radiotherapy protocols for
advanced disease, as well as the application of partial versus total laryngectomy
procedures in selected patients with laryngeal cancer, are all based on the recognition that the exact nature of the treatment modality dictates the functional
impairments the head and neck cancer patient will suffer posttreatment.

Principles of Tumor Management in the Larynx

Tumors in the larynx may be managed primarily by radiotherapy or surgery, with
chemotherapy as an adjuvant treatment. For smaller tumors, particularly on the
true vocal cord, radiotherapy is the more frequent treatment choice. Cure rates
for these small tumors are usually equal with radiotherapy or surgery, with radiotherapy considered the less ablative treatment. Combined treatment—that is,
radiotherapy plus surgery or high-dose chemotherapy plus radiation therapy (i.e.,
organ preservation protocol)—is used in larger tumors (Goepfert, Lindberg, &
Jesse, 1981; U.S. Department of Health, Education, and Welfare, 1979).

   Tumors in the larynx are also staged, as in the oral cavity, following the
tumor–node–metastasis (TNM) classification system. For the purposes of staging, the larynx is divided into three areas: the supraglottis, the glottis, and the
subglottis, as shown in Figure 8.1. Approximately 60% of malignant laryngeal
tumors occur in the glottic area, 35% in the supraglottic area, and 5% in the subglottic area. In staging of laryngeal tumors, the T followed by a number (1 to 4)
represents the size of the tumor, T1 being the smallest and T4 the largest. There
are specific definitions of tumor size for each of the three areas of the larynx.
The N followed by a number indicates the status of disease in the nodes of the
head and neck, with the number following the N indicating the number of
nodes involved with tumor. An N0 indicates that no nodes are involved with
tumor. The M stands for metastasis at distant sites, such as the lung or liver. An
M1 indicates one metastatic site outside of the region. Thus, a T1N0M0 lesion
is a small lesion with no nodal or distant metastasis. The primary physician diag-

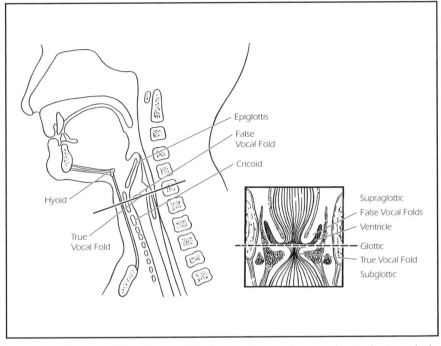

Figure 8.1. Lateral and frontal views of the larynx, showing the supraglottic, glottic, and subglottic divisions of the larynx.

nosing the patient, usually an otolaryngologist or general surgeon, will stage the patient's tumor before treatment, so the results of treatment can be compared with results of other treatments on patients presenting with the same site and stage of disease.

In the larynx, the extent of normal tissue resected along with the tumor depends on the site of the malignancy. Much is known about the lymphatic drainage system and the pattern of spread of tumors in the larynx (U.S. Department of Health, Education, and Welfare, 1979). For example, because of the way in which the lymph system drains in the supraglottic larynx, a tumor of the supraglottic larynx (Figure 8.2) will not spread downward to the true vocal cord and/or subglottic larynx unless the tumor is located at the base of the epiglottis. Thus, a lesion on the supraglottic larynx can be removed with a minimum of normal tissue at the inferior edge because tumor cells are known not to spread in that direction. In the larynx, then, the rule of a 1½- to 2-cm normal margin that is used for oral cancers is not always followed because of the knowledge of the lymphatic system in the larynx. However, at the superior end of a laryngeal resection, a 2-cm margin of normal tissue must be maintained.

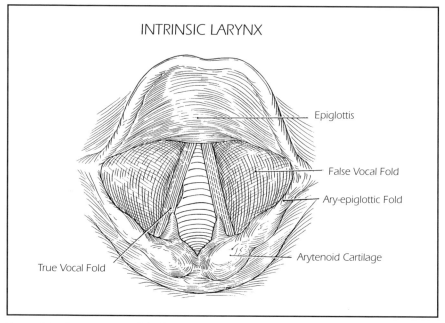

Figure 8.2. Superior view of the larynx.

Typical Tumor Locations and Resections in the Larynx and Associated Swallowing Disorders

As with resections of the oral cavity, the swallowing therapist must discuss with the surgeon each laryngeal cancer patient's surgical resection and reconstruction. Standard names for surgical procedures can be misleading. Each resection may vary somewhat, as may the reconstruction. The surgeon should be asked to describe the exact structures included in the resection and the details of the reconstruction. Providing the surgeon with anatomic drawings of the larynx and asking him or her to circle the resected structures can also be helpful.

Supraglottic Tumors

Smaller lesions on the supraglottic larynx, predominantly involving the epiglottis (anterior or posterior surface), the aryepiglottic fold, or the false vocal folds, are frequently treated with a partial laryngectomy procedure known as a *horizontal or supraglottic laryngectomy* (Ogura, Biller, Calcaterra, & Davis, 1969; Powers, Ogura, & Holtz, 1963; Shumrick & Keith, 1968). A lesion extending below the false vocal cord usually requires a different management procedure. Figure 8.3 illustrates the typical extent of this resection, which generally includes

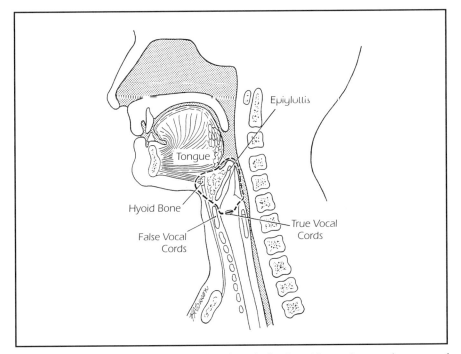

Figure 8.3. Lateral view of the head and neck, with the dotted line indicating the extent of resection in supraglottic laryngectomy.

a part or all of the hyoid bone and epiglottis superiorly, the aryepiglottic folds, and the false vocal folds inferiorly. Even if a tumor extends onto the false vocal fold, the supraglottic procedure will take only the upper half of the ventricle, clearly not taking a full 2-cm margin of normal tissue. Again, this is because of the pattern of normal lymphatic drainage in the larynx and typical tumor spread, which is lateral rather than inferior in a supraglottic tumor. The resection shown in Figure 8.3 might be called a standard supraglottic laryngectomy. This procedure clearly removes the structures contributing to airway protection during swallowing: (1) the epiglottis and the aryepiglottic folds and (2) the false vocal folds. It leaves the base of the tongue, the arytenoids, and the true vocal folds as the only protective mechanism.

In reconstruction, the surgeon usually elevates the remaining larynx and tucks it under the tongue base for additional protection during the swallow. To relearn to swallow postoperatively, the patient must completely occlude the airway entrance, that is, by retracting the tongue base to make contact with the anteriorly tilting arytenoid (Logemann et al., 1994), which prevents material from entering the airway during the swallow (Aguilar, Olson, & Shedd, 1979; Sessions, Zill, & Schwartz, 1979; Staple & Ogura, 1966). Laryngeal elevation, another contributor to airway protection by bringing the arytenoid closer to

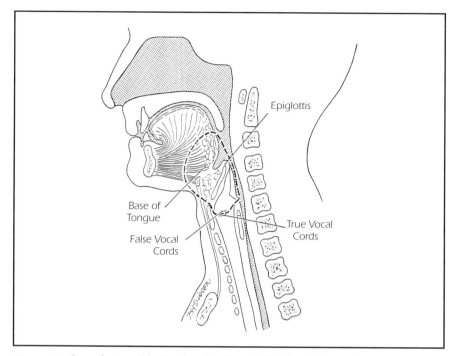

Figure 8.4. Lateral view of the head and neck, with the dotted line indicating supraglottic resection with extension into the base of the tongue.

the tongue base, is also damaged. With the hyoid bone partially or completely removed, laryngeal suspension and elevation are damaged. The super-supraglottic swallow can serve both as a range-of-motion exercise for the tongue base and arytenoid and as a swallow procedure for these patients. The tongue base is also a major pressure generator in the pharynx and must make complete contact with the posterior pharyngeal wall during the pharyngeal swallow. If complete contact is not made, there will be residue in the pharynx that will fall directly into the airway after the swallow, because the patient with a supraglottic laryngectomy has no valleculae and smaller pyriform sinuses than normal.

The supraglottic laryngectomy procedure is sometimes extended either inferiorly or superiorly, depending on the exact location and size of the tumor. If the tumor invades the anterior surface of the epiglottis and extends into the base of the tongue, the supraglottic laryngectomy procedure may be extended up onto and into the base of the tongue, as shown in Figure 8.4, the superior limits of resection being at the foramen cecum. Patients who have had the supraglottic laryngectomy extended into the base of the tongue have a more precipitous drop-off from the tongue into the airway. Thus, food and liquid tend to fall onto the closed airway entrance or, if the airway entrance fails to close, onto the closed true vocal cords (Litton & Leonard, 1969; Staple & Ogura, 1966; Weaver & Fleming, 1978). Also, the elevation of the larynx must be intact so the larynx can adequately deflect material (Ogura, Kawasaki, & Takenouchi, 1964). Jabaley and Hoopes (1969) described a technique for suspending the larynx after resection of the hyomandibular complex. Occasionally, patients with such extended resections may experience reduced lingual movement and control of the bolus so that range-of-motion and bolus control exercises are necessary. Sometimes, the sensation in the larynx is reduced because of the sacrifice of one superior laryngeal nerve, with the cough reflex reduced and the patient unaware of any aspiration that does occur. Occasionally, the pharyngeal swallow may also be delayed.

As shown in Figure 8.5, the supraglottic laryngectomy can also be extended inferiorly to include part of one vocal cord (Ogura & Mallen, 1965). On occasion, this inferior extension may include part or all of one arytenoid cartilage. Because the arytenoids are a major contributor to airway entrance closure in the patient who has undergone a supraglottic laryngectomy, as this inferior extension includes larger amounts of a vocal fold and the arytenoid cartilage, the patient's chances for recovery of normal swallowing without significant chronic

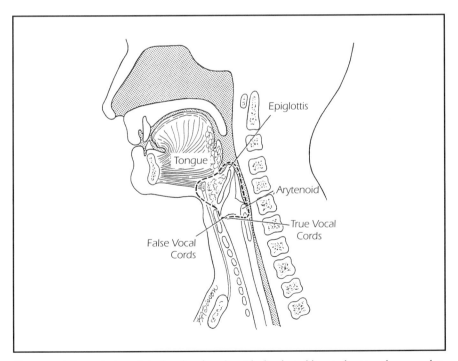

Figure 8.5. Lateral view of the head and neck, with the dotted line indicating the supraglottic resection with extension inferiorly to include an arytenoid cartilage.

aspiration are diminished (Jenkins, Logemann, Lazarus, & Ossoff, 1981; Padovan & Oreskovic, 1975). Long-term follow-up of 25 patients after supraglottic laryngectomy revealed that those patients with a standard supraglottic resection (i.e., a resection that had not been extended into the base of the tongue or the arytenoid cartilages) were able to regain normal swallowing without aspiration *during or after* the swallow (Jenkins et al., 1981). They were able to swallow a normal diet, including liquids and a full range of solid foods, at an average of 1 month after surgery, with some patients taking 3 to 6 months to recover oral intake. In contrast, those patients whose resection was extended to include part or all of the arytenoid cartilage spent a minimum of 2 months and more frequently 6 to 12 months attempting rehabilitation. Several were never able to drink liquids without significant aspiration and always required a tracheostomy tube.

Those patients with extension of the surgery into the tongue base also take significantly longer to return to oral intake (often 6 months or more). Those with larger resections of the tongue base may never be able to gain enough tongue base movement to protect the airway entrance and may need to be converted to a total laryngectomee. Those supraglottic laryngectomy patients who do not have complete closure of the airway entrance at the time swallowing is evaluated postoperatively, may be put on a program of tongue base and arytenoid range-of-motion exercises in an attempt to improve muscle function. In general, these exercises will have an effect within the first 2 to 4 weeks after initiation. If adequate closure of the airway entrance is not attained after 2 to 4 weeks, exercises can be continued, if even slow progress is demonstrated. Some patients will attain successful airway protection 3 to 4 months after surgery if they continue to exercise (Rademaker et al., 1993). Those patients with good tongue base action who are able to learn the sequence of instructions for the super-supraglottic swallow will be rehabilitated and swallow normally, usually within 1 month postoperatively.

One of the criteria for selection of patients to receive a supraglottic laryngectomy is that they must have the capability of relearning a swallowing sequence. Those patients who have mental disorders or who are not able to relearn or follow a sequence of instructions should not be candidates for the supraglottic surgical procedure. If the swallowing therapist questions the patient's learning ability during the preoperative counseling and evaluation procedures, the therapist should ask the patient to go through a series of instructions similar to those for a supraglottic swallow and assess the patient's ability to handle them. If a serious question remains regarding the patient's competence after this trial attempt, the swallowing therapist should speak with the surgeon regarding this patient's candidacy for the procedure.

In a study of recovery of swallow after partial laryngectomy, Rademaker et al. (1993) found that patients who had not achieved oral intake before beginning radiotherapy took significantly longer to attain oral intake. If possible, the onset of postoperative radiotherapy should be delayed until oral intake is reinstated.

Unilateral Laryngeal Tumors

Tumors located on the free margin of one vocal fold with only local extension are usually treated with a *vertical laryngectomy* or *hemilaryngectomy*, or an *extended hemilaryngectomy* (Ogura et al., 1969; Padovan & Oreskovic, 1975; Shumrick & Keith, 1968; Som, 1951). The hemilaryngectomy involves physical removal of one vertical half of the larynx, as shown in Figure 8.6. This resection includes one false vocal fold, one ventricle, and a true vocal fold, usually excluding the arytenoid cartilage, as well as a portion of the thyroid cartilage on the side of the resection. The hyoid bone and epiglottis are usually left intact. The patient who has undergone a typical hemilaryngectomy should experience few difficulties with swallowing postoperatively because some tissue bulk is reconstructed on the

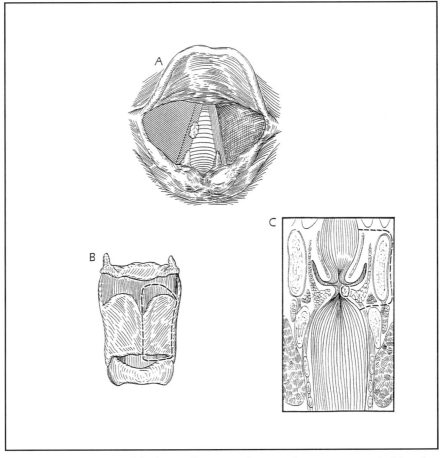

Figure 8.6. Three views of the larynx illustrating the tumor location in a standard hemilaryngectomy (A) and the extent of the surgical resection (B and C).

operated side, against which the unoperated side can attain normal laryngeal clo-sure during swallowing. For normal swallowing, the reconstructed side must be at the same level as the normal vocal fold (Schoenrock, King, Everts, Schnei-der, & Shumrick, 1972; Sessions et al., 1979). Occasionally, these patients expe-rience some temporary difficulty with aspiration during the swallow (Jenkins et al., 1981; Weaver & Fleming, 1978). Usually, tipping the patient's head for-ward to push the epiglottis more posteriorly and narrow the airway entrance (Welch, Logemann, Rademaker, & Kahrilas, 1993) provides sufficient added air-way protection to eliminate all aspiration and allow the patient to resume nor-mal eating. If there is still aspiration with the chin down, head rotation to the operated side may further improve laryngeal closure. The two postures may be combined for best airway protection. Patients usually need to use this chin-down posture for only a few weeks postoperatively.

In many instances, the tumor requires that the hemilaryngectomy procedure be extended either anteriorly or posteriorly. The hemilaryngectomy is known as a vertical laryngectomy because one vertical half of the larynx is removed. How-ever, if the lesion is located anteriorly on one vocal fold, as shown in Figure 8.7, the surgical resection needs to include part or all of the anterior commissure of the larynx. In this case, the hemilaryngectomy becomes a frontolateral laryngec-tomy including approximately one third of the anterior portion of the larynx on both sides. These patients are usually reconstructed with some bulk of tissue on the operated side, possibly taken from the strap muscles, so there is something for the normal true and false vocal folds to contact against. The epiglottis and hyoid bone remain, as do most of the strap muscles, for suspension and elevation of the larynx. Both arytenoid cartilages are present so the constricter mechanism at the level of the true vocal fold is intact. Therefore, these patients will prob-ably be rehabilitated quickly also (within 2 to 3 weeks postoperatively) (Conley, 1960). However, more of them will initially need the chin-down head posture to prevent aspiration during the swallow than patients who have undergone the lesser resection.

The hemilaryngectomy may also be extended further anteriorly into the other vocal cord if the lesion is located even more anteriorly. As shown in Fig-ure 8.8, the resection can be extended along the anterior commissure to include approximately one half of the other side of the larynx. This becomes a three-fourths laryngectomy. Because these patients have their arytenoid cartilages intact, a normal epiglottis and hyoid bone, and tissue bulk placed on the oper-ated side to add bulk, there is usually sufficient constriction at the level of the true vocal folds and at the airway entrance to prevent aspiration. As is true of the extended procedure described previously, these patients often need the chin-down and head rotated postures to regain normal swallowing. Some may also need adduction exercises and/or the super-supraglottic swallow to improve the sphincteric action for airway protection.

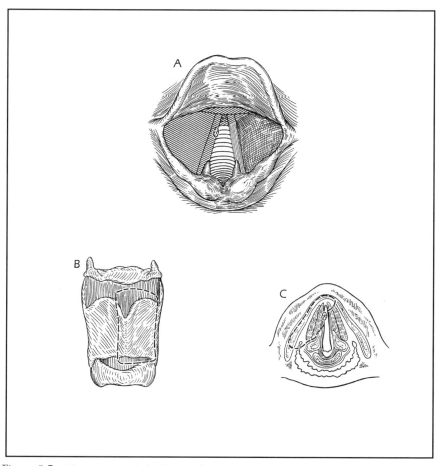

Figure 8.7. Three views of the larynx illustrating the tumor location (A) and resection (B and C) in a hemilaryngectomy extended to include the anterior commissure.

The hemilaryngectomy may also be extended posteriorly to include the arytenoid cartilage if the location of the tumor so dictates, as shown in Figure 8.9. When the arytenoid cartilage is included in the resection, the patient's chances of returning to normal swallowing with no aspiration are greatly decreased (Jenkins et al., 1981; Sessions & Zill, 1979). A long-term follow-up study of 25 patients who had undergone hemilaryngectomy revealed that those patients with a limited resection resumed normal swallowing within 1 week after initiation of oral feeding postoperatively (Jenkins et al., 1981). In contrast, those patients who had undergone extended hemilaryngectomy including arytenoid cartilage, experienced a much longer period of rehabilitation. Several of them were never able to drink liquids by mouth because of aspiration *during* the

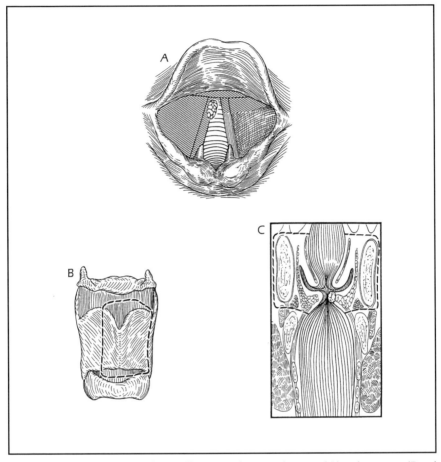

Figure 8.8. Three views of the larynx illustrating the tumor location (A) and resection (B and C) in a frontolateral partial laryngectomy extended to include the anterior commissure and the anterior half of the opposite vocal fold.

swallow and needed a permanent tracheostomy. Patients with an arytenoid included in the resection typically require adduction exercises, as well as a chin-down and head rotated posture to facilitate swallowing without aspiration during the swallow.

A number of other partial laryngectomy procedures involving extensive resection of the vocal folds have been reported (Pearson, 1981; Pearson, Woods, & Hartman, 1980). No physiologic descriptions of these patients' swallowing have been recorded other than surgeons' comments that the patients "swallow adequately." Preventing aspiration is a major problem in any extended partial laryngectomy procedure. If aspiration is controlled by reconstructing a narrow

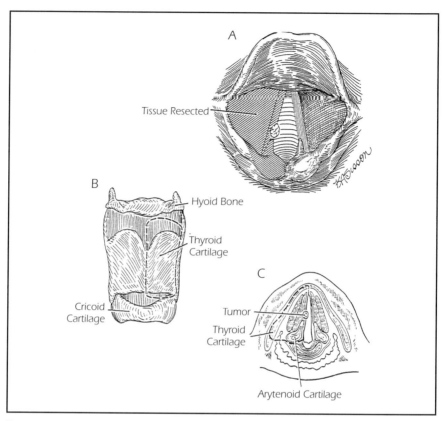

Figure 8.9. Three views of the larynx illustrating the tumor location (A) and resection (B and C) in a hemilaryngectomy extended to include the arytenoid cartilage posteriorly.

glottic chink, the airway is usually compromised and the functional tradeoff for elimination of aspiration is a permanent tracheostomy.

Large Lesions or Those Involving More than One Region of the Larynx

Large lesions (T3 or T4) or lesions involving more than one region of the larynx usually require *total laryngectomy* or *high-dose radiation with or without chemotherapy*. Patients who have undergone total laryngectomy, resulting in physical separation of the gastrointestinal tract from the respiratory tract, do not run the risk of aspiration of food or liquid. However, several types of swallowing problems are reported in total laryngectomy patients. The first appears to relate to the nature of closure of the surgical defect. Postoperatively, some patients have a fold of tissue at the base of the tongue, often called a pseudo-epiglottis, which Davis, Vincent, Shapshay, and Strong (1982) correlated with vertical closure of the surgical defect. These authors hypothesized that the pouchlike recess occurred because the tongue must be stretched in a vertical direction to attain a vertical closure at its base. When, in this case, tension is released, the suture folds on itself, possibly leading to the formation of the pseudoepiglottis. Kirchner, Scatliff, Dey, and Shedd (1963) proposed a second explanation: The suture line at the base of the tongue may break down from tension on the wound edges created by pull of tongue muscles in one direction and of pharyngeal constrictors in the other. Either of these two hypotheses may be correct. However, other factors in the pharyngeal reconstruction may need to be taken into account. Further research is necessary to define the etiology of this fold of tissue.

On lateral fluoroscopy this tissue fold appears as a pseudoepiglottis that forms a pocket at the base of the tongue, collecting food and liquid during swallowing. The effect of this tissue must be examined during deglutition, as it can look deceptively benign when examined at rest when it lies against the tongue base. During swallowing, the contraction of the pharyngeal constrictor muscles pulls the pseudoepiglottic tissue posteriorly, widening the gap at the base of the tongue, and forming a large pocket where food can collect. Thus, a structure that looks deceptively small on mirror examination of the base of the tongue at rest, can widen to essentially occlude the pharynx and prevent material from passing when the patient attempts to swallow. Often, the greater the struggle reaction of the patient, the greater the widening of the pocket and the more severe the difficulty in swallowing. Some total laryngectomees are restricted to a liquid food consistency because of this problem. Treatment is generally surgical resection of the tissue fold.

The second type of swallowing problem that can occur in the total laryngectomee relates to the tightness of the surgical closure. Patients with lesions in the pyriform sinus or extending into the hypopharynx require more extensive resection of pharyngeal mucosa as a part of their total laryngectomy, thus necessitating a tighter closure. Some patients form scar tissue strictures in the esophagus after surgery, which narrow the esophagus sufficiently to prevent any large amount of material or material of thick consistency from passing through the esophagus. The major treatment for this condition in the past has been dilatation. In the dilatation procedure, patients are asked to swallow increasingly larger sized, mercury-filled rubber catheters, which gradually stretch the stricture. However, this treatment has generally been only temporarily successful and has had to be repeated at regular intervals (often monthly). Singer and Blom (1981) described a procedure of pharyngoesophageal myotomy after total laryngectomy to release this scar tissue stricture and permit more normal swallowing. According to Singer and Blom, this procedure may also impact on the patient's ability to put air in and out of the esophagus to produce esophageal voice. There are no exercises to improve such a stricture. Sometimes, however, changing head positions such as head rotation will stretch and open a strictured or narrow area if dilatation or surgery is not feasible. Both a pseudoepiglottis and a stricture can result in backflow of food as the patient struggles to swallow.

If total laryngectomy includes pharyngectomy or esophagectomy with reconstruction by distal flap, stomach pull-up, or jejunal graft, greater swallowing problems can occur, including backflow of food upward into the nose or mouth (Logemann, 1983b; McConnel, Hester, Mendelsohn, & Logemann, 1988). These disorders can sometimes be managed by postural change (i.e., extending the neck or head rotation to stretch the reconstructed tissues). If a total laryngectomy patient has not returned to full preoperative diet at 2 months postoperation, a radiographic study of the oropharyngeal and cervical esophageal aspects of swallow should be completed to identify any structural abnormalities. A pseudoepiglottis may be surgically removed while a stricture may be dilated. It is critical that these disorders be assessed physiologically as they can appear quite benign on anatomic examination. If a total laryngectomy patient complains of swallowing problems months or years after surgery, particularly if he or she had been eating well, the person should return to the surgeon immediately, as this may be a sign of recurrence of the disease. Differing functional deficits clearly result from partial laryngectomy, total laryngectomy, or radiotherapy for laryngeal cancer (Logemann, 1983a, 1989, 1993; McConnel et al., 1988; McConnel, Mendelsohn, & Logemann, 1986; Ogura et al., 1964; Rademaker et al., 1993).

Over the years, a number of surgical and prosthetic voice rehabilitation techniques have been attempted on total laryngectomy patients (Rush, 1981; Shedd & Weinberg, 1980; Woods & Pearson, 1980). In all of these procedures, some method of reconnecting pulmonary airflow to the pharyngoesophagus was attempted. A major problem with most of these techniques has been the aspiration of food into the trachea from the esophagus. One of these procedures, the Staffieri neoglottis procedure (Leipzig, Griffiths, & Shea, 1980; Staffieri, 1981), resulted in aspiration in a majority of patients, so the procedure has essentially been discontinued.

The most continuously successful surgical prosthetic procedure, the tracheoesophageal puncture procedure (Blom, Singer, & Hamaker, 1982; Singer & Blom, 1980), involves placement of a small flexible prosthesis into a puncture wound made at 12 o'clock on the patient's stoma that connects the trachea with the esophagus below the level of the vibratory segment. The small prosthesis placed in the puncture wound prevents the backflow of material from the esophagus into the trachea, so aspiration is eliminated. In addition, the trachealus muscle tends to form a tight seal at the puncture site around the prosthesis, diminishing backflow of material into the trachea from the esophagus around the outside of the prosthesis. Because aspiration is eliminated, the tracheoesophageal puncture procedure and a similar technique, the Panje procedure

(Panje, 1981), are the most uniformly successful procedures that have been attempted to rapidly restore optimum voice to total laryngectomy patients post-operatively. If patients who have undergone any of these procedures aspirate, there is generally no exercise program that will change their aspiration. In the case of Singer and Blom's (1980) procedure, the surgeon can cauterize the puncture site to narrow it so the prosthesis better fills the puncture tract.

Patients who are candidates for the Singer–Blom procedure may need a myotomy for prevention of pharyngospasm. This type of myotomy involves a much broader cutting of the pharyngeal musculature than the cricopharyngeal myotomy described later in this book. After the cricopharyngeal myotomy procedure, the patient may experience diffuse pharyngeal residue, whereas those who receive a neurectomy may have residue limited to the tongue base (Pauloski, Blom, Logemann, & Hamaker, 1995). A neurectomy involves cutting the innervation to the pharyngeal wall musculature rather than cutting the musculature itself. Both procedures are utilized to eliminate pharyngospasm or contraction of the pharyngeal musculature in response to airflow introduced below it. Pharyngospasm is a functional phenomenon and is not structural; that is, it is not present except when air is introduced into the pharynx from below.

After total laryngectomy, the patient will experience some minor changes in swallowing (Logemann, 1983b) and perceive some increase in lingual effort. In fact, after total laryngectomy, patients do increase lingual pressures to compensate for the absence of the larynx and reduced pharyngeal wall function post-operatively (McConnel et al., 1986). Usually, this change is minor and patients resume a full diet within 1 to 2 months postoperatively.

Radiotherapy

If treated with radiotherapy for a small (T1 or T2) tumor, laryngeal cancer patients may experience only temporary voice change, including hoarseness or vocal roughness, which improves in the month or two following completion of radiotherapy. Patients may also experience very small changes in saliva flow, depending upon the exact focus of the radiotherapy. Rarely do these patients complain of swallowing disorders.

Currently, some patients who would otherwise receive a total laryngectomy are receiving high-dose radiation therapy (6,000 to 7,000 cGy), with or without chemotherapy. The radiation field in these patients is usually similar to that delivered to the patient with a tonsil or base of tongue tumor (i.e., the field extends from the oropharynx to the top of the esophagus). After these combined aggressive protocols with radiotherapy and chemotherapy, advanced laryngeal cancer patients often exhibit significantly reduced laryngeal elevation and reduced pharyngeal wall motion during swallow, which impair both the efficiency and safety of their swallow. Laryngeal movement up and forward is critical to normal closure of the laryngeal entrance and opening of the upper esophageal sphincter (UES) (Kahrilas, Dodds, Dent, Logemann, & Shaker, 1988; Logemann et al., 1992). These effects may begin during the course of radiotherapy or any time thereafter, including years later. These changes are believed to occur because of the process of fibrosis resulting from damage to capillaries feeding muscle fibers in the radiated area. The severity of these disorders will vary from patient to patient. Patients may be taught exercises to improve laryngeal motion (the falsetto exercise and the Mendelsohn maneuver) and to take volitional control over airway closure and UES opening (Kahrilas, Logemann, Krugler, & Flanagan, 1991; Lazarus et al., 1996; Logemann, 1993). Exercise programs can improve laryngeal elevation after radiotherapy, sometimes years later, and can restore oral intake to patients who have been forced to eliminate thicker foods from their diet or to resort to nonoral feeding. In some cases, however, severe dysphagia remains. To date we are unable to predict which patients will respond well to exercise programs.

General Guidelines for Swallowing Therapy with Treated Laryngeal Cancer Patients

Laryngeal cancer patients should be counseled prior to treatment by the speech and swallowing therapist. The therapist should ensure that the patient is aware that posttreatment changes may occur in his or her voice and swallowing. The exact nature of these changes is often not known until after surgery or radiotherapy, but the patient should be told to anticipate the need for some swallowing therapy postoperatively, and helped to realize the importance of his or her participation in any exercise program that may be needed posttreatment. Rehabilitation is much more difficult if the patient is unaware of his or her ultimate responsibility and the need to work actively to rehabilitate his or her swallowing as well as his or her communication. It is usually advisable for the radiated patient to begin range-of-motion exercises for the tongue base and laryngeal elevation before or at the beginning of radiotherapy and to do the exercises 5 to 10 times daily for 10 minutes each time. Patients should continue these exercises throughout radiotherapy and for a good while afterward to maintain as much movement as possible.

Postoperatively, the swallowing therapist should review the patient's chart and determine the exact extent of the resection and the nature of the reconstruction and/or the exact plan for radiotherapy. As indicated previously, the resection and reconstruction will determine the patient's functional capacity after surgery. In the case of the surgically treated patient, an exercise program can begin when the surgeon indicates that the suture lines will withstand the pressure of swallowing. First, a videofluoroscopic examination of swallowing should be conducted to assess the patient's functioning and define the optimal therapy regimen. Based on this fluoroscopic study, many patients will be able to resume normal eating within the same day if their swallowing is found to be functional or normal. If, despite all trial therapy attempts to increase the force and coordination of muscle function, pharyngeal and/or laryngeal physiology is still abnormal and aspiration is significant *before, during, and/or after* the swallow, an exercise program will be necessary before actual oral feeding is begun. Usually, the duration of the exercise program should be no more than 2 to 4 weeks before maximum function is attained. However, some patients will slowly improve over many months and be able to resume oral feeding 1 to 2 years after surgery (Staple & Ogura, 1966). Patients should be seen daily in the hospital for swallowing therapy and be followed weekly after hospital discharge as necessary. Throughout this therapy regimen it is important for the entire team of professionals seeing the patient to cooperate in the swallowing rehabilitation. It is necessary to continually reinforce the patient's swallowing practice. Consistent support of the nursing service and the physicians involved with the patient is very important. Difficulties arise if two or three different professionals give the patient different advice about his or her problems. The best swallowing rehabilitation occurs when a single set of instructions is given to the patient and reinforced by all professionals caring for the patient.

References

Aguilar, N. V., Olson, M. L., & Shedd, D. P. (1979). Rehabilitation of deglutition problems in patients with head and neck cancer. *American Journal of Surgery, 138*, 501–507.

Alonso, J. (1947). Conservative surgery of cancer of the larynx. *Transactions American Academy Ophthalmology, 51*, 633–642.

Blom, E., Singer, M., & Hamaker, R. A. (1982, May). *Tracheostoma valve for postlaryngectomy voice rehabilitation.* Paper presented at the American Broncho-esophagological Association annual meeting, Palm Beach, FL.

Conley, J. (1960). Swallowing dysfunctions associated with radical surgery of the head and neck. *Archives of Surgery, 80*, 602–612.

Davis, R., Vincent, M., Shapshay, S., & Strong, M. (1982). The anatomy and complications of "T" versus vertical closure of the hypopharynx after laryngectomy. *Laryngoscope, 92*, 16–22.

Goepfert, H., Lindberg, R., & Jesse, R. (1981). Combined laryngeal conservation surgery and irradiation: Can we expand the indications for conservation therapy? *Otolaryngology—Head and Neck Surgery, 89*, 974–978.

Jabaley, M., & Hoopes, J. (1969). A simple technique for laryngeal suspension after partial or complete resection of the hyomandibular complex. *American Journal of Surgery, 118*, 685–690.

Jenkins, P., Logemann, J., Lazarus, C. & Ossoff, R. (1981). *Functional changes after hemilaryngectomy.* Paper presented at the American Speech-Language-Hearing Association annual meeting, Los Angeles.

Kahrilas, P., Dodds, W., Dent, J., Logemann, J., & Shaker, R. (1988). Upper esophageal sphincter function during deglutition. *Gastroenterology, 95*, 52–62.

Kahrilas, P. J., Logemann, J. A., Krugler, C., & Flanagan, E. (1991). Volitional augmentation of upper esophageal sphincter opening during swallowing. *American Journal of Physiology, 260 (Gastrointestinal Physiology, 23)*, G450–G456.

Kirchner, J., Scatliff, J., Dey, F., & Shedd, D. (1963). The pharynx after laryngectomy. *Laryngoscope, 73*, 18–33.

Lazarus, C. L., Logemann, J. A., Pauloski, B. R., Colangelo, L. A., Kahrilas, P. J., Mittal, B. B., & Pierce, M. (1966). Swallowing disorders in head and neck cancer patients treated with radiotherapy and adjuvant chemotherapy. *Laryngoscope, 106*, 1157–1166.

Leipzig, B., Griffiths, C., & Shea, J. (1980). Neoglottic reconstruction following total laryngectomy. *Annals of Otolaryngology, 89*, 204–208.

Litton, W., & Leonard, J. (1969). Aspiration after partial laryngectomy: Cineradiographic studies. *Laryngoscope, 79*, 888–908.

Logemann, J. (1983a). *Evaluation and treatment of swallowing disorders*. Austin, TX: PRO-ED.

Logemann, J. A. (1983b). Speech therapy after extensive surgery for post cricoid carcinoma. In Y. Edels (Ed.), *Vocal rehabilitation after laryngectomy* (pp. 233–248). London: Croom Helm.

Logemann, J. (1989). Deglutition disorders in cancer of the head and neck. In A. R. Kagan & J. Miles (Eds.), *Head and neck oncology* (pp. 155–161). Elmsford, NY: Pergamon Press.

Logemann, J. (1993). *Manual for the videofluoroscopic study of swallowing* (2nd ed.). Austin, TX: PRO-ED.

Logemann, J. A., Gibbons, P., Rademaker, A. W., Pauloski, B. R., Kahrilas, P. J., Bacon, M., Bowman, J., & McCracken, E. (1994). Mechanisms of recovery after supraglottic laryngectomy. *Journal of Speech and Hearing Research, 37*, 965–974.

Logemann, J. A., Kahrilas, P. J., Cheng, J., Pauloski, B. R., Gibbons, P. J., Rademaker, A. W., & Lin, S. (1992). Closure mechanisms of the laryngeal vestibule during swallow. *American Journal of Physiology, 262 (Gastrointestinal Physiology, 25)*, G338–G344.

McConnel, F. M. S., Hester, T. R., Mendelsohn, M. S., & Logemann, J. A. (1988). Manofluorography of deglutition after total laryngopharyngectomy. *Plastic and Reconstructive Surgery, 81*, 346–351.

McConnel, F. M. S., Mendelsohn, M. S., & Logemann, J. A. (1986). Examination of swallowing after total laryngectomy using manofluorography. *Head & Neck Surgery, 9*, 3–12.

Ogura, J. (1955). Surgical pathology of cancer of the larynx. *Laryngoscope, 65*, 868–926.

Ogura, J., Biller, H., Calcaterra, T., & Davis, W. (1969). Surgical treatment of carcinoma of the larynx, pharynx, base of tongue and cervical esophagus. *International Surgery, 52*, 29–40.

Ogura, J., Kawasaki, M., & Takenouchi, S. (1964). Neurophysiologic observations on the adaptive mechanism of deglutition. *Annals of Otology, Rhinology, and Laryngology, 73*, 1062–1081.

Ogura, J., & Mallen, R. (1965). Partial laryngectomy for supraglottic and pharyngeal carcinoma. *Transactions of the American Academy of Ophthalmology and Otolaryngology, 69*, 832–845.

Padovan, I. F., & Oreskovic, M. (1975). Functional evaluation after partial resection in patients with carcinoma of the larynx. *Laryngoscope, 85*, 626–638.

Panje, W. (1981). Prosthetic vocal rehabilitation following laryngectomy: The voice button. *Annals of Otology, Rhinology and Laryngology, 90*, 116–120.

Pauloski, B. R., Blom, E. D., Logemann, J. A., & Hamaker, R. C. (1995). Functional outcome after surgery for prevention of pharyngospasms in trachoesophageal speakers: Part II. Swallow characteristics. *Laryngoscope, 105,* 1104–1110.

Pearson, B. (1981). Subtotal laryngectomy. *Laryngoscope, 91,* 1904–1912.

Pearson, B., Woods, R., & Hartman, D. (1980). Extended hemilaryngectomy for T3 glottic carcinoma with preservation of speech and swallowing. *Laryngoscope, 90,* 1950–1961.

Pfister, D. G., Strong, E. W., Harrison, L. B., Haines, I. E., Pfister, D. A., Sessions, R., Spiro, R., Shah, J., Gerold, F., McLure, T., Vikram, B., Fass, D., Armstrong, J., & Bosl, G. J. (1991). Larynx preservation with combined chemotherapy in advanced but resectable head and neck cancer. *Journal of Clinical Oncology, 9,* 850–859.

Powers, W., Ogura, J., & Holtz, S. (1963). Contrast examination of the larynx and pharynx. *New York State Journal of Medicine, 63,* 1163–1173.

Pressman, J. (1954). Cancer of the larynx: Laryngoplasty to avoid laryngectomy. *Archives of Otolaryngology, 59,* 355–412.

Rademaker, A. W., Logemann, J. A., Pauloski, B. R., Bowman, J., Lazarus, C., Sisson, G., Milianti, F., Graner, D., Cook, B., Collins, S., Stein, D., Beery, Q., Johnson, J., & Baker, T. (1993). Recovery of postoperative swallowing in patients undergoing partial laryngectomy. *Head & Neck, 15,* 325–334.

Rush, B. (1981). New voices for old: Attempts to create a new larynx in the post-laryngectomy patient. *Surgical Rounds, 4,* 16–22.

Schoenrock, L., King, A., Everts, E., Schneider, H., & Shumrick, D. (1972). Hemilaryngectomy: Deglutition evaluation and rehabilitation. *Transactions of the Academy of Ophthalmology and Otolaryngology, 76,* 752–757.

Sessions, D., Zill, R., & Schwartz, J. (1979). Deglutition after conservation surgery for cancer of the larynx and hypopharynx. *Otolaryngology—Head and Neck Surgery, 87,* 779–796.

Shedd, D., & Weinberg, B. (Eds.). (1980). *Surgical and prosthetic approaches to speech rehabilitation.* Boston: G. K. Hall Medical.

Shumrick, D., & Keith, R. (1968). *Conservation surgery of the larynx.* Scientific exhibit at the American Speech-Hearing Association, annual meeting, Denver.

Singer, M., & Blom, E. (1980). An endoscopic technique for restoration of voice after laryngectomy. *Annals of Otology, Rhinology and Laryngology, 89,* 529–533.

Singer, M., & Blom, E. (1981). Selective myotomy for voice restoration after total laryngectomy. *Archives of Otolaryngology, 107,* 670–673.

Som, M. (1951). Hemilaryngectomy—A modified technique for cordal carcinoma with extension posteriorly. *Archives of Otolaryngology, 54,* 524–533.

Staffieri, M. (1981). Phonatory neoglottis surgery. *Ear, Nose and Throat Journal, 60,* 254–258.

Staple, T., & Ogura, J. (1966). Cineradiography of the swallowing mechanism following supraglottic subtotal laryngectomy. *Radiology, 87,* 226–230.

U.S. Department of Health, Education, and Welfare. (1979). *Management guidelines for head and neck cancer.* Washington, DC: Author.

U.S. Department of Veterans Affairs Laryngeal Cancer Study Group. (1991). Induction chemotherapy plus radiation in patients with advanced laryngeal cancer. *New England Journal of Medicine, 324,* 1685–1690.

Weaver, A., & Fleming, S. (1978). Partial laryngectomy: Analysis of associated swallowing disorders. *American Journal of Surgery, 136*, 486–489.

Weiss, M. H. (1993). Head and neck cancer and the quality of life [Editorial]. *Otolaryngology—Head and Neck Surgery, 108*, 311–312.

Welch, M. V., Logemann, J. A., Rademaker, A. W., & Kahrilas, P. J. (1993). Changes in pharyngeal dimensions effected by chin tuck. *Archives of Physical Medicine and Rehabilitation, 74*, 178–181.

Woods, R., & Pearson, B. (1980). Alaryngeal speech and development of an internal tracheopharyngeal fistula. *Otolaryngology—Head and Neck Surgery, 88*, 64–73.

INTRODUCTION TO CHAPTERS 9 AND 10: SWALLOWING DISORDERS CAUSED BY NEUROLOGIC IMPAIRMENTS

Two types of neurologic disorders affect swallowing: conditions that occur suddenly and from which the patient can be expected to recover at least in part, such as stroke, head trauma, or spinal cord injury, and conditions that are degenerative in nature and will cause gradual deterioration in swallowing ability over time. Management questions for the two groups of patients differ. In the case of patients whose swallowing disorder can be expected to improve, questions to be answered include the following: What treatment should be initiated to normalize the patient's swallowing physiology? Will the patient be able to eat a normal diet, and, if so, when? Is the patient's recovery typical for individuals with this type of lesion? What other factors may interact with the neurologic damage to worsen the dysphagia?

In cases of degenerative disease, the questions include the following: Are there typical changes in swallowing that occur at the onset of each disease and that can be used to identify the disease entity? Are there progressive and predictable changes in swallowing physiology characteristic of each lesion location? How long can the patient continue to eat by mouth before nonoral feeding may be necessary? What techniques can prolong oral feeding for the patient?

General Considerations in Management of Patients with Swallowing Disorders Due to a Neurologic Disorder

In all patients with a neurologic disorder, sensitivity to aspiration appears to be significantly reduced, as indicated by their frequent failure to cough. If they do cough, the coughing may not be productive in clearing aspirated material. Many of these patients of all etiologies are unaware of their swallowing disturbances and deny any swallowing problem, yet videofluoroscopy may reveal that the patient is aspirating a significant portion of every bolus swallowed. Apparently, many neurologic conditions affect the patient's sensory feedback regarding position of food in the vocal tract and entry of food into the airway. Whereas many other types of patients are aware of residual material in the pharynx, many patients with neurologic impairments do not have this awareness. They often do not dry swallow to clear this material. Thus, in assessing and treating the patient with neurologic impairment, the swallowing therapist must be constantly aware of the potential for silent aspiration.

A study by Aviv and colleagues (1996) indicates that dysphagic stroke patients exhibit reduced pharyngeal and supraglottic sensation as compared with age-matched normal controls. It is quite likely that dysphagic patients with other types of neurologic disorders, whether of sudden onset or degenerative nature, also have poor sensation in the upper aerodigestive tract. Unfortunately, direct sensory testing of many of these patients is not possible because of their cognitive and/or language problems. Indirect evidence of sensory loss is available from the patient's reaction to the presence of residual food in the pharynx after the swallow. If the patient does not display the normal reaction to residual food (i.e., to dry swallow quickly to clear the food out of the pharynx), this is an indirect indicator of reduced pharyngeal sensory awareness. Reduced reaction to aspiration or residue may also occur because of desensitization by the presence of aspiration and/or residue chronically.

Fatigue throughout the day or throughout a meal may also affect swallowing function in a patient with dysphagia of neurogenic etiology. Observation of the patient at various times of the day may be important, as different strategies for dysphagia management may be needed. If significant changes in function related to fatigue are suspected, the clinician should complete the fatigue test as a part of a modified barium swallow. If the patient fatigues easily, use of swallow maneuvers may not be appropriate as they will usually increase the patient's fatigue. More frequent, smaller meals can often be helpful. Other therapy procedures, such as postural changes, heightening preswallow sensory input, and diet changes, may also be appropriate.

Evaluation of the Neurologic Patient in the Intensive Care Unit

In many instances, the swallowing therapist will be asked to evaluate patients with neurologic impairments while they are still in the intensive care unit. If the patient is intubated, swallowing assessment should wait until the patient is extubated. One study indicates that it may take up to 1 week for the pharyngeal swallow to be triggered normally after extubation (DeLarminat, Montravers, Dureuil, & Desmonte, 1995). Occasionally, patients need to be evaluated when they are comatose. Several techniques can be used to assess the swallowing function of the patient with severe impairment while putting the patient at minimal risk for aspiration or pulmonary complications. First, the swallowing therapist can evaluate the frequency of swallowing and the apparent strength of the pharyngeal swallow by resting a hand lightly on the submandibular and laryngeal areas of the neck. This is described in the section of Chapter 5 on evaluating the pharyngeal swallow at the bedside. Resting the fingers on these structures for a period of 5 or 10 minutes allows the swallowing therapist to assess the frequency of swallowing and the strength of laryngeal elevation that indicates triggering of the pharyngeal swallow. Alternatively, the clinician can use surface electromyography to assess frequency of swallowing. A surface electrode can be placed over the submandibular muscles under the chin and/or on the neck above the thyroid cartilage, over the laryngeal elevator muscles. These electrodes record muscle activity during the swallow and enable the clinician to observe swallowing frequency over a longer period.

Simultaneous with observation of swallowing frequency, the therapist can assess how the patient handles his or her own secretions. If necessary, the therapist can then open the patient's mouth and attempt thermal–tactile stimulation of the pharyngeal swallow using the ice cold laryngeal mirror, size 00. Any muscle contractions in response to the stimulation may be evaluated. After repeated thermal–tactile stimulation to the base of the anterior faucial arch, the swallowing therapist may position a very small amount of liquid, generally iced ginger ale, with a straw at the base of the anterior arch. The therapist then assesses the reaction of the mechanism to the presentation of liquid and determines whether the pharyngeal swallow is triggered. If the patient is able to follow directions, a complete bedside examination can be carried out, including assessment of the functional status of each vocal tract structure during volitional and reflexive movement.

On the basis of the results of this examination, the swallowing therapist may ask the patient to repeat several more swallows of small amounts of material. If the patient is unable to follow directions, the swallowing therapist may be able to perform some informal observational assessments of vocal tract function. This full examination involves giving the patient less than ⅓ teaspoon of liquid and should not increase the patient's risk of pulmonary complications. It is not recommended that the patient be given any larger amount of material until a radiographic examination can confirm the success of the swallowing pattern. Although some clinicians recommend an aggressive swallowing rehabilitation program to reinitiate oral feeding with very ill or comatose patients in the intensive care unit, the present state of the art in bedside assessment of the functional status of these patients makes the chances for success of such an assessment in this patient population particularly poor and may place the patient at unwarranted risk. These patients can be given a radiographic study if they can be positioned in the fluorographic equipment while positioned on a gurney (cart) with their back elevated and supported, and if a nurse, resident, or physician accompanies them to the study in case of any medical complications. My colleagues and I at Northwestern University have successfully assessed over 500 noncomatose patients from intensive care in this way, including those on mechanical ventilation, and have had no complications.

References

Aviv, J. E., Martin, J. H., Sacco, R. L., Zagar, D., Diamond, B., Keen, M. S., & Blitzer, A. (1996). Supraglottic and pharyngeal sensory abnormalities in stroke patients with dysphagia. *Annals of Otology, Rhinology, and Laryngology, 105*, 92–97.

DeLarminat, V., Montravers, P., Dureuil, B., & Desmonte, J. M. (1995). Alteration in swallowing reflex after extubation in intensive care unit patients. *Critical Care Medicine, 23*, 486–488.

C H A P T E R 9

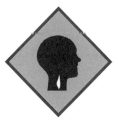

SWALLOWING DISORDERS CAUSED BY NEUROLOGIC LESIONS FROM WHICH SOME RECOVERY CAN BE ANTICIPATED

A number of types of sudden-onset neurologic conditions may result in swallowing disorders, from which some degree of recovery can be anticipated: stroke, closed head trauma, cervical spinal cord injury, anterior cervical fusion, neurosurgical procedures affecting the brainstem and cranial nerves, poliomyelitis, Guillain-Barré syndrome, and congenital neurologic damage.

Swallowing Problems After Stroke

Swallowing problems have been reported in patients who have suffered unilateral or bilateral brainstem, cortical, and subcortical strokes (Donner, 1974; Kilman & Goyal, 1976; Logemann et al., 1993; Meadows, 1973; Robbins & Levine, 1988). Typically, patients who have suffered an infarct limited to the posterior cortex with no motor component will not experience swallowing difficulties unless the posterior lesion creates sufficient edema to affect the anterior cortex.

There is indirect evidence from videofluorographic studies of oropharyngeal swallowing and direct evidence from initial studies of pharyngeal sensation that stroke patients have some degree of sensory loss in the pharynx (Aviv et al., 1996; Horner, Massey, Riski, Lathrop, & Chase, 1988). On videofluorographic studies, stroke patients often do not respond normally to oral and/or pharyngeal residue (i.e., they do not attempt to dry swallow in response to residue). When asked if there is any food left in their pharynx, they often indicate that they do not feel anything there.

Swallow Disorders by Site of Lesion

Knowledge of swallow abnormalities resulting from stroke at specific sites in the central nervous system is still evolving (Barer, 1989; Celifarco, Gerard, Faegenburg, & Burakoff, 1990; Delgado, 1988; Logemann & Kahrilas, 1990; Meadows, 1973; Robbins & Levine, 1988; Smith & Dodd, 1990; Wade & Hewer, 1987). However, there is adequate information to begin to understand the types of swallow disorders exhibited by patients with isolated lesions in the brainstem, subcortical regions, and left and right hemispheres of the cerebral cortex. The following discussion is based on data from studies of patients at 3 weeks poststroke at Northwestern Memorial Hospital and the Rehabilitation Institute of Chicago who suffered a single infarct with no prior history of stroke or other neurologic disorders or damage to the head and neck, and who have been otherwise apparently healthy until their stroke. Medical complications, preexisting medical problems, and medications can affect the severity of swallowing problems poststroke, as discussed in the later section titled Effects of Other Factors on Swallowing Function and Recovery in the Stroke Patient.

Effects of Lesions in the Lower Brainstem (the Medulla)

Lesions in the lower brainstem (medullary region) generally result in significant oropharyngeal swallow impairment because of the location of the major swallow centers (nucleus tractus solitarius and nucleus ambiguous) within the medulla (Jean & Car, 1979; Miller, 1982). Patients with unilateral medullary lesions typically exhibit functional or near-normal oral control with significantly impaired triggering and neuromotor control of the pharyngeal swallow. Specifically, these patients often exhibit what appears to be an absent pharyngeal swallow in the first week poststroke. In fact, this may be a very weak pharyngeal swallow, so weak it is not recognized as a swallow. As the pharyngeal swallow begins to appear (usually in the second week poststroke), there is a significant delay in triggering the pharyngeal swallow (often 10 to 15 seconds or more). Thermal–tactile stimulation can be helpful (Lazzara, Lazarus, & Logemann, 1986). If lingual function is relatively normal, the patient can propel material from the mouth into the pharynx using tongue movement. Material then falls into the valleculae or pyriform sinuses and rests there unless it dislodges and falls into the open airway. These patients may exhibit much voluntary submandibular, tongue base, and hyoid bone movement in their efforts to propel material from the oral cavity with the tongue. These efforts can be highly misleading when evaluating the triggering of the pharyngeal swallow clinically and can occasionally be mistaken for the hyoid and laryngeal movement that occurs as a result of triggering of the pharyngeal swallow.

When the pharyngeal swallow triggers, these patients usually exhibit (1) reduced laryngeal elevation and anterior motion, which contributes to reduced opening of the cricopharyngeal region, with the symptom of residual food collecting in the pyriform sinuses, particularly on one side, and (2) unilateral pharyngeal weakness, which further contributes to the residual food remaining in the pyriform sinus on one side and reduced cricopharyngeal opening because bolus pressure contributes to cricopharyngeal opening. Some patients also exhibit unilateral adductor vocal fold paresis (Jacob, Kahrilas, Logemann, Shah, & Ha, 1989; Kahrilas, Logemann, Krugler, & Flanagan, 1991). Whereas these patients often exhibit significant dysphagia requiring nonoral intake at 1 to 2 weeks poststroke, but by 3 weeks poststroke their swallow has often recovered sufficiently to be functional and allow full oral intake. In general, the more severe the swallow abnormalities at 2 to 3 weeks postictus and the more medical complications present, the longer the swallow recovery period. After medullary stroke, some patients with a number of complicating factors will not recover functional swallowing for 4 to 6 months poststroke. Therapeutically, these patients benefit from thermal–tactile stimulation for the absent or delayed pharyngeal swallow, head rotation to the side of the pharyngeal weakness, and the Mendelsohn maneuver (Logemann, Kahrilas, Kobara, & Vakil, 1989). They also benefit from range-of-motion exercises for laryngeal elevation (Logemann & Kahrilas, 1990; Robbins & Levine, 1993).

Sometimes, brainstem stroke patients are considered for cricopharyngeal myotomy. This procedure is discussed in Chapter 11. In general, patients who have suffered a brainstem stroke should not be considered for cricopharyngeal myotomy until at least 6 months after their stroke so that adequate time is allotted for recovery. The vast majority of patients with a cricopharyngeal problem following brainstem stroke have a reduction in laryngeal motion rather than any spasticity in the cricopharyngeal muscle portion of the cricopharyngeal or upper esophageal sphincter.

Examination of pharyngeal swallow measures at 12 and 24 weeks poststroke in medullary stroke patients whose swallow was functional at 3 weeks postictus at Northwestern Memorial Hospital reveals that, although their swallow is functional (i.e., they are eating a full, normal diet orally with no aspiration and only small amounts of residue in the pyriform sinuses), their measures of pharyngeal movement during swallow are outside the normal range for individuals of their age and gender.

Effects of High Brainstem (Pontine) Stroke

A high brainstem stroke in the region of the pons generally leaves the patient with severe hypertonicity. This hypertonicity manifests itself in the pharynx as a delay in triggering of the pharyngeal swallow or an absent pharyngeal swallow, a unilateral spastic pharyngeal wall paresis or paralysis, and reduced laryngeal elevation with a severe cricopharyngeal dysfunction. These patients often do not respond typically to head rotation. The rotation may need to be tried toward each side to define which works best. Also, thermal–tactile stimulation may be helpful but may also increase oropharyngeal muscle tone. Recovery in these patients can be quite slow and difficult. Massage to reduce muscle tone in the buccal musculature and in the neck may be helpful prior to initiating swallowing therapy in each session.

Effects of Subcortical Stroke

Subcortical lesions may affect motor as well as sensory pathways to and from the cortex. Subcortical stroke usually results in mild delays (3 to 5 seconds) in oral transit time, mild delays (3 to 5 seconds) in triggering the pharyngeal swallow, and mild to moderate impairments in timing of the neuromuscular components of the pharyngeal swallow (Logemann et al., 1993). A small number of these patients exhibit aspiration before the swallow as a result of the pharyngeal swallow delay or after the swallow because of the impairment in neuromuscular control in the pharynx. Their recovery of full oral intake may take 3 to 6 weeks poststroke if no medical complications are present, and longer if medical problems, such as diabetes or pneumonia, are present. Swallowing therapy directed at improving the triggering of the pharyngeal swallow and improving range of motion of the larynx and tongue base is usually beneficial.

Effects of Stroke in the Cerebral Cortex

Patients with lesions in the left or right hemisphere of the cerebral cortex display differences in swallow function. Swallowing disorders characteristic of various areas within each hemisphere have not been well defined to date. Stroke within the *anterior left hemisphere* of the cerebral cortex can result in apraxia of swallow, which can range from mild to severe, and usually, but not always, accompanies some degree of oral apraxia. Apraxia of swallow is characterized by delay in initiating the oral swallow with no tongue motion in response to presentation of a bolus in the mouth or by mild to severe searching motions of the tongue prior to initiating the swallow. Generally, patients with swallow apraxia exhibit better swallow function when feeding themselves and eating automatically without any verbal commands to swallow. Left cortical stroke patients also usually exhibit mild oral transit delays (3 to 5 seconds) and mild delays in triggering the pharyngeal swallow (2 to 3 seconds). Usually, the pharyngeal swallow itself is motorically normal in these patients. Sensory enhancement procedures, such as increasing bolus taste, increasing pressure of the spoon on the tongue, and thermal–tactile stimulation, are frequently most helpful in speeding the swallow in patients with swallow apraxia.

In contrast to the left cortical stroke patient, the patient who has suffered a stroke in the *right hemisphere* usually exhibits mild oral transit delays (2 to 3 seconds) and slightly longer pharyngeal delays (3 to 5 seconds). When the pharyngeal swallow triggers in these patients, laryngeal elevation may be slightly delayed, contributing to aspiration before or as the pharyngeal swallow is triggering. Therapeutically, these patients benefit from the chin-down posture and thermal–tactile stimulation for the pharyngeal delay. Some of these patients can use a supraglottic or super-supraglottic swallow to protect the airway during the delay. They may also need range-of-motion exercises to improve laryngeal elevation. Despite both verbal and physical prompting, the right hemisphere patient may have difficulty integrating therapy or compensatory strategies into oral feeding, including postural compensations such as the chin-down position, because of cognitive disorders and relative inattention. For this reason, patients suffering right cortical strokes may be later in returning to oral intake than patients who have suffered left cortical strokes.

Effects of Multiple Strokes

Patients who have suffered multiple strokes often exhibit more significant swallowing abnormalities. Their oral function may be slower, with many repetitive tongue movements and oral transit times of over 5 seconds. Delay in triggering the pharyngeal swallow is also usually more severe, taking over 5 seconds. When the pharyngeal swallow triggers, these patients may exhibit reduced laryngeal elevation and reduced closure of the laryngeal vestibule/entryway, resulting in penetration of food into the laryngeal entrance, as well as unilateral weakness of the pharyngeal wall, resulting in residual food remaining on the pharyngeal wall and in the pyriform sinus on the affected side. Often, their attention is affected and their ability to utilize therapy strategies and to focus on the task of eating and swallowing is also impaired. The increased severity of swallowing disorders in the multistroke patient may result because the mechanism does not return to normal swallow function after their first stroke, as described in the next section.

Recovery of Swallow Poststroke

Little data exist on recovery of swallow after stroke in specific locations in the brainstem, subcortical regions, or cortex (Barer, 1989; Wade & Hewer, 1987). An ongoing study of recovery in first-time stroke patients (infarct only), recently completed at Northwestern University and the Rehabilitation Institute of Chicago (NU–RIC), indicates that in the noncomplicated stroke patients, recovery was steady, vigorous, and rapid, with over 95% of the stroke subjects returning to full oral intake by 9 weeks postictus, regardless of site of lesion. All of the patients in the NU–RIC study had active swallowing therapy. However, even when these patients returned to full oral intake within 3 weeks, their temporal measures of swallow physiology, such as duration of airway closure and cricopharyngeal opening, and the temporal relationship between these neuro-muscular actions, did not return to entirely normal values as compared with age-matched controls. Their swallow was functional; that is, they did not aspi-rate, but they exhibited a longer pharyngeal delay and slightly more oral and/or pharyngeal residue than their normal age-matched controls. This would indi-cate that the swallowing mechanism is never quite the same poststroke, and may help to explain why swallowing dysfunction is more severely affected following a second or third stroke.

Recovery is most rapid in the first 3 weeks poststroke, indicating the need to evaluate the patient's swallow function in the first week, and reevaluate at 3 to 4 weeks poststroke. This is particularly important if nonoral feeding is inserted in the first few days poststroke. The patient may no longer need this nonoral nutritional support at 3 to 4 weeks postonset.

Because the criteria for entry into the NU–RIC investigation were very nar-row, excluding patients with a history of any factors that might affect swallow function, as outlined in the next section, the population of stroke patients stud-ied represented only approximately 10% of the total stroke admissions to the two institutions in any 1 year. However, the resulting data represent, as much as pos-sible, the "pure" effect of the infarct on the patients' swallow function. Prelimi-nary analyses of the data from this study indicate that the patient's prior medical history and any complications that arise in the patient's poststroke care are more important contributors to the patient's poststroke swallow function and recov-ery than previously acknowledged.

Effects of Other Factors on Swallowing Function and Recovery in the Stroke Patient

A number of other factors in the patient's medical history or medical manage-ment can affect his or her swallowing ability poststroke (Wright, 1985). *Tra-cheostomy* during the acute stroke phase may worsen the patient's swallowing problem, particularly if the tracheostomy cuff is kept inflated. Inflating the tra-cheostomy cuff for long periods of time can create tracheal irritation, but also produces a greater friction on the tracheal wall as the larynx tries to elevate, potentially reducing laryngeal elevation more than does a tracheostomy tube with the cuff deflated (Buckwalter & Sasaki, 1984; Nash, 1988). Particularly in older patients (over age 80), whose larynges normally rest lower in the neck, tra-cheostomy may contribute to reducing laryngeal elevation and closure during the swallow. Long-term tracheostomy (more than 6 months) can contribute to reduced closure of the airway during the swallow, because the sensory receptors under the vocal folds are not stimulated by airflow. In addition, an open tracheostomy tube does not permit the buildup of subglottic pressure during swallow, which is thought to facilitate airway closure. When the patient who is tracheotomized is swallowing, he or she should be taught to lightly cover the external end of the tracheostomy tube during the swallow to facilitate more normal vocal fold closure and airway protection *if* the modified barium swallow indicates that light coverage of the tube improves the patient's swallow.

Some *medications* given to stroke patients may worsen their poststroke swallowing disorders. Antidepressant medications, in particular, may slow swallow coordination and increase the severity of swallowing disorders. Medications or the interaction of medications may also cause xerostomia (dry mouth), which makes swallowing more difficult (Hughes et al., 1987).

Other *concurrent medical problems*, such as long-standing insulin-dependent diabetes, can increase the severity or prolong the recovery of swallowing function because of the potential for myopathies and neuropathies, which may affect pharyngeal muscle coordination and range of motion. Any prior history of transient ischemic attacks (TIAs), prior strokes, or other neurologic damage may increase the stroke patient's chances for significant swallowing problems or worsen their severity. It is important that the speech–language pathologist investigate the patient's medical history carefully from chart review and family and/or patient interview to identify factors that may pertain to the patient's dysphagia and recovery. In this way, patient and/or family counseling regarding recovery can be more realistic.

To date, no *age* effects on swallowing function poststroke have been identified. The age of the stroke patient does not appear to affect potential for recovery of functional swallow. Minor differences in oropharyngeal swallowing function have been identified in older normal subjects (ages 60 to 80) (Robbins, Hamilton, Lof, & Kempster, 1992; Tracy et al., 1989), as described in Chapter 2. These older subjects exhibited a significantly longer pharyngeal delay time than younger subjects, although the difference was only a fraction of a second. No differences in amount of residue were observed between the older and the younger subjects. Studies of oropharyngeal swallow physiology in normal male subjects over age 80 indicate a significant reduction in range of hyoid and laryngeal movement as compared with young men ages 21 to 30 (Logemann, 1993).

Treatment/Management Strategies

Management strategies may include postural changes, changes in sensory input prior to attempts to swallow, including controlling the characteristics of the bolus itself such as volume and taste, or active exercises.

Changes in Sensory Input via the Bolus

Changing bolus volume can improve swallow physiology in some stroke patients (Bisch, Logemann, Rademaker, Kahrilas, & Lazarus, 1991, 1994; Lazarus et al.,

1993). Many first-time stroke patients exhibit significant difficulty swallowing small bolus volumes, such as saliva (1 to 3 ml), or large bolus volumes (10 to 20 ml), as in cup drinking. Providing a variety of liquid bolus volumes during the radiographic study will enable the clinician to identify the bolus volume most effective for each patient. Larger bolus volumes may provide increased sensory input for the patient.

Changes in bolus viscosity can also change the speed of bolus flow (normal transit times are slower on thicker foods), and thus some viscosities are more easily swallowed in the presence of particular swallowing abnormalities. For example, the stroke patient with a delay in triggering the pharyngeal swallow typically exhibits greater difficulty, as sometimes evidenced by coughing, on thin liquids than on pudding and purees. This difference occurs because thin liquids move more rapidly and splash into the pharynx and potentially into the open airway during the pharyngeal delay, whereas thicker foods slide more slowly from the mouth into the pharynx and often remain in the valleculae during the pharyngeal delay, not entering the airway. Stroke patients with other swallowing disorders may find purees more difficult. For example, the patient who has suffered a brainstem stroke with reduced laryngeal elevation, causing a cricopharyngeal dysfunction, has greater difficulty with thick foods, such as purees, and can more easily handle thin liquids. In this case, thin liquids drain through even a small cricopharyngeal opening, whereas thicker foods tend to get caught in the opening, clogging and preventing flow. Thicker foods may also heighten the patient's sensory awareness of the food. The techniques for feeding dysphagic patients and the factors affecting treatment selection described in Chapter 6 are applicable to many stroke patients.

Changes in bolus taste are another factor that may affect swallow physiology. Presenting a strongly flavored bolus, particularly sour, may improve the stroke patient's awareness of the bolus, the oral onset time, and the pharyngeal delay time (Logemann et al., 1995). Care must be taken, however, as aspiration of an acidic bolus may create more pulmonary reaction.

Active Exercises

Patients with a lingual hemiparesis may experience reduction in tongue control of the bolus during oral preparation for the swallow and disturbed lingual propulsion of the bolus during oral transit. If a unilateral pharyngeal paralysis is present, the pharyngeal wall contraction in the pharynx may be reduced on the affected side, resulting in residue remaining in the pyriform sinus and valleculae on the side of the paresis (Donner, 1974; Kilman & Goyal, 1976). If the larynx is also involved in the hemiparesis, laryngeal elevation and airway protection during the swallow may be reduced.

In patients with paresis or paralysis of muscles affecting movements of structures in the upper aerodigestive tract, it is important to initiate therapy to improve range and precision of oral tongue and tongue base movement, laryngeal elevation, adduction of the vocal folds, closure of the airway entrance, and stimulation of the pharyngeal swallow simultaneously (Crary, 1995). It is often best to work on these motor skills *first* in preparation for swallowing, before requiring the patient to incorporate them into a successful swallowing pattern.

There are a small number of brainstem stroke patients for whom cricopharyngeal dysfunction is the major problem in swallowing and it remains unchanged for 6 months postictus. In these patients, a cricopharyngeal myotomy may be appropriate (Buchholz, 1995; Robbins & Levine, 1993). This assumes that spontaneous recovery has taken place and that the residual dysfunction will not change without intervention. In these patients, the myotomy alone may not allow them to eat but may allow them to use a Mendelsohn maneuver to be able to swallow efficiently enough to eat (Robbins & Levine, 1993).

Swallowing Problems Following Closed Head Trauma

Many patients suffer severe swallowing disturbances following closed head trauma or neurosurgical procedures involving the cortex or brainstem after head injury, although the exact frequency of occurrence of oropharyngeal dysphagia in these populations has not been assessed. Delay in triggering of the pharyngeal swallow, the swallowing problem that occurs most frequently in the stroke population, is also the most prevalent in head trauma and neurosurgical patients.

The swallowing problems of patients who have suffered closed head trauma can be quite complex because of the various types of neurologic injuries these patients may sustain during the accident, including structural injuries to other parts of the body, in addition to the head injury and the nature of their emergency care. It is critical for the swallowing therapist to carefully explore the patient's history relative to the exact nature and extent of damage during the accident that caused the head trauma, as well as the care provided in the first few weeks after the injury. An early study on head injury and swallowing disorders revealed an apparent relationship between length of coma and severity of swallowing problems, with swallowing problems becoming more severe in patients whose coma lasted longer (Lazarus & Logemann, 1987).

The neurogenic damage resulting from head injury can occur because of the direct head injury, the effects of contra-coup damage (i.e., the effect of the brain bouncing against the opposite side of the brain case), and the effects of twisting on the brainstem that can occur. The injury causing the neurologic damage may also have caused puncture wounds in the neck if the patient landed on a sharp object; laryngeal fracture if the patient did not wear a seatbelt and went forward against the dashboard of an automobile; or penetration wounds to the chest, affecting the esophagus.

In emergency care, sometimes tracheostomy is performed at the site of the injury and the tracheostomy may be placed too high, creating scar tissue in the larynx. Also, severely injured patients are often intubated and may remain intubated for periods of several weeks. Intubation itself can cause laryngeal damage, as described in Chapter 5. Thus, all of these factors must be taken into account when assessing the patient with head injury and potential swallowing problems.

Patients with head injuries exhibit a variety of oral disorders, including reduced lip closure; reduced range of tongue motion with poor bolus control; abnormal oral reflexes, such as the bite reflex; a delay in triggering the pharyngeal swallow or even an absent pharyngeal swallow; and a number of neuromuscular abnormalities in the control of the pharyngeal stage of swallow, including reduced laryngeal elevation, reduced closure of the airway entrance, reduced tongue base motion, reduced airway closure, reduced cricopharyngeal opening (generally related to reduced laryngeal motion), unilateral or bilateral pharyngeal wall paresis or paralysis, tracheoesophageal fistula, and/or reduced velopharyngeal closure. In general, reduced closure of the larynx and reduced cricopharyngeal opening relate to changes in laryngeal motion and usually are caused by physical damage to the patient's neck during the accident in which the head injury occurs. Usually airway closure disorders and cricopharyngeal disorders in this population do not relate to the neurologic damage. If the clinician is first seeing the patient with a head injury at 3 months or more after the injury, the clinician may have a difficult time reconstructing the various types of damage that could create the patient's swallowing disorders, but it is critical that the clinician attempt to do so in order to understand the patient's deglutition.

The patient with a head injury has a number of characteristics in addition to the actual physical swallowing disorders that can make return to oral intake more difficult. These include impulsiveness and a tendency to put too much food in the mouth; cognitive difficulties, which make the understanding of some swallow therapy procedures, such as swallow maneuvers, quite difficult; and reduced sensation, which makes the awareness of swallowing disorders less than optimal.

The recovery of swallow after head injury has not been well documented. However, in one study based on bedside observations, the frequency of apparent swallowing difficulties diminished significantly from the acute care setting through the initial and final rehabilitation stages, indicating a pattern of consecutive improvement in swallowing disorders (Yorkston, Honsingner, Mitsuda, & Hammen, 1989). However, because this study was based only on bedside assessment of swallowing evaluation, this study may have underestimated those with swallowing disorders and overestimated their recovery.

Compliance with dietary recommendations and swallowing therapy can be a difficult problem in some patients with head injuries, especially if they did not receive good assessment of their swallow in the acute care period. It is important that the patient receive swallowing assessment during the acute care stage, as soon as anyone detects that a swallowing problem might be present. If the family and patient are counseled about the nature of any swallowing problems and the ways in which they can be managed, patients and families are usually quite compliant, in my experience. However, if the swallowing problems are ignored or not assessed and the patient is allowed to eat in acute care and then moves to the rehabilitation phase, where swallow is assessed and found to be unsafe or inefficient, and feeding patterns are changed on this basis, family and patient may become angry and noncompliant. Because swallowing problems are often not evident from external examination, the family and patient do not understand why eating should be restricted in any way and usually the patient will not comply. Many young adult patients with head injuries can continue to aspirate, particularly on liquids, with no immediately apparent pulmonary consequences. However, over a period of a year or more, if the patient continues to aspirate and does not recover his or her swallowing function, the patient will usually develop pneumonia and may require prolonged hospitalization.

Counseling of the patient with head injury and his or her family after the radiographic study of swallowing is critical to help them understand why diet changes or other treatment strategies may be necessary. However, even with use of the videofluoroscopic study as an educational tool, many of these patients and families are unwilling to accept a recommendation to avoid thin liquids or any other kind of dietary change since the patient shows no external signs of struggling or difficulty when eating. Because many of these patients are young, healthy men prior to injury, their pulmonary function is generally good and they can apparently tolerate prolonged aspiration without pulmonary consequences. However, if they are chronically aspirating, they are at higher risk to develop pneumonia than other individuals.

Patients with head injuries, if they also have cognitive deficits, need compensatory strategies such as postural changes and enhanced sensory input as initial treatment strategies, as appropriate. Many can also cooperate with resistance and range-of-motion exercises. However, swallow maneuvers may be much too difficult for them to learn. Luckily, most of them do not require swallow maneuvers because of the nature of their most frequent swallowing problems (i.e., reduced range and/or coordination of tongue motion and delayed or absent pharyngeal swallow). Often, family members can be enlisted to provide additional therapy to a patient using range-of-motion exercises and thermal–tactile stimulation. These techniques can be taught to the family, who can increase the frequency of therapy with these procedures beyond the time available from the swallowing therapist. However, when using family, it is critical to give them the goal for the procedure (e.g., "We need to gain one inch of vertical tongue motion" or "We need to reduce the pharyngeal delay to one second"). If family or significant others do not have a goal to the exercises they are practicing with the patient, they may become inappropriately excited over very small gains and expect the patient to be able to eat based on a very slight improvement.

Changing diet is another option in management of swallowing disorders in the patient with head injury. If the patient has particular difficulty with thin liquids because of the delayed pharyngeal swallow, the patient may be able to safely manage thicker liquids and foods. These various viscosities should be introduced during the diagnostic radiographic study to define the improvements seen in the swallow and the ability to manage these particular foods.

Some patients who are severely dysphagic may plateau in their progress and appear to have reached their maximum gains at a point where they are still unable to eat because they are aspirating or having tremendously inefficient swallowing. These patients may remain on nonoral feeding or on limited oral intake. However, they should be reassessed every 6 months to 1 year in order to determine whether recovery may have taken place. Many clinicians have seen patients with head injuries who have been discharged from treatment still requiring nonoral feeding but who regain swallow function a year or two later. It is critical that swallowing therapists identify this recovery in order to remove unnecessary nonoral feeding.

Swallowing Problems After Cervical Spinal Cord Injury

Cervical spinal cord injury can result in swallowing problems whether or not a head injury is also present. If there is no head injury, the patient's swallowing problems are usually pharyngeal in nature and may include a delay in triggering the pharyngeal swallow, reduced laryngeal elevation and anterior movement causing reduced cricopharyngeal opening, reduced tongue base motion, and unilateral or bilateral pharyngeal wall dysfunction. There is a tendency for poor laryngeal movement and consequent reduced cricopharyngeal opening to occur more often when damage occurs at cervical vertebrae 4, 5, or 6. Patients with injuries to cervical vertebrae 1 or 2 may have no sensory awareness of their swallowing difficulty. Occasionally, patients who have sustained a cervical spinal cord injury also exhibit problems in closing the airway entrance. Often, these problems are secondary to the reduction in anterior and laryngeal movement. Problems with closure at the vocal folds occur infrequently in these patients and are usually related to direct laryngeal damage in the trauma or the emergency airway management (e.g., tracheostomy placement or intubation) or to prolonged tracheostomy (6 months or more) which can result in reduced vocal fold closure. These disorders may be exacerbated by the presence of a tracheostomy tube with the cuff of the tube inflated. The inflated cuff may further restrict laryngeal movement. Many of these patients will also be in a cervical brace and on mechanical ventilation, especially in acute care or if their lesion is at the level of cervical vertebra 3 or above. If mechanical ventilation is present, a cuffed tracheostomy tube with cuff inflated is frequently also present to facilitate operation of the ventilator, because many ventilators operate on positive pressure principles.

The presence of a mechanical ventilator and/or a tracheostomy tube makes accurate bedside assessment even more difficult because the clinician will have more difficulty feeling any laryngeal elevation during the patient's swallow attempt and because of the high incidence of pharyngeal stage swallowing problems in the vast majority of dysphagic patients who have suffered a spinal cord injury at cervical vertebra 5 or above. If the patient with a cervical spinal cord injury complains of any swallowing disorder or exhibits any of the symptoms of dysphagia, he or she requires an in-depth physiologic assessment, usually a radiographic study.

During the videofluoroscopic study of oropharyngeal swallow, patients with spinal cord injuries may not be able to be elevated to a complete vertical position, or may be elevated only when some type of neck and/or chin brace is present. If the patient is unable to be elevated, the radiographic study should be completed in the position in which the patient is usually fed. This may be at 30° or 60° from horizontal.

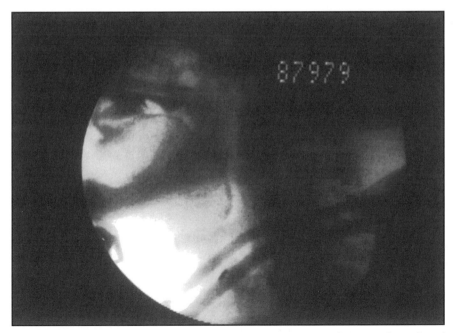

Figure 9.1. Lateral radiographic view of a patient who has sustained a cervical spinal cord injury wearing a SOMI brace. The shoulder portions of the brace can be seen in the lower portion of the X-ray. The mandibular support hardware can be seen under the chin.

If the patient has head and neck bracing in place, certain parts of the oral cavity or pharynx may be shadowed or covered by the brace, as shown in Figure 9.1. If this is the case, the patient's wheelchair or cart may need to be angled slightly to reveal all of the oropharyngeal structures. Usually, angling the chair or cart 15° to 30° from straight lateral will sufficiently move the shadow of the bracing away from critical anatomic elements of the pharynx. Although the radiographic view will not be strictly lateral with the cart or wheelchair at an angle, the oropharyngeal swallow physiology can be examined.

During the radiographic study, the introduction of therapy procedures is critical to facilitating faster return to oral intake. Because these patients may also be wearing some form of cervical bracing, with no ability to move the head or neck, postural changes are usually not possible. Instead, sensory enhancement therapies and swallow maneuvers are often most helpful. Because the patient with cervical spinal cord injury but no head injury does not have cognitive difficulties, he or she is frequently able to utilize swallow maneuvers quite productively.

Cervical Bracing

The effects of bracing of the neck and head for patients with cervical spinal cord injuries have not been clearly defined. Many patients report a worsening of their swallow when they have been placed in a SOMI or a halo brace. However, no studies have examined whether physiology of swallow changes in these two bracing conditions in patients with spinal cord injuries. A study presented at the American Speech-Language-Hearing Association in 1992 examined the effects of SOMI bracing worn by 10 young adult normal men (Bisch, Logemann, Rademaker, & Quigley, 1992). The swallow physiology was measured in all subjects with and without the brace, and they were asked to report any subjective changes in their perception of swallowing safety. Subjects were given only 15 minutes to accommodate to the brace prior to participating in the radiographic study of swallowing. All subjects felt that swallowing was less comfortable when wearing a SOMI brace. However, only one measure of swallowing changed significantly with the brace condition. That was the duration of airway closure, which was prolonged in the bracing condition. This may well have resulted from the subjects' feelings of discomfort and wishes to protect themselves should the swallow be less successful. Although these data indicate that there may be no negative effects of bracing on oropharyngeal swallow, patients with cervical spinal cord injury may react quite differently to the bracing than do young adult normal subjects. More research is needed to understand whether and how various types of bracing affect swallowing and/or whether certain bracing positions affect swallow differently than other positions. Generally, if the patient is braced in such a way that the chin is pulled back and the chin or head is retracted on the neck or the patient's head is extended, patients will have greater complaints of swallowing difficulty.

Anterior Cervical Fusion

Patients with cervical injuries, degenerative disc disease, and so forth, may have cervical fusion to stabilize their cervical vertebrae. The approach to the fusion may be anterior or posterior. Data on the percentage of patients who receive anterior or posterior fusion who have some degree of postoperative dysphagia are not available (Martin, Neary, & Diamant, 1997). These patients may have a significant amount of hardware or bone implanted in and between the vertebrae to accomplish the fusion (Figure 9.2). Postoperatively, swelling in the posterior pharyngeal wall is often seen, which may contribute to dysphagia. Patients usually exhibit reduced laryngeal elevation and anterior movement, with consequent reduced closure of the airway entrance and reduced cricopharyngeal opening. Reduced unilateral or bilateral pharyngeal wall movement is often seen, as

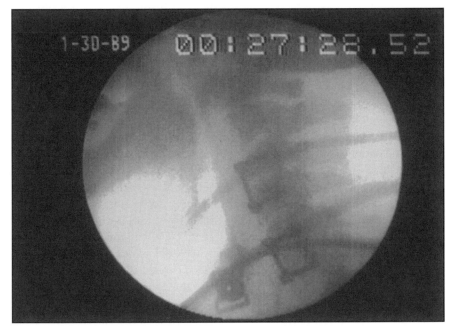

Figure 9.2. Lateral radiographic view of the head and neck in a patient who has received anterior cervical fusion with hardware (screws and bolts) implanted between two different sets of vertebrae.

well. Patients may also exhibit oral stage problems and a delay in triggering the pharyngeal swallow. These disorders may occur for a variety of reasons, including trauma to peripheral nerves, pharyngeal swelling postoperatively, and reaction to the hardware in the neck. Generally, these patients will experience significant recovery of their swallow within 3 months postoperatively. The duration of recovery generally reflects the number of complications. In the interim, a modified barium swallow can define the nature of the patient's swallowing disorder and, perhaps, define intervention strategies that enable the patient to eat safely by mouth. Most frequently, swallowing maneuvers are helpful to these patients, particularly the Mendelsohn maneuver and the supraglottic or super-supraglottic swallow.

Swallowing Problems After Neurosurgical Procedures Affecting the Brainstem and/or Cranial Nerves

Neurosurgical procedures affecting the medulla often result in significant swallowing problems, sometimes a complete inability to trigger a pharyngeal swallow. The patient may exhibit oral tongue, tongue base, and laryngeal struggling motions but no true pharyngeal swallow. In these cases, thermal–tactile stimulation and suck–swallow can be utilized to heighten stimulation to the central nervous system in an attempt to lower the threshold of the swallowing center and enable the patient to trigger a pharyngeal swallow. If the surgical procedure is unilateral, the effects may be similar to surgical procedures affecting cranial nerves on one side, as described below.

After surgical removal of an acoustic neuroma or other tumor from a cranial nerve, the patient may exhibit unilateral damage to cranial nerves IX, X, XII, and possibly VII. Damage to these cranial nerves may occur from surgical trauma or from actual cutting of these nerves in order to resect a tumor of nerve VIII or other cranial nerve. The extent of damage depends upon the size of the acoustic neuroma or other tumor and the difficulty of resection. Patients tend to exhibit one or more of the following: unilateral facial weakness, unilateral pharyngeal wall paresis or paralysis, unilateral vocal fold adductor paralysis, unilateral soft palate weakness, and unilateral tongue paresis. With damage to cranial nerve IX, there is often a delay in triggering the pharyngeal swallow. Because this damage is unilateral, these patients often benefit from postural strategies, including head rotation to the damaged side of the pharynx and the chin-down posture to improve airway protection and help prevent aspiration because of a delayed pharyngeal swallow. These patients usually benefit from aggressive range-of-motion and resistance exercises for the lips, oral tongue, tongue base, and larynx. These exercises include the falsetto exercise for laryngeal elevation as well as the effortful swallow, and the super-supraglottic swallow or the super-supraglottic breath-hold. Patients who are cognitively intact can practice these exercises independently 10 times a day for approximately 5 minutes each time to improve range of motion.

Swallowing Problems Resulting from Poliomyelitis

Disturbances in the oral stage of the swallow in poliomyelitis patients may include reduced lingual control of the bolus in chewing and a disturbed pattern of lingual bolus propulsion during the oral stage of swallow. In addition, many of these patients exhibit reduced pharyngeal contraction. Pharyngeal disorders resulting from poliomyelitis include (1) reduced velopharyngeal closure during swallowing, causing nasal regurgitation; (2) reduced pharyngeal contraction; and (3) unilateral pharyngeal paralysis (Bosma, 1953; Kaplan, 1951; Kilman & Goyal, 1976). A discussion of postpolio syndrome is included in Chapter 10.

Swallowing Problems Associated with Guillain–Barré

Guillain–Barré is a viral-based disease causing rapid onset of paresis, which may progress to complete paralysis requiring tracheostomy and mechanical ventilation (Chen, Donofrio, Frederick, Ott, & Pikna, 1996). The general weakness and paralysis usually begin within a day or two after the swallowing problem is noticed. Radiographic studies of swallowing usually reveal a generalized weakness in the oral and pharyngeal swallow, resulting in reduced range of motion of the oral tongue, tongue base, and larynx. Although the progressive paralysis is rapid (i.e., over a period of several days), recovery can be very slow, lasting a period of months or years. Respiration is often unstable for a period of time in these patients, so swallowing therapy that affects duration of airway closure, such as swallow maneuvers, should be used carefully or not at all until respiratory control has stabilized. Even manipulation of a tracheostomy tube, such as cuff deflation, can be problematic and should not be done without medical approval.

Generally, therapy begins with gentle resistance and range-of-motion exercises, increasing effort as the patient improves. When respiratory control has improved, the patient may benefit from swallow maneuvers, particularly the supraglottic swallow and the Mendelsohn maneuver. Occasionally, the first sign of Guillain–Barré is swallowing difficulty.

Swallowing Problems Associated with Cerebral Palsy

Much has been written about the oral dysfunctions of individuals with cerebral palsy (Arvedson, Rogers, Buck, Smart, & Msall, 1994; Gisel, Applegate-Ferrante, Benson, & Bosma, 1996; Larnert & Ekberg, 1995; McPherson et al., 1992; Rogers, Arvedson, Msall, & Demerath, 1993; Rudolph, 1994; Sloan, 1977). The degree of involvement of oral musculature varies widely from one child to the next. Children may exhibit inappropriate oral reflexive behaviors; inability to hold material in a cohesive bolus, especially if the material is being masticated; and/or disorganized lingual movements that do not contribute to a smooth peristaltic action of the tongue in moving the material posteriorly. Often, as the individual is chewing, particles of food break away and spread throughout the oral cavity. Some of these pieces may fall into the pharynx and then into the open airway. Only rarely does the pharyngeal swallow trigger when these small amounts fall into the airway, possibly because the voluntary oral stage of swallow has not been initiated.

Less information is available on the occurrence of swallowing disturbances in the pharyngeal and esophageal stages of swallowing in individuals with cerebral palsy. Based on a review of the records of 150 children with cerebral palsy between the ages of 5 and 12 assessed at Northwestern University Medical School, the children were placed into three categories of swallowing disorders: (1) those with moderate to severe oral function problems, including reduced lip closure and tongue thrust, as well as reduced tongue coordination; (2) those with the same moderate to severe oral problems and a delay in triggering the pharyngeal swallow; and (3) those with moderate to severe oromotor problems, pharyngeal delay, and neuromuscular abnormalities in their pharyngeal swallow, including reduced tongue base retraction and reduced laryngeal elevation, resulting in significant residue in the pharynx after the swallow and increased risk of aspiration after the swallow. Many children in Group 3 aspirate on every food consistency. The largest number of the children with cerebral palsy were in Group 2, as were a group of 15 children classified as having largely spastic quadriplegia, studied by Gartenberg (1991). These children, ages 5 to 12, exhibited a range of oral problems, including tongue thrust, poor lateralization of the tongue, and discoordinated front-to-back tongue movement. They also exhibited a delay in triggering the pharyngeal swallow. All of these problems are typical of children in Group 2. Children in Group 2 have swallowing difficulty with foods requiring chewing because of oromotor difficulty, and with liquids because of the pharyngeal delay if they are given large amounts of liquids at one time. Therefore, syringe feeding or the dumping of large amounts of liquid down the child while in a supine position are not appropriate. Management strategies may include oromotor therapy, thermal–tactile stimulation of the pharyngeal swallow, and diet change, including thickened liquids and purees. Diet change should be the last choice for management because it is less appealing to the child and family.

Cricopharyngeal dysfunction or abnormal opening of the upper esophageal sphincter is rarely a problem in an individual with cerebral palsy. Any surgical procedure, such as cricopharyngeal myotomy, should be delayed in favor of swallowing therapy and growth effects. As the child grows and the laryngeal position changes (lowers), opening of the upper esophageal sphincter may normalize. In general, laryngeal closure during swallow is adequate, so that no aspiration is seen *during* the swallow. Most aspiration in children and adults with cerebral palsy occurs *before* the swallow, usually because of reduced tongue control for chewing or because of delayed pharyngeal swallow, or *after* the swallow, because of poor tongue base action or poor laryngeal elevation creating inefficient swallowing with residue left in the pharynx. Developmental changes in these aspects of swallowing have not been assessed.

Some evidence indicates that some individuals with severe developmental delay and cerebral palsy may need chronic therapy (e.g., thermal–tactile stimulation) to maintain their function (Helfrich-Miller, Rector, & Straka, 1986). In this situation, the swallowing therapist should define the optimal therapy and eating strategies, teach them to the caregivers, and monitor the caregivers at regular intervals.

Swallowing Problems Associated with Dysautonomia (Riley–Day Syndrome)

Familial dysautonomia is an inherited disease with widespread effects, including autonomic imbalance, sensory deficits, motor incoordination, and certain episodic phenomena. Some of these children exhibit only minimal disturbances with oropharyngeal swallowing, possibly mild reduction in oral tongue coordination of the bolus and reduced tongue base and pharyngeal wall contraction. Other children demonstrate more severe oral involvement and a delay in triggering the pharyngeal swallow sufficient so that these children cannot handle liquids safely and receive a gastrostomy for liquid intake (Brunt, Marguiles, Coburn, Donner, & Hendrix, 1967; Gyepes & Linde, 1968; Sparberg, Knudsen, & Frank, 1968). These children also usually exhibit a dysfunctional lower esophageal sphincter, which also allows reflux, greater on thin liquids, and contributes to a need for a gastrostomy for liquid intake. Reduced tongue base action and reduced pharyngeal contraction can also be problems. Occasionally, difficulty with opening of the cricopharyngeal sphincter is also observed (Brunt et al., 1967; Kilman & Goyal, 1976; Linde & Westover, 1962; Marguiles, Brunt, Donner, & Silbiger, 1968; Pearson, 1979). In addition, manometry has revealed abnormal esophageal motility (i.e., an almost total lack of normal peristaltic waves). These children also benefit from oromotor exercises to improve oral tongue function and thermal–tactile stimulation to improve triggering of the pharyngeal swallow.

References

Arvedson, J., Rogers, B., Buck, G., Smart, P., & Msall, M. (1994). Silent aspiration in children with dysphagia. *International Journal of Pediatric Oto-Rhino-Laryngology, 28,* 173–181.

Aviv, J. E., Martin, J. H., Sacco, R. L., Zagar, D., Diamond, B., Keen, M. S., & Blitzer, A. (1996). Supraglottic and pharyngeal sensory abnormalities in stroke patients with dysphagia. *Annals of Otology, Rhinology, and Laryngology, 105,* 92–97.

Barer, D. H. (1989). The natural history and functional consequences of dysphagia after hemispheric stroke. *Journal of Neurology, Neurosurgery and Psychiatry, 52,* 236–241.

Bisch, E. M., Logemann, J. A., Rademaker, A. W., Kahrilas, P. J., & Lazarus, C. (1991, November). *Pharyngeal effects of bolus temperature.* Paper presented at the American Speech-Language-Hearing Association annual convention, Atlanta.

Bisch, E. M., Logemann, J. A., Rademaker, A. W., Kahrilas, P. J., & Lazarus, C. L. (1994). Pharyngeal effects of bolus volume, viscosity and temperature in patients with dysphagia resulting from neurologic impairment and in normal subjects. *Journal of Speech and Hearing Research, 37,* 1041–1049.

Bisch, E. M., Logemann, J. A., Rademaker, A. W., & Quigley, J. (1992). *Swallow effects of the SOMI brace.* Abstracts of the 1992 ASHA convention, p. 130.

Bosma, J. (1953). Studies of disability of the pharynx resultant from poliomyelitis. *Annals of Otology, Rhinology and Laryngology, 64,* 529–547.

Brunt, P. W., Marguiles, S. I., Coburn, W. M., Donner, N. W., & Hendrix, T. R. (1967). The oesophagus in dysautonomia: A manometric and cinefluorographic study. *Journal of the British Society of Gastroenterology, 167,* 636–637.

Buchholz, D. (1993). Clinically probable brainstem stroke presenting primarily as dysphagia and nonvisualized by MRI. *Dysphagia, 8,* 235–238.

Buchholz, D. W. (1995). Cricopharyngeal myotomy may be effective treatment for selected patients with neurogenic oropharyngeal dysphagia. *Dysphagia, 10,* 255–258.

Buckwalter, J. A., & Sasaki, C. T. (1984). Effect of tracheostomy on laryngeal function. *Otolaryngologic Clinics of North America, 17,* 41–48.

Celifarco, A., Gerard, G., Faegenburg, D., & Burakoff, R. (1990). Dysphagia as the sole manifestation of bilateral strokes. *American Journal of Gastroenterology, 85,* 610–613.

Chen, M. Y. M., Donofrio, P. D., Frederick, M. G., Ott, D. J., & Pikna, L. A. (1996). Videofluoroscopic evaluation of patients with Guillain–Barré syndrome. *Dysphagia, 11,* 11–13.

Crary, M. A. (1995). A direct intervention program for chronic neurogenic dysphagia secondary to brainstem stroke. *Dysphagia, 10,* 6–18.

Delgado, J. J. (1988). Paralysis, dysphagia and balance problems associated with stroke. *Journal of Neuroscience Nursing, 20*(4), 260.

Donner, M. (1974). Swallowing mechanism and neuromuscular disorders. *Seminars in Roentgenology, 9*, 273–282.

Gartenberg, T. (1991). *Swallowing disorders in children with cerebral palsy.* Unpublished doctoral dissertation, Northwestern University, Evanston, IL.

Gisel, E. G., Applegate-Ferrante, T., Benson, J., & Bosma, J. F. (1996). Oral motor skills following sensorimotor therapy in two groups of moderately dysphagic children with cerebral palsy: Aspiration versus non-aspiration. *Dysphagia, 11*, 59–71.

Gyepes, M., & Linde, L. (1968). Familial dysautonomia: The mechanism of aspiration. *Radiology, 91*, 471–475.

Helfrich-Miller, K. R., Rector, K. L., & Straka, J. A. (1986). Dysphagia: Its treatment in the profoundly retarded patient with cerebral palsy. *Archives of Physical Medicine and Rehabilitation, 67*, 520–525.

Horner, J., Massey, E. W., Riski, J. E., Lathrop, D. L., & Chase, K. N. (1988). Aspiration following stroke: Clinical correlates and outcomes. *Neurology, 38*, 1359–1362.

Hughes, C. V., Baum, B. J., Fox, P. C., Marmary, Y., Yeh, C. K., & Sonies, B. C. (1987). Oral-pharyngeal dysphagia: A common sequelae of salivary gland dysfunction. *Dysphagia, 1*, 173–177.

Jacob, P., Kahrilas, P., Logemann, J., Shah, V., & Ha, T. (1989). Upper esophageal sphincter opening and modulation during swallowing. *Gastroenterology, 97*, 1469–1478.

Jean, A., & Car, A. (1979). Inputs to the swallowing medullary neurons from the peripheral afferent fibers and the swallowing cortical area. *Brain Research, 178*, 567–572.

Kahrilas, P. J., Logemann, J. A., Krugler, C., & Flanagan, E. (1991). Volitional augmentation of upper esophageal sphincter opening during swallowing. *American Journal of Physiology, 260*, G450–G456.

Kaplan, S. (1951). Paralysis of deglutition: A post poly-poliomyelitis complication treated by section of the cricopharyngeus muscle. *Annals of Surgery, 133*, 572–573.

Kilman, W., & Goyal, R. (1976). Disorders of pharyngeal and upper esophageal sphincter motor function. *Archives of Internal Medicine, 136*, 592–601.

Larnert, G., & Ekberg, O. (1995). Positioning improves the oral and pharyngeal swallowing function in children with cerebral palsy. *Acta Pædiatrica, 84*, 689–692.

Lazarus, C., & Logemann, J. A. (1987). Swallowing disorders in closed head trauma patients. *Archives of Physical Medicine and Rehabilitation, 68*, 79–87.

Lazarus, C. L., Logemann, J. A., Rademaker, A. W., Kahrilas, P. J., Pajak, T., Lazar, R., & Halper, A. (1993). Effects of bolus volume, viscosity and repeated swallows in non-stroke subjects and stroke patients. *Archives of Physical Medicine and Rehabilitation, 74*, 1066–1070.

Lazzara, G., Lazarus, C., & Logemann, J. A. (1986). Impact of thermal stimulation on the triggering of the swallowing reflex. *Dysphagia, 1*, 73–77.

Linde, L., & Westover, J. (1962). Esophageal and gastric abnormalities in dysautonomia. *Pediatrics, 29*, 303–306.

Logemann, J. A. (1993, July). *Aging effects on swallow in young and old men.* Paper presented at the International Congress on Aging, Budapest, Hungary.

Logemann, J. A., & Kahrilas, P. J. (1990). Relearning to swallow post CVA: Application of maneuvers and indirect biofeedback—A case study. *Neurology, 40*, 1136–1138.

Logemann, J., Kahrilas, P., Kobara, M., & Vakil, N. (1989). The benefit of head rotation on pharyngoesophageal dysphagia. *Archives of Physical Medicine & Rehabilitation, 70,* 767–771.

Logemann, J. A., Pauloski, B. R., Colangelo, L., Lazarus, C., Fujiu, M., & Kahrilas, P. J. (1995). Effects of a sour bolus on oropharyngeal swallowing measures in patients with neurogenic dysphagia. *Journal of Speech and Hearing Research, 38,* 556–563.

Logemann, J. A., Shanahan, T., Rademaker, A. W., Kahrilas, P. J., Lazar, R., & Halper, A. (1993). Oropharyngeal swallowing after stroke in the left basal ganglion/internal capsule. *Dysphagia, 8,* 230–234.

Marguiles, S., Brunt, P., Donner, M., & Silbiger, M. (1968). Familial dysautonomia: A cineradiographic study of the swallowing mechanism. *Radiology, 90,* 107–112.

Martin, R. E., Neary, M. A., & Diamant, N. E. (1997). Dysphagia following anterior cervical spine surgery. *Dysphagia, 12,* 2–8.

McPherson, K. A., Kenny, D. J., Koheil, R., Bablich, K., Sochaniwskyj, A., & Milner, M. (1992). Ventilation and swallowing interactions of normal children and children with cerebral palsy. *Developmental Medicine and Child Neurology, 34,* 577–588.

Meadows, J. (1973). Dysphagia in unilateral cerebral lesions. *Journal of Neurology, Neurosurgery, and Psychiatry, 36,* 853–860.

Miller, A. J. (1982). Deglutition. *Physiologic Review, 62,* 129–184.

Nash, M. (1988). Swallowing problems in the tracheotomized patient. *Otolaryngologic Clinics of North America, 21,* 701–709.

Pearson, J. (1979). Familial dysautonomia (A brief review). *Journal of the Autonomic Nervous System, 1,* 119–126.

Robbins, J., Hamilton, J. W., Lof, G. L., & Kempster, G. B. (1992). Oropharyngeal swallowing in normal adults of different ages. *Gastroenterology, 103,* 823–829.

Robbins, J., & Levine, R. (1988). Swallowing after unilateral stroke of the cerebral cortex: Preliminary experience. *Dysphagia, 3,* 11–17.

Robbins, J. A., & Levine, R. (1993). Swallowing after lateral medullary syndrome plus. *Clinics in Communication Disorders, 3*(4), 45–55.

Rogers, B. T., Arvedson, J., Msall, M., & Demerath, R. (1993). Hypoxemia during oral feeding of children with cerebral palsy. *Developmental Medicine and Child Neurology, 35,* 3–10.

Rudolph, C. D. (1994). Feeding disorders in infants and children. *Journal of Pediatrics, 125,* S116–S124.

Sloan, R. (1977). The cinefluorographic study of cerebral palsy deglutition patterns. *Journal of Osaka Dental University, 11,* 58–73.

Smith, D. S., & Dodd, B. A. (1990). Swallowing disorders in stroke. *The Medical Journal of Australia, 153,* 372–373.

Sparberg, M., Knudsen, K., & Frank, S. (1968). Dysautonomia and dysphagia. *Neurology, 18,* 504–506.

Tracy, J., Logemann, J., Kahrilas, P., Jacob, P., Kobara, M., & Krugler, C. (1989). Preliminary observations on the effects of age on oropharyngeal deglutition. *Dysphagia, 4,* 90–94.

Wade, D., & Hewer, R. (1987). Motor loss and swallowing difficulty after stroke: Frequency, recovery, and prognosis. *Acta Neurology Scandinavia, 76,* 50–54.

Wright, A. (1985). An unusual but easily treatable cause of dysphagia and dysarthria complicating stroke. *British Medical Journal, 291,* 1412–1413.

Yorkston, K. M., Honsingner, M. J., Mitsuda, P. M., & Hammen, V. (1989). The relationship between speech and swallowing disorders in head-injured patients. *Journal of Head Trauma Rehabilitation, 4*(4), 1–16.

C H A P T E R   1 0

SWALLOWING PROBLEMS
ASSOCIATED WITH
DEGENERATIVE DISEASE

Many degenerative diseases are characterized by swallowing problems that may begin early or later in the disease process and that generally worsen over the course of the disease. Currently, relatively little information is available on (1) the progression of these swallowing disorders in each diagnosis and (2) whether the progression is predictable in all patients with similar conditions. Most research has been done in the area of neurologic disease. Early studies that examined the swallowing problems associated with neurologic disease assessed a variety of patients from a number of diagnoses rather than a homogeneous group of patients with the same diagnosis. More recently, investigators have examined more homogeneous groups of patients with a particular disease but have not always categorized patients according to the stage of deterioration of their neurologic systems. Those who have done so have found inconclusive results regarding the association between the disease stage and the severity or nature of the resultant dysphagia. There is need for more research that follows patients from the onset of their neurologic symptoms to determine the progression of swallowing dysfunction. Such research would offer the potential for designing optimum management programs at specific times in the disease process. At present, the armamentarium of treatments for the patient with progressive disease varies with the specific diagnosis.

Management of swallowing problems in the patient with a degenerative disease often involves progressively changing strategies, shifting and often restricting the nature (usually the viscosity) of the diet, and, in some cases, eventually recommending a shift from oral feeding to a combination of oral and nonoral feeding and then complete nonoral feeding. Often, some oral intake for pleasure is possible while reducing the pressure to take all calories orally by introducing nonoral intake to follow the patient's oral intake. It is important that the patient's swallowing be regularly evaluated so that (1) progressively worsening function can be compensated for as much as possible, (2) the patient is put at minimal risk of serious aspiration and pulmonary problems, and (3) an optimal nutrition and hydration status is maintained by initiation of appropriate non-oral feeding methods when needed.

Counseling of the patient regarding these goals and their general progress is critical. The patient and significant others should be informed of the risks and benefits of all procedures recommended. The patient is the ultimate decision maker regarding nature and continued use of oral intake.

Swallowing Problems Associated with Neurologic or Neuromuscular Disease

A large number of degenerative neurologic and neuromuscular diseases result in swallowing problems, as described in the following text.

Alzheimer's Disease

Alzheimer's disease is a progressive dementia that causes a number of feeding and swallowing disorders. Initially, patients often develop an agnosia for food; that is, they cannot visually recognize food as food when it is placed in front of them. For example, if asked to recognize something to eat by discriminating between a sandwich, a pencil, and a pair of scissors, the patients cannot identify the sandwich as something to eat. This makes it difficult for them to accept food into the mouth and swallow it and explains their slowness in opening their mouth and accepting food. As the dementia progresses, these patients often develop an apraxia for both feeding and swallowing. The feeding apraxia makes it difficult for them to use utensils to feed themselves. The patients may be observed to pick up a spoon or fork and turn it around in their hand as if trying to figure out which end to use. The swallowing apraxia makes it difficult to initiate the oral stage of swallowing. The patients may move the food around the mouth in searching motions as if trying to determine what to do with it and how to begin the swallow, or they may hold the food in the mouth for several minutes with no tongue motion. These patients also develop an oral tactile agnosia for food. When food is not recognized in the mouth, there is no reason for the patients to initiate the oral stage of swallow. This contributes to holding the food in the mouth without swallowing it.

In addition to the swallowing apraxia, the patient with Alzheimer's disease may exhibit physiologic changes in the swallow, including reduction in lateral tongue motion for chewing, a delay in triggering the pharyngeal swallow, and motor abnormalities in the pharynx, which include bilateral pharyngeal weakness, reduced laryngeal elevation, and reduced posterior motion of the tongue base (Horner, Alberts, Dawson, & Cook, 1994). Often, the agnosia and swallowing apraxia present first and gradually worsen until they cause a significant delay in a patient's oral intake, threatening the adequacy of his or her intake for nutrition and hydration (Suski & Nielsen, 1989). Some patients may take 3 or 4 minutes to initiate a single swallow.

On this basis, a critical aspect of feeding and swallowing assessment in patients with Alzheimer's disease involves measuring the length of time it takes them to accept food into the mouth and initiate the oral stage of the swallow. How long do the caregivers spend feeding the patient? The slowness in this activity may be so severe that it compromises both nutrition and hydration. Often, procedures to heighten sensory input prior to placing food in the mouth and/or as food is being placed in the mouth will speed both oral acceptance and initiation of the oral stage of swallow, as described in Chapter 6. Because all of the sensory enhancement procedures are under the control of the caregiver or feeder, they can be used quite successfully for a time with patients who have dementia. Alzheimer's dementia can be a slowly progressing process or it can result in more rapid deterioration. In either case, there will be a point at which the patient will have deteriorated beyond the ability of the swallowing therapist to significantly improve either feeding or swallowing. The swallowing therapist must be willing to identify when the patient can no longer benefit from swallowing therapy and withdraw from the patient's care.

Effects of Other Types of Dementia on Oropharyngeal Swallowing

Other types of dementia may also affect oropharyngeal swallowing ability. Currently, no studies have definitively distinguished swallowing patterns in patients with various types of dementia. However, in my experience, some patients with dementia, usually with organic brain syndrome or multistroke dementia, exhibit a separation in the cortically and brainstem (medullary) controlled aspects of the swallow (i.e., the oral preparatory and oral stages of swallow and the pharyngeal aspects of the swallow). The behavior that these patients exhibit is to initiate a swallow on command, propelling the bolus from the oral cavity with good lingual motion, but the pharyngeal swallow does not trigger. Repeated requests for the patient to swallow generally result in the patient's responding with a comment such as, "I did swallow." Although the patient did initiate the voluntary, cortically controlled aspects of the swallow, apparently there is a disconnection in the neural pathways between the cortex, which controls the oral stages of swallow, and the medulla, which controls the pharyngeal stage of swallow. Generally, after several minutes, with the bolus resting in various locations in the pharynx, a motorically normal pharyngeal swallow triggers in these patients. The problem seems to be the continuity and/or speed of transmission of neural signals from the cortex to the brainstem. These patients may benefit from heightened sensory input via a stronger tasting bolus or a larger bolus, or from techniques to heighten oral sensation, such as thermal–tactile stimulation, described in Chapter 6.

Amyotrophic Lateral Sclerosis

Amyotrophic lateral sclerosis (ALS) is a progressive disease. It usually involves progressive upper and lower motor neuron degeneration, and it can affect predominantly the corticobulbar tracts or the corticospinal tracts, or both. In patients with predominantly corticobulbar involvement, swallowing impairment often begins with reduction in tongue mobility, so patients become less able to lateralize food to chew and less able to control material in the oral cavity (Dworkin & Hartman, 1979; Kilman & Goyal, 1976). They are unable to increase the pressure generated by their tongue as needed when food viscosity increases; thus, they have increasing difficulty as food increases in thickness. Patients often naturally begin to avoid eating thicker foods and foods requiring chewing. Lip closure is often reduced, causing drooling and spillage of food from the mouth. Velar function may become involved so that anterior velar bulging to keep food in the oral cavity while holding a bolus and velar elevation during swallowing is reduced (Robbins, Logemann, & Kirshner, 1982). When laryngeal elevation is reduced, usually somewhat later in the disease progression, complete closure of the airway entrance is impaired, allowing penetration of food into the airway during the swallow, with aspiration of this material after the swallow. Earlier in the progression of the disease, tongue base posterior movement and pharyngeal contraction are reduced, so residual material remains in the pharynx after the swallow. This material may then be aspirated when the patient inhales after the swallow. Usually at the same time that tongue base retraction and pharyngeal contraction are affected, the triggering of the pharyngeal swallow becomes delayed. At this time, thermal–tactile stimulation is often helpful for a period of approximately 6 to 12 months. Patients can be taught to do the technique to themselves. At some point, however, the effectiveness of the procedure is reduced as the nervous system continues to deteriorate. As long as laryngeal function remains adequate to protect the airway, the patient can feed orally by gradually changing the viscosity of the diet to liquids and thin paste consistencies.

Twenty ALS patients with predominantly corticobulbar involvement were followed at Northwestern University Medical School from the initiation of their swallowing disorders until the termination of oral feeding. In all of these patients, the disease began with involvement of oral musculature and later progressed to involve neuromuscular control of respiration and the extremities. The progression of deterioration in neuromuscular control of deglutition observed in 16 of these ALS patients began with reduction in oral lingual control, tongue base movement, and pharyngeal contraction, followed by a delay in triggering the pharyngeal swallow. A few patients developed cricopharyngeal disorders, usually as a result of poor laryngeal movement (Smith, Mulder, & Code, 1957). Cricopharyngeal myotomy is not usually successful in these patients, probably because the cricopharyngeal problems are usually related to poor laryngeal movement and because of the severity of pharyngeal, laryngeal, and oral aspects of the swallow, including the triggering of the pharyngeal swallow. The patients are unable to generate adequate pressure to propel food through the upper digestive tract, even if the upper esophageal sphincter is open.

Patients with predominantly corticospinal involvement often do not experience swallowing changes until a number of years after their initial diagnosis. The nature of their swallowing disorders is frequently quite different from that of patients with predominantly corticobulbar involvement, often characterized by reduced velar movement and reduced pharyngeal wall contraction. The first sign of dysphagia in these patients may be a slowly progressive weight loss. The patients themselves may not be aware of any swallowing problem.

Swallowing management in patients with ALS usually involves use of compensatory procedures rather than active exercise, which may simply cause fatigue. Swallowing disorders may be the first sign of motor neuron disease. They may be accompanied by fasciculations in the tongue and concomitant changes in speech.

Pediatric Motor Neuron Disease: Werdnig–Hoffmann Disease

Werdnig–Hoffmann disease is an aggressive form of pediatric motor neuron disease that is usually diagnosed when the infant begins missing motor milestones at approximately 12 to 18 months of age. Usually the child is essentially paralyzed from the shoulders down by 3 to 3½ years of age. The pharyngeal stage of the swallow often begins to be affected at approximately 18 to 24 months of age in the presence of normal oral function for both speech and swallowing. Six children with this disease were followed longitudinally at Northwestern Memorial Hospital. All maintained normal articulation and oromotor function for chewing and oral transit during swallowing, even when they were completely paralyzed from the shoulders down and mechanically ventilated, usually at some point in the third year of life. At that point, the pharyngeal swallow was completely nonfunctional because of a delayed pharyngeal swallow, severely reduced pharyngeal wall contraction unilaterally or bilaterally, and reduced laryngeal elevation. The latter disorders caused chronic aspiration after the swallow.

Management strategies for the swallowing problems associated with this disease generally involve compensatory strategies, including postural changes and sensory enhancement techniques, such as thermal–tactile stimulation. Aggressive exercise generally caused fatigue. A gentle supraglottic swallow can also be helpful. However, as in adults with motor neuron disease, all of these strategies will eventually fail as the nervous system continues to deteriorate. Even when these children are fed nonorally, use of head posture changes may help with management of secretions.

Parkinson's Disease

Patients with Parkinson's disease may exhibit a number of swallowing disorders in all three stages of deglutition (Blonsky, Logemann, Boshes, & Fisher, 1975; Donner & Silbiger, 1966; Hurwitz, Nelson, & Haddad, 1975; Kilman & Goyal, 1976; Leopold & Kagel, 1996; Logemann, Blonsky, & Boshes, 1975; Nowack, Hatelid, & Sohn, 1977; Robbins et al., 1982, 1986). In the oral phase of the swallow, patients with Parkinson's disease often exhibit a typical repetitive anterior–posterior rolling pattern in lingual propulsion of the bolus. The bolus is held in a normal position when the swallow is begun. Then the midline of the tongue rolls the bolus posteriorly. However, the back tongue often does not lower and the bolus rolls back anteriorly. This backward–forward movement of the bolus may be repeated a number of times until, finally, one single anterior–posterior movement of the tongue is sufficient to propel the bolus and the back tongue lowers to allow the bolus to pass (Blonsky et al., 1975; Massengill & Nashold, 1969a). This type of "festination" in the lingual musculature may involve some degree of muscle rigidity—the patient is unable to lower the back of his or her tongue once it has been elevated to hold the bolus in the preparatory position for swallowing.

Some patients with Parkinson's disease exhibit a delay in the triggering of the pharyngeal swallow, although it is usually mild (2 to 3 seconds). Once the pharyngeal swallow triggers, pharyngeal wall contraction and posterior motion of the tongue base are often reduced, resulting in residue of material in the valleculae and pyriform sinuses after each swallow (Donner & Silbiger, 1966; Silbiger, Pikielney, & Donner, 1967). This residue may increase with each consecutive swallow, particularly if material is of a thick paste or pudding consistency. In the later stages of the disease, patients may experience sufficient involvement of laryngeal musculature so that laryngeal elevation and laryngeal closure during the swallow are incomplete, and some material enters the airway during the swallow. More frequently, aspiration in these patients is caused by the material remaining in the pharynx *after* the swallow because of poor tongue base and pharyngeal wall function. This residue falls into the open airway when the patient inhales after the swallow. Occasionally, patients with Parkinson's disease exhibit a disorder of the cricopharyngeal juncture or upper esophageal sphincter, usually related to both reduced laryngeal elevation and poor tongue base and/or pharyngeal wall motion. Some authors have reported a higher incidence of cricopharyngeal disorder in these patients (Donner & Silbiger, 1966) and indicate a problem with relaxation of the cricopharyngeal muscular portion of the sphincter.

In my experience, the progression of swallowing dysfunction in the patient with Parkinson's disease begins with reduction in tongue base retraction and the repetitive rocking–rolling motion of the tongue. Triggering of the pharyngeal swallow may then become delayed. As the disease progresses, the reduction in tongue base movement and pharyngeal contraction may worsen, and laryngeal elevation and closure during swallowing may also become inadequate. A cricopharyngeal dysfunction may also occur. It is important to note that not all patients with Parkinson's disease exhibit severe swallowing problems, even at advanced stages of the disease, and that there is some variability in disorders and progression among patients.

Many patients with Parkinson's disease exhibit tremors at rest in various structures in the head and neck. Tremors may occur in the mandible, oral tongue or tongue base, soft palate, and/or larynx. When beginning a radiographic study with a patient with Parkinson's disease or any movement disorder, before placing food in the patient's mouth, the clinician should turn on the videofluoroscopy and observe the patient's mouth and pharynx at rest, looking for any tremor activity. In contrast to patients with Parkinson's disease, individuals with essential tremor have been found to exhibit no swallowing disorders (Blonsky et al., 1975), but they may also exhibit some tremors in head and neck structures.

Oropharyngeal swallowing problems may be the first sign of Parkinson's disease. The rocking–rolling tongue motion described earlier is a particularly pathognomonic sign of this disease. If the swallowing therapist suspects Parkinson's disease as a possible cause of a patient's oropharyngeal swallowing disorder, referral to a neurologist is needed. If the diagnosis is not confirmed, the swallowing therapist and neurologist should follow the patient for reevaluation in 6 months to 1 year for a possible increase or change in symptoms.

End-stage Parkinson's disease may also result in dementia, which can make feeding and swallowing management difficult (Bine, Frank, & McDade, 1995). The patient may not be able to follow directions to use some therapy strategies. Use of compensatory procedures may be most effective. Patients may also have severe rigidity, which makes use of some of the postural changes difficult. In some cases, modification of diet or nonoral feeding may be needed.

Patients with dysphagia resulting from Parkinson's disease may exhibit improvement in their swallowing function when placed on medication as newly diagnosed patients or when given a new medication. Before beginning swallowing therapy with a newly diagnosed patient with dysphagia resulting from Parkinson's disease, the clinician may wish to wait several weeks to determine the effects of the medications on the patient's swallow. In some patients with Parkinson's disease, dysphagia is significantly improved to functional levels with no aspiration when they reach optimal medication doses (Bushmann, Dobmeyer, Leeker, & Perlmutter, 1989; Fonda, Schwarz, & Clinnick, 1995).

Longitudinal studies of medication effects on swallowing in Parkinson's disease are needed. Patients with Parkinson's disease often respond well to very active range-of-motion exercises for the tongue, lips, and laryngeal elevation. In addition to lip and tongue exercises, the effortful swallow, Mendelsohn maneuver, effortful breath-hold, and falsetto exercise can all be used. Patients are usually advised to do these exercises in the morning and at night for a total of 10 to 12 minutes each time.

Postpolio Syndrome

Patients who had polio during the epidemic of the 1950s are now often suffering increasing muscle weakness, including swallowing problems, particularly those who suffered bulbar polio (Bosma, 1953; Buchholz, 1994c). Interestingly, these patients may not have had swallowing problems in their initial bout of polio (Ivanyi, Phoa, & deVisser, 1994; Sonies & Dalakas, 1991). The swallowing problems displayed by these patients include unilateral and bilateral pharyngeal wall weakness, reduced tongue base retraction, and reduced laryngeal elevation resulting in reduced closure of the laryngeal vestibule. All of these disorders cause residue to remain in various areas of the pharynx, with the risk of aspiration after the swallow. Often, postural changes selected to match the patient's swallow physiology will facilitate a better swallow with reduced risk of aspiration. Interestingly, however, many of these patients do not perceive the improvements in their swallow efficiency as a result of the postural change and must be convinced of its worth by review of the videotape and discussion with the clinician. In most cases, aggressive exercise will fatigue the mechanism more than strengthen it. Compensatory strategies are, therefore, usually the procedures of choice.

Multiple Sclerosis

Patients with multiple sclerosis (MS) usually have multiple plaques in the neurologic system from the cortex to the brainstem and cerebellum to the corticospinal tracts. The disorders that these patients have in swallowing may relate to any of their neurologic lesions from the cortex to the brainstem and the cranial nerve–innervated peripheral nerves. Because these lesions may affect single or multiple cranial nerves, the patient with MS can exhibit swallowing disorders of various types (Daly, Code, & Andersen, 1962; Kilman & Goyal, 1976). If the hypoglossal nerve is affected, the patient's lingual control of bolus manipulation, chewing, and oral transit will be reduced to some extent. If cranial nerve X is involved, the patient's tongue base movement, pharyngeal wall movement, and laryngeal function will be reduced. If cranial nerve IX is involved, the triggering of the pharyngeal swallow may be delayed (Silbiger et al., 1967). If all three of these or any other combination of nerves is involved, the patient will exhibit multiple swallowing problems.

In the 150 patients with MS studied at Northwestern University Medical School, delayed pharyngeal swallow and reduction in pharyngeal wall contraction occurred most frequently in this population. A study of two groups of MS patients, one group with swallowing complaints and the other without complaints, revealed that all had swallowing disorders (Fabiszak, 1987). The patients without complaints exhibited milder swallowing problems. The most common swallowing disorders in the patients in this study were a delay in triggering the pharyngeal swallow and reduced tongue base retraction and pharyngeal wall contraction, leaving residue in the valleculae. Patients with bulbar involvement tended to have a reduction in lingual function and laryngeal adduction as well. However, these latter disorders were far less common and were not seen in all patients with advanced disease. Patients with MS respond well to therapy procedures designed to heighten sensory input, such as thermal–tactile stimulation to improve triggering of the pharyngeal swallow (Sorensen, Brown, Logemann, Wilson, & Herndon, 1994).

Improvements in swallowing function are often seen when MS patients are given new medications, but no studies have systematically examined effects of medications on swallowing in these patients. Some patients with MS develop cognitive impairments and dementia. In these patients, the compensatory strategies are quite important, particularly postures and sensory enhancement procedures.

Myasthenia Gravis

Myasthenia gravis, a neurologic disease causing biochemical changes in the myoneural junction, generally presents as a fatiguing of the involved musculature with repeated use (Carpenter, McDonald, & Howard, 1979; Donner, 1974; Silbiger et al., 1967). Most frequently, cranial nerves are initially involved. Although ocular muscles are most often affected first, causing ptosis, any other musculature innervated by cranial nerves may also be involved as the initial symptom (Aronson, 1971, 1980; Carpenter et al., 1979; Donner, 1974; Donner & Silbiger, 1966). Aronson (1974) reported a case of laryngeal dysfunction as the first symptom of myasthenia gravis. Two patients have been seen at Northwestern University Medical School with initial pharyngeal wall involvement that was exhibited only during deglutition at mealtime. In these patients, pharyngeal contraction was progressively reduced with use until no pharyngeal contraction could be seen. Pharyngeal constrictor involvement as the sole initial symptom of myasthenia gravis is relatively rare, and often difficult to document without fluoroscopy completed at the beginning of the patient's feeding and after approximately 15 to 20 minutes of consecutive swallowing. Patients with myasthenia gravis may be misdiagnosed as having an emotionally based swallowing disorder and referred for psychotherapy or psychotherapeutic treatment. One such patient received 6 months of electroshock therapy for a myasthenic swallowing disorder that was misdiagnosed as a psychiatric disturbance. Thus, it is important for the swallowing therapist to keep myasthenia gravis in mind as a potential etiology for swallowing disturbance, particularly in the presence of a history of difficulty with swallowing that worsens with use and improves with rest. I have also seen patients whose myasthenia gravis affected only the tongue musculature or velar function, usually resulting in both nasality during speech and backflow of food into the nasal cavity during swallowing, or the muscles of mastication, affecting the patient's ability to chew.

Diagnostic evaluation for myasthenia gravis may involve a tensilon test, with swallowing, speech, or other function evaluated before and after administration of tensilon. Similarly, the modified barium swallow can be used to assess effects of fatigue by repeating the test before and after the patient eats for 15 to 20 minutes. Generally, medication for the disease results in swallowing improvement. Use of compensatory swallowing management strategies is usually best because active exercise may only contribute to fatigue. Patients should also be advised as to the diet they can swallow best, depending on their particular muscle involvement, and eating more small meals per day may be better than eating three large meals.

Muscular Dystrophy

A number of types of muscular dystrophy affect the swallowing mechanism. *Myotonic dystrophy*, characterized by prolonged contraction and difficulty in relaxation of involved muscles, frequently affects the sternocleidomastoid, the muscles of mastication, and the cricopharyngeal (upper esophageal) sphincter so that the muscular portion of the sphincter, the cricopharyngeal muscle, will not relax adequately to allow the larynx to move and open the sphincter during swallowing (Casey & Aminoff, 1971; Donner & Silbiger, 1966; Hughes, Swann, Gleeson, & Lee, 1965; Kilman & Goyal, 1976; Siegel, Hendrix, & Collins, 1966). These patients can exhibit aspiration because the material that cannot pass through the cricopharyngeal juncture overflows the pyriform sinuses and enters the airway. If careful assessment reveals a hypertonic cricopharyngeal muscle, a cricopharyngeal myotomy may be appropriate.

Oculopharyngeal dystrophy, a muscular dystrophy affecting the ocular and pharyngeal muscles selectively, may result in reduced pharyngeal contraction and dysfunction of the muscular portion of the cricopharyngeal juncture (Aarli, 1969; Duranceau, Letendre, Clermont, Levisque, & Barbeau, 1978; Kilman & Goyal, 1976). These patients often cannot propel material through the pharynx because of the reduced strength of the pharyngeal constrictors and, in addition, cannot move material through the cricopharyngeal sphincter because the muscular portion does not relax and allow the larynx to move up and forward and open the sphincter.

Other types of muscular dystrophy may also affect the pharynx and cause a reduction in strength of the pharyngeal constrictors. This is the most common swallowing dysfunction in patients with muscular dystrophy of any type (Silbiger et al., 1967). Generally, compensatory strategies are best for management of the swallowing disorders in various forms of muscular dystrophy.

Dystonia

Dystonia is a relatively rare chronic disease characterized by involuntary, irregular chronic contortions of muscles of the head, neck, trunk, and extremities, which may affect speech and/or swallowing. Bosma et al. (1982) completed a detailed study of swallowing in one patient with medication-induced dystonia. According to Bosma, dystonia may worsen with volitional attempts to manipulate food in preparation for the swallow. As the dystonic movements worsen, the labial seal worsens and food is lost from the mouth. Collecting the bolus to initiate the swallow may be severely impaired, and some material may fall over the base of the tongue prematurely. Oral transit times are slowed, with disorganized lingual propulsion of the bolus. Once the pharyngeal swallow is initiated, the motor control of the pharyngeal stage of the swallow is usually normal.

Dermatomyositis

Dermatomyositis is a collagen disease in which polymyositis or multiple muscle involvement is one distinguishing characteristic. The polymyositis usually causes dysphagia (Dietz, Logemann, Sahgal, & Schmid, 1980; Metheny, 1978). Reduced pharyngeal contraction and dysfunctioning of the cricopharyngeus muscle are two of the main swallowing problems observed in these patients.

Oropharyngeal Swallowing Problems as a First Sign of Neurologic Disease

In some patients with progressive neurologic disease, dysphagia is the first symptom. Parkinson's disease, myasthenia gravis, amyotrophic lateral sclerosis (ALS), and Guillain–Barré may all initially present with swallowing disorders (Buchholz, Neumann, Jones, & Ravich, 1995). The patient with Parkinson's disease may exhibit rocking–rolling tongue motion alone or in combination with reduced tongue base movement and/or reduced lip closure and poor laryngeal elevation. The patient with myasthenia gravis usually presents with fatigue on use of selected muscles during swallowing. Use of the fatigue test during videofluoroscopy—that is, repeating the test before and after eating—is also recommended. The patient with ALS may exhibit reduced lip closure, reduced fine tongue control, and chewing with or without fasciculations in the tongue. Soft palate involvement may also be present. The patient with Guillain–Barré may exhibit a generally weak swallow with reduced range of motion of all pharyngeal structures. The patient with a brainstem tumor may also exhibit slowly progressive swallowing problems, usually affecting triggering of the pharyngeal swallow, reduced laryngeal elevation, and reduced tongue base action.

When a patient with no identified medical diagnosis exhibits any significant oropharyngeal dysphagia on videofluorographic study, the movement patterns in the mouth and pharynx during the oropharyngeal swallow should be carefully observed and compared to swallow movement patterns seen in patients with specific neurologic diagnoses. In addition, the swallowing therapist should observe the patient's posture, gait, and fine motor control. These often reflect changes in the patient's motor control critical to a neurologic diagnosis. In addition, a careful history should be taken to determine whether the problem is progressive. In general, the first referral for such a patient should be to a neurologist. In addition to sending the report of the swallow study to the neurologist, the swallowing therapist should talk with the neurologist before the patient meets the doctor to alert the neurologist to the nature of the patient's dysphagia as a possible indicator of neurologic disease or damage (Buchholz, 1994a, 1994b). Stroke, particularly a small brainstem stroke, may also cause only swallow dysfunction (Buchholz, 1993).

Other Degenerative Diseases Causing Swallowing Problems

Other degenerative diseases or conditions characterized by deterioration may cause swallowing problems. These include rheumatoid arthritis and chronic obstructive pulmonary disease.

Rheumatoid Arthritis

Rheumatoid arthritis (RA) can affect several structures involved in swallowing. It can invade the cricoarytenoid joint, thereby restricting arytenoid movement during swallowing. Because the arytenoid cartilage rotates to bring the vocal folds into adduction, and tilts anteriorly to contribute to closure of the airway entrance, movement of the arytenoid cartilage on the cricoid cartilage is critical to normal swallowing. A flare-up of rheumatoid arthritis can cause swelling in the cricoarytenoid joint and in the arytenoid cartilage, resulting in a collection of food around the arytenoid and/or in the airway entrance, with aspiration after the swallow. One of our patients exhibited such significant swelling in the arytenoid cartilage that she received a biopsy to rule out laryngeal cancer. Results of the biopsy were inflammatory changes consistent with rheumatoid arthritis.

Rheumatoid arthritis may also cause swelling in the cervical vertebrae, which may impinge on the posterior pharyngeal wall (Ekberg, Redlund-Johnell, & Sjoblom, 1987). These arthritic changes in the vertebrae may also make use of postural changes to improve swallowing more difficult. Rheumatoid arthritis can also damage the temporomandibular joint, making chewing painful. Usually, if the patient with rheumatoid arthritis is in a flare-up of the disease, medication is changed or increased to counteract the problem. The medication should reduce edema and improve swallowing. The swallowing therapist simply needs to introduce compensatory strategies, if possible, to facilitate oral intake until the inflammation in involved structures is eliminated.

Chronic Obstructive Pulmonary Disease

Because respiration and swallowing are closely coordinated, it is likely that changes in respiratory function, such as occur with chronic obstructive pulmonary disease (COPD), may result in swallowing problems. COPD is a generic term for physiologic abnormalities causing chronic airflow limitation (Coelho, 1987; Gold, 1985). Few investigators have examined the swallowing problems in patients with COPD, and the incidence of swallowing disorders in this population has not been well defined. However, the few discussions of dysphagia in COPD have found a difficulty with airway closure and aspiration during the swallow. Whether the airway closure problem results from the chronic obstructive pulmonary disease or is the contributing cause of the pulmonary disease is unknown. Typically, in these patients, compensatory strategies are best because other types of exercises may put further stress and work on the respiratory system and be unproductive. Compensatory changes, such as postural changes, diet changes, and use of sensory enhancement procedures, typically do not increase muscular effort or the duration of airway closure, which is a particular problem with patients who have respiratory disease.

References

Aarli, J. (1969). Oculopharyngeal muscular dystrophy. *Acta Neurologica Scandinavia, 45*, 484–492.

Aronson, A. (1971). Early motor unit disease masquerading as psychogenic breathy dysphonia: A clinical case presentation. *Journal of Speech and Hearing Disorders, 36*, 116–124.

Aronson, A. (1980). *Clinical voice disorders: An interdisciplinary approach.* New York: Thieme-Stratton.

Bine, J. E., Frank, E. M., & McDade, H. L. (1995). Dysphagia and dementia in subjects with Parkinson's disease. *Dysphasia, 10*, 160–164.

Blonsky, E., Logemann, J., Boshes, B., & Fisher, H. (1975). Comparison of speech and swallowing function in patients with tremor disorders and in normal geriatric patients: A cinefluorographic study. *Journal of Gerontology, 30,* 299–303.

Bosma, J. (1953). Studies of disability of the pharynx resultant from poliomyelitis. *Annals of Otology, Rhinology and Laryngology, 64,* 529–547.

Bosma, J., Geoffrey, V., Thach, B., Weiffenbach, J., Kavanagh, J., & Orr, W. (1982). A pattern of medication induced persistent bulbar and cervical dystonia. *The International Journal of Orofacial Myology, 8,* 5–19.

Buchholz, D. W. (1993). Clinically probable brainstem stroke presenting primarily as dysphagia and nonvisualized by MRI. *Dysphagia, 8,* 235–238.

Buchholz, D. W. (1994a). Dysphagia associated with neurologic disorders. *Acta Oto-Rhino-Laryngologica Belgica, 48,* 143–155.

Buchholz, D. W. (1994b). Neurogenic dysphagia: What is the cause when the cause is not obvious? *Dysphagia, 9,* 245–255.

Buchholz, D.W. (1994c). Postpolio dysphagia. *Dysphagia, 9,* 99–100.

Buchholz, D., Neumann, S., Jones, B., & Ravich, W. (1995). Neurogenic dysphagia: Results of swallowing center neurologic evaluation of 228 cases [Abstract]. *Dysphagia, 10,* 137.

Bushmann, M. M., Dobmeyer, S. M., Leeker, L., & Perlmutter, J. S. (1989). Swallowing abnormalities and their response to treatment in Parkinson's disease. *Neurology, 39,* 1309–1314.

Carpenter, R., McDonald, T., & Howard, F. (1979). The otolaryngologic presentation of myasthenia gravis. *Laryngoscope, 89,* 922–927.

Casey, E., & Aminoff, M. (1971). Dystrophia myotonica presenting with dysphagia. *British Medical Journal, 2* (Suppl.), 443.

Coelho, C. (1987). Preliminary findings on the nature of dysphagia in patients with chronic obstructive pulmonary disease. *Dysphagia, 2,* 28–31.

Daly, D., Code, C., & Andersen, H. (1962). Disturbances of swallowing and esophageal motility in patients with multiple sclerosis. *Neurology, 12,* 250–256.

Dietz, F., Logemann, J., Sahgal, V., & Schmid, F. (1980). Cricopharyngeal muscle dysfunction in the differential diagnosis of dysphagia in polymyositis. *Arthritis and Rheumatism, 23,* 491–495.

Donner, M. (1974). Swallowing mechanisms and neuromuscular disorders. *Seminars in Roentgenology, 9,* 273–282.

Donner, M., & Silbiger, M. (1966). Cinefluorographic analysis of pharyngeal swallowing in neuromuscular disorders. *American Journal of Medical Science, 251,* 600–616.

Duranceau, C., Letendre, J., Clermont, R., Levisque, H., & Barbeau, A. (1978). Oropharyngeal dysphagia in patients with oculopharyngeal muscular dystrophy. *Canadian Journal of Surgery, 21,* 326–329.

Dworkin, J., & Hartman, D. (1979). Progressive speech deterioration and dysphagia in amyotrophic lateral sclerosis: Case report. *Archives of Physical Medicine and Rehabilitation, 60,* 423–425.

Ekberg, O., Redlund-Johnell, I., & Sjoblom, K. G. (1987). Pharyngeal function in patients with rheumatoid arthritis of the cervical spine and temporomandibular joint. *Acta Radiologica, 28,* 35–39.

Fabiszak, A. (1987). *Swallowing patterns in neurologically normal subjects and two subgroups of multiple sclerosis patients.* Unpublished doctoral dissertation, Northwestern University, Evanston, IL.

Fonda, D., Schwarz, J., & Clinnick, S. (1995). Parkinsonian medication one hour before meals improves symptomatic swallowing: A case study. *Dysphagia, 10*, 165–166.

Gold, P. M. (1985). Chronic obstructive pulmonary disease. In R. Conn (Ed.), *Current diagnosis* (pp. 339–343). Philadelphia: W. B. Saunders.

Horner, J., Alberts, M. J., Dawson, D. V., & Cook, G. M. (1994). Swallowing in Alzheimer's disease. *Alzheimer Disease and Associated Disorders, 8*(3), 177–189.

Hughes, D., Swann, J., Gleeson, J., & Lee, F. (1965). Abnormalities in swallowing associated with dystrophia myotonica. *Brain, 88*, 1037–1042.

Hurwitz, A., Nelson, J., & Haddad, J. (1975). Oropharyngeal dysphagia: Manometric and cineesophagraphic findings. *Digestive Disease, 20*, 313–324.

Ivanyi, B., Phoa, S. S. K. S., & deVisser, M. (1994). Dysphagia in postpolio patients: A videofluorographic follow-up study. *Dysphagia, 9*, 96–98.

Kilman, W., & Goyal, R. (1976). Disorders of pharyngeal and upper esophageal sphincter motor function. *Archives of Internal Medicine, 136*, 592–601.

Leopold, N. A., & Kagel, M. A. (1996). Prepharyngeal dysphagia in Parkinson's disease. *Dysphagia, 11*, 14–22.

Logemann, J., Blonsky, E., & Boshes, B. (1975). Dysphagia in Parkinsonism. *Journal of the American Medical Association, 231*, 69–70.

Massengill, R., & Nashold, B. (1969a). Cinefluorographic evaluation of swallowing in patients with involuntary movements. *Confinia Neurologica, 31*, 269–272.

Metheny, J. (1978). Dermatomyositis: A vocal and swallowing disease entity. *Laryngoscope, 88*, 147–161.

Nowack, W., Hatelid, J., & Sohn, R. (1977). Dysphagia in Parkinsonism. *Archives of Neurology, 34*, 320.

Robbins, J., Logemann, J., & Kirshner, H. (1982). *Velopharyngeal activity during speech and swallowing in neurologic disease*. Paper presented at the American Speech-Language-Hearing Association annual meeting, Toronto.

Robbins, J., Logemann, J., & Kirshner, H. (1986). Swallowing and speech production in Parkinson's disease. *Annals of Neurology, 19*, 283–287.

Siegel, C., Hendrix, T., & Collins, J. (1966). The swallowing disorder in myotonia dystrophica. *Gastroenterology, 50*, 541–549.

Silbiger, M., Pikielney, R., & Donner, M. (1967). Neuromuscular disorders affecting the pharynx: Cineradiographic analysis. *Investigative Radiology, 2*, 442–448.

Smith, A., Mulder, D., & Code, C. (1957). Esophageal motility in amyotrophic lateral sclerosis. *Mayo Clinic Proceedings of the Staff Meetings, 32*, 438–441.

Sonies, B. C., & Dalakas, M. C. (1991). Dysphagia in patients with the postpolio syndrome. *New England Journal of Medicine, 324*, 1162–1167.

Sorensen, P., Brown, S., Logemann, J. A., Wilson, K., & Herndon, R. (1994). MS Care: Communication disorders and dysphagia. *Journal of Neurologic Rehabilitation, 8*(3), 137–143.

Suski, N. S., & Nielsen, C. C. (1989). Factors affecting food intake of women with Alzheimer's type dementia in long-term care. *Journal of the American Dietetic Association, 89*, 1770–1773.

MEDICAL TREATMENT
FOR SWALLOWING DISORDERS

Several types of medical procedures are used in the management of swallowing disorders, including techniques designed to improve specific anatomic or physiologic swallowing disorders; procedures designed to eliminate or control unremitting, prolonged aspiration; procedures to provide nutrition and hydration nonorally; and medications to improve swallowing disorders.

Techniques Designed To Improve Specific Swallowing Disorders

Although several medical procedures are designed to improve specific types of swallowing disorders, none are used broadly. These techniques include surgical reduction of osteophytes; vocal fold medialization, or injection of Teflon or similar material into a reconstructed or damaged vocal fold to improve vocal fold closure during swallowing; laryngeal suspension for reduced laryngeal elevation; dilatation for scar tissue in the cricopharyngeal region; cricopharyngeal myotomy to cut a spastic cricopharyngeal muscle; and botulinum toxin injection into a spastic cricopharyngeal muscle.

Surgical Reduction of Osteophytes

Cervical osteophytes are boney overgrowths on the cervical vertebra that displace the posterior pharyngeal wall anteriorly. If the pharyngeal narrowing is severe, surgical reduction can be performed by entering the paraesophageal space through an incision in the side of the neck (Blumberg, Prapote, & Viscomi, 1977; Parker, 1989; Valadka, Kubal, & Smith, 1995). The vertebral periosteum is reflected back and the excess bone removed. There is some difference of opinion on the effect of cervical osteophytes on swallowing. There is no doubt that if a cervical osteophyte is large enough, the mass of bone can significantly diminish the pharyngeal space, making the passage of a large or thick bolus of food difficult. Also, as Press and Leffall (1972) reported, the boney overgrowth may press on the cervical nerve roots, producing the sense of dysphagia. However, entering the neck can have negative side effects, such as creation of scar tissue or damage to nerves innervating structures involved in swallowing, which can create dysphagia.

Procedures To Improve Airway Closure at the Vocal Folds

Injection of an inert substance into a damaged vocal fold is designed to add bulk to one vocal fold or to whatever tissue is located at the top of the airway in order to improve closure at the vocal folds and airway protection during swallowing. The additional mass is added to the damaged or reconstructed vocal fold and is thought to improve contact with the other, movable, more normal vocal fold, thus facilitating closure (Arnold, 1962; Lewy, 1963; Sessions, Zill, & Schwartz, 1979; Ward, Hanson, & Abermayor, 1985; Yarington & Harned, 1971). The technique is usually used in patients whose laryngeal adduction for airway protection has not been sufficiently improved with an exercise program. It has been used in head and neck surgical patients, particularly partial laryngectomy patients whose remaining tissues in the larynx are insufficient to adduct and protect the airway. One limitation to the procedure is the denseness of the tissue into which the injection is made. There must be enough tissue space to accept the injected material. Such injections have also been used in neurologic patients with inadequate vocal fold closure, including individuals with Parkinson's disease and amyotrophic lateral sclerosis. Glycerin, gel foam, or some other *temporary* substance can be injected to simulate the effect of a more permanent injection.

If the swallowing disorder causing aspiration is reduced closure of the larynx at the vocal fold level, such an injection may be a successful treatment. If, however, the procedure is done on patients whose swallowing has not been carefully evaluated radiographically, and who are aspirating because of failure of closure of the airway entrance, not at the vocal fold level, or because of reduced lingual control, delayed or absent pharyngeal swallow, reduced pharyngeal wall contraction, or reduced tongue base movement, adding bulk to the adductor mechanism will not improve the swallow or reduce the aspiration. Unfortunately, some of the literature on swallowing describes aspiration in such a way that it sounds as if poor vocal fold closure is the most frequent cause. Our experience is that 10% or less of aspiration is caused by inadequate vocal fold closure. Vocal fold medialization procedures have also been used to move the damaged vocal fold to midline (Koufman, 1986).

Laryngeal Suspension for Reduced Laryngeal Elevation

If the patient's larynx does not lift and move forward adequately, airway entrance closure and cricopharyngeal opening are negatively affected. Occasionally, laryngeal suspension is attempted surgically (Calcaterra, 1971; Edgerton & Duncan, 1959; Goode, 1976). A suture is placed from the middle of the mandible to the laryngeal cartilage, and the larynx is raised and tilted under the tongue base. This is done occasionally in head and neck cancer patients but rarely in neurologic patients.

Dilatation of Scar Tissue in the Cricopharyngeal Region

Dilatation of scar tissue of the cricopharyngeal region involves the passage of mercury-filled soft rubber tubes (bougies) of increasing diameter through the cricopharyngeal region to gradually stretch it open and to tear any scar tissue that might be present. Most clinicians have found the effects of dilatation to be temporary, lasting approximately 1 to 3 months (Calcaterra, Kadell, & Ward, 1975; Palmer, 1974; Zinninger, 1966). Because of the increased resistance at the upper esophageal sphincter in these patients, it may be difficult to pass the bougie, and a perforation can occur (Duranceau, Letendre, Clermont, Levisque, & Barbeau, 1978). Dilatation will generally not help a patient with cricopharyngeal dysfunction related to neurologic damage.

Cricopharyngeal Myotomy

Cricopharyngeal myotomy involves an external incision through the side of the neck (usually the left side) into the cricopharyngeal muscle, slitting the fibers of the muscle from top to bottom, usually at the posterior midline, to permanently open the sphincter. Usually the incision extends upward to include some of the inferior constrictor fibers, and downward into the esophageal musculature (Calcaterra et al., 1975). The patient frequently can begin to eat within 1 week after the myotomy (Mitchell & Armanini, 1975). Studies of the success of this procedure have sometimes reported improvement rates of 60% to 78% (Lebo, Sang, & Norris, 1976; Mills, 1973). When the criteria used for selection of patients in these studies are carefully examined, it is often clear that patients with swallowing disorders other than cricopharyngeal dysfunction have been treated with this surgery; the success of a cricopharyngeal myotomy in those patients would be negligible and thus affect the success rate of the procedure. Success rates for myotomy climb when patients are carefully selected for the procedure using the following criteria: (1) a cricopharyngeal muscle dysfunction must be the predominant problem; (2) the patient must be able to move material through the oral and pharyngeal stages of the swallow up to the cricopharyngeal region; and (3) the patient must be able to voluntarily close the airway during the swallow (Aki & Blakeley, 1974; Blakeley, Garety, & Smith, 1968; Wilkins, 1964).

Historically, cricopharyngeal myotomy has been used as a generic treatment for swallowing disorders in a number of types of patients, including those with Parkinson's disease, amyotrophic lateral sclerosis, and occulopharyngeal dystrophy (Aki & Blakeley, 1974; Asherson, 1973; Calcaterra et al., 1975; Chodosh, 1975; Cruse, Edwards, Smith, & Wyllie, 1979; Dayal & Freeman, 1976; Duranceau et al., 1978; Ellis, Schlegel, Lynch, & Payne, 1969; Henderson & Marryatt, 1977; Mills, 1964; Mladick, Horton, & Adamson, 1971; Palmer, 1974; Stevens & Newell, 1971; Wilkins, 1964). At this time, this procedure has limited use, that is, in a small subset of patients with a cricopharyngeal dysfunction whose muscular portion of the upper esophageal sphincter (i.e., the cricopharyngeal muscle) is in spasm and does not allow the larynx to move up and forward. This is a small proportion of patients. Many more patients with cricopharyngeal dysfunction have difficulty with the anterior superior laryngeal movement component of cricopharyngeal opening in the presence of an apparently normally relaxing cricopharyngeal muscle. These latter patients need exercise programs to improve laryngeal movement.

In general, a cricopharyngeal myotomy should *not* be performed early in the recovery course of a patient who has suffered a stroke, head injury, or spinal cord injury. Most of these patients will recover well. A few patients do not recover well and at 6 months after a brainstem stroke are still experiencing severe swallowing problems because of difficulty in opening the cricopharyngeal region. Several clinicians have questioned whether a myotomy would improve the swallow, or at least allow the patient to do a more successful Mendelsohn maneuver (Buchholz, 1995; Robbins & Levine, 1993). Patients for the procedure would need to be carefully selected.

Cricopharyngeal myotomy has often been done as a prophylactic treatment to potentially improve swallowing in patients undergoing supraglottic laryngectomy or tongue base resection (Mladick, Horton, & Adamson, 1961). In a clinical trial conducted by the Radiation Therapy Oncology Group (RTOG, Philadelphia), patients of these two types were randomized to receive or not receive a cricopharyngeal myotomy as a part of their oncologic surgical procedure. No difference was found in oral pharyngeal swallowing efficiency between the two groups, indicating that myotomy, at the time of the oncologic surgical procedure, does not improve postoperative swallowing in patients who receive a supraglottic laryngectomy or a tonsil/base of tongue resection (Jacobs et al., 1997; T. Pajak, personal communication, October 5, 1996).

Some patients who have received a myotomy may not benefit from it unless a postural assist or the Mendelsohn maneuver is also used. The patient is usually asked to turn his or her head toward the unoperated side, thus directing material through the pyriform sinus on the operated and, presumably, the more open side. Some patients need to use both head rotation and the Mendelsohn maneuver.

Patients with multiple dysfunctions in the vocal tract, including reduced lingual control, delayed pharyngeal swallowing, or reduced pharyngeal contraction, in addition to cricopharyngeal dysfunction, are generally poor candidates for the procedure. If the pharyngeal swallow does not trigger, the larynx will stand open to receive any material that drains over the base of the tongue into the pharynx. Complications of the procedure may include hemorrhage or recurrent laryngeal nerve damage, as well as complications inherent in surgically opening the neck (Lund, 1968).

Botulinum Toxin Injection

Botulinum toxin injection into the cricopharyngeal muscle has been reported in one case study to have resulted in significantly improved swallowing (Kostas, Karam, Langhans, & Vasquez, 1995). There is great difficulty in accurately placing the injection because the cricopharyngeal muscle is hidden behind the cricoid cartilage. Inaccurate injection could paralyze other muscles in the area, resulting in a potentially worse dysphagia.

Procedures Designed To Control Unremitting Aspiration

A number of surgical procedures described in the literature are designed to improve or control unremitting aspiration. These include epiglottic pull-down, suturing the vocal folds together, suturing the false vocal folds together, laryngeal bypass, tracheostomy, and total laryngectomy (Baredes, Blitzer, Krespi, & Logemann, 1992; Habal & Murray, 1972; Mendelsohn, 1993a, 1993b). Most of these procedures require a tracheotomy, and voice production is changed significantly. None of these procedures should be done until an adequate trial of swallowing therapy has been attempted.

- **Epiglottic Pull-Down**—There are a number of versions of the epiglottic pull-down procedure. The most common version involves making an incision around the epiglottis, aryepiglottic folds, arytenoids, and interarytenoid area, and suturing the epiglottis to the arytenoids. The procedure is potentially reversible. It is not uncommon, however, for the epiglottis to pull away from this attachment, making the procedure unsuccessful.

- **Suturing the Vocal Folds Together**—This procedure usually involves stripping the epithelium from the vocal folds and suturing them together (Montgomery, 1975). Unfortunately, the vocal folds often tear apart, making the procedure unsuccessful. Also, it is usually nonreversible.

- **Suturing the False Vocal Folds Together**—This procedure involves stripping the epithelium from the false vocal folds and suturing them together (Kitahara et al., 1993). The advantages of this procedure are that it is reversible and the false vocal folds are less apt to tear apart.

- **Laryngeal Bypass or Tracheoesophageal Diversion**—This procedure involves separating the air and food passages by cutting the trachea at about the third or fourth tracheal ring and suturing the proximal end into the cervical esophagus (Lindeman, 1975). The distal end is bent forward and brought to the skin, where an opening is made to the skin. This is a relatively permanent procedure.

- **Tracheostomy**—Tracheostomy is often described as a procedure to prevent aspiration and improve pulmonary toilet (Baredes et al., 1992). To prevent aspiration, a cuffed tracheostomy tube is used and the cuff inflated. As discussed in Chapter 5, this is not a good procedure to eliminate aspiration as there is often still leakage around the cuff and cuff inflation can irritate the trachea.

- **Total Laryngectomy**—Total laryngectomy involves removal of the hyoid bone and entire larynx. The tracheal stump is bent forward and sutured to the patient's neck skin to form a tracheostoma. This is a permanent procedure, resulting in complete separation of the eating and respiratory tracts. It should not be used unless there is no other solution for the patient's aspiration. It has usually been used in patients who have undergone partial laryngectomy and cannot relearn to swallow (Baredes et al., 1992).

Techniques for Nonoral Feeding

Several procedures can be used to feed patients who are unable to take nutrition and hydration by mouth. These include nasogastric feeding or the variants, pharyngostomy, esophagostomy, percutaneous or surgical gastrostomy, and percutaneous or surgical jejunostomy (Bergstrom, Larson, Zinmeister, Sarr, & Silverstein, 1995; Heine, Reddihough, & Catto-Smith, 1995; Kirby, 1995; Park et al., 1992). All of these nonoral feeding procedures have a higher rate of gastroesophageal reflux than oral feeding (Heine et al., 1995). With proper care, however, this complication can be kept to a minimum. All of these procedures are temporary and can be removed at any time. Patients and families and significant others usually do not understand that all nonoral feeding procedures are temporary or can be. If this is the intent of the dysphagia team, this should be communicated to the patient and significant others. Counseling regarding the exact nature of the nonoral feeding to be used or recommended and what it will provide the patient (i.e., good nutrition and hydration) should be emphasized rather than the loss of oral feeding.

Nasogastric Feeding

The nasogastric feeding technique utilizes a tube placed through the nose, pharynx, and esophagus into the stomach (see Figure 11.1). The tubes vary in diameter; however, a narrow tube is preferred to create minimal irritation in the pharynx, particularly as the tube passes through the cricopharyngeal juncture at the top of the esophagus. Food is passed through the tube into the stomach. The number of feedings per day and the amount of food given per feeding vary from one setting to another. However, each feeding is usually followed by at least 120 to 240 cc of water to cleanse the feeding tube and provide proper hydration (Sessions et al., 1979). In general, patients should be kept upright for 1 hour after a meal to reduce the risk of gastroesophageal reflux.

Disadvantages of the nasogastric tube are its physical presence in the nose, pharynx, and esophagus, and the potential for reflux of food from the stomach

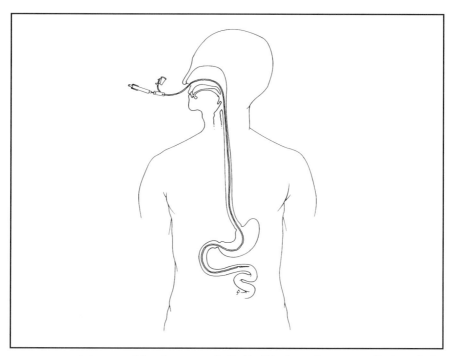

Figure 11.1. A drawing of the placement of a Dobhoff feeding tube transnasally through the stomach and into the jejunum.

up the esophagus and into the pharynx. Also, the feeding usually consists of pre-pared liquid diets, which can be expensive. The Dobhoff tube is designed to reduce the potential for reflux and aspiration by extending into the jejunum. It is of a small diameter and, presumably, creates less irritation in the nose and pharynx. There are still no data indicating any swallowing changes resulting from the presence of the nasogastric tube. Studies of swallowing in dysphagic patients with and without a nasogastric tube in place are needed. Although no major effects have been reported in patients with a properly positioned nasogas-tric tube, there may be more subtle effects that have not been observed.

Nasogastric feeding is generally considered a temporary solution to problems with oral feeding, and is usually replaced with a more permanent procedure after 3 to 4 months if the patient remains dysphagic. However, some types of patients may have a nasogastric tube in place for 5 or 6 months, or longer. These patients or their families can be taught to place the nasogastric tube for each meal and to remove it after feeding.

Pharyngostomy

A pharyngostomy involves creation of a hole or stoma from the skin into the pharynx, through which a tube is placed into the esophagus and, then, the stom-ach. The advantage of the pharyngostomy over the nasogastric tube is the elimi-nation of the tube through the nose, which is irritating and socially less accept-able to many patients. Its disadvantage is the creation of a hole that may need to be closed surgically and may create pharyngeal scarring. Some head and neck cancer patients develop a pharyngostomy spontaneously.

Esophagostomy

An esophagostomy is a hole from the skin into the cervical esophagus through which a feeding tube is passed, which extends into the esophagus and stomach. Its advantages and disadvantages are similar to those of the pharyngostomy.

Gastrostomy

The gastrostomy can be performed as a general surgical procedure with general anesthetic or can be done percutaneously under local anesthetic with an endo-scope. The latter procedure is called percutaneous endoscopic gastrostomy, or PEG. Either procedure creates an external opening in the abdomen leading into the stomach (see Figure 11.2). The patient wears a light dressing on the open-ing, designed to close in sphincteric fashion around a soft tube. For feeding, food is passed through the tube directly into the stomach. The patient can take blenderized table food through the tube.

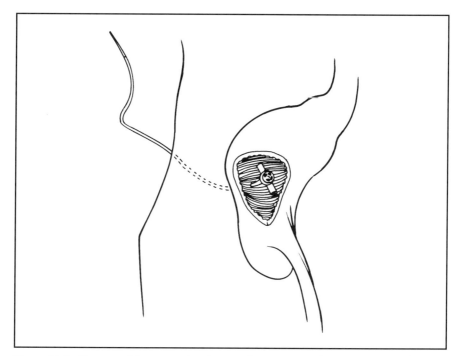

Figure 11.2. Diagram of the internal and external positioning of a percutaneous endoscopic gastrostomy (PEG).

The procedure is generally considered a long-term solution to a severe swallowing disorder because it removes the risk of nasal and pharyngeal irritation that may result from a nasogastric tube. It can be reversed should the patient regain the ability to eat by mouth. Its disadvantage is that the stoma site can leak, or can become infected, sore, or uncomfortable.

Jejunostomy

In jejunostomy, an external opening is created on the abdominal wall that leads into the jejunum. Like a gastrostomy, jejunostomy can be performed as a general surgical procedure with a general anesthetic or under local anesthetic with an endoscope and percutaneous approach. Because the jejunum enters the digestive tract below the stomach, a jejunostomy of either type requires prepared feedings, which further increase the cost of nonoral nutrition. A jejunostomy is often placed to reduce the risk of reflux. However, patients can still have gastroesophageal reflux, even when fed through a jejunostomy.

Fundoplication—Antireflux Surgery

In children who receive gastrostomy or jejunostomy, and in adults with a history of reflux disease who receive these nonoral feeding procedures, a fundoplication is often done to reduce the risk of reflux of nonoral feedings. A fundoplication is a general surgical procedure that involves twisting the top of the stomach around the lower esophageal sphincter to reinforce it and thereby reduce reflux (Little, 1996). If wrapped too tightly, the patient may have difficulty getting food into the stomach.

Criteria for Implementation of a Nonoral Feeding Procedure

Use of a nonoral feeding procedure should satisfy a patient's nutritional and hydration needs. Any patient who is aspirating significantly (more than 10% of all food consistencies) despite therapeutic interventions or who is taking longer than 10 seconds to swallow a single bolus of all types of foods, regardless of consistency, is a candidate for a nonoral feeding technique to at least supplement nutritional intake. In general, if the patient's swallowing disorder is thought to be short term in nature (1 month or less), a nasogastric tube is the treatment of choice. If swallowing rehabilitation is anticipated to take more than 1 month, a PEG may be more appropriate, unless the patient can be taught to place the nasogastric tube for each meal and remove it between meals. Currently, in some facilities, PEGs are used even in short-term dysphagia.

Medications

Although there are no medications at this time that will improve specific oral or pharyngeal swallowing problems, there are a number of medications designed to improve esophageal disorders. Some patients with dysphagia resulting from neurologic disease, such as Parkinson's disease, myasthenia gravis, and multiple sclerosis, may gain improved swallowing when put on medications for their disease.

References

Aki, B., & Blakeley, W. (1974) Late assessment of results of cricopharyngeal myotomy for cervical dysphagia. *American Journal of Surgery, 128*, 818–821.

Arnold, G. (1962). Vocal rehabilitation of paralytic dysphonia: IX technique of intracordal injection. *Archives of Otolaryngology, 76*, 358–368.

Asherson, N. (1973). Dysphagia in pharyngeal paralysis treated by cricopharyngeal sphincterotomy. *Lancet, 1*, 722.

Baredes, S., Blitzer, A., Krespi, Y., & Logemann, J. A. (1992). Swallowing disorders and aspiration. In A. Blitzer, M. F. Brin, C. T. Sasaki, S. Fahn, & K. S. Harris (Eds.), *Neurological disorders of the larynx* (pp. 201–213). New York: Thieme Medical.

Bergstrom, L. R., Larson, D. E., Zinmeister, A. R., Sarr, M. G., & Silverstein, M. D. (1995). Utilization and outcomes of surgical gastrostomies and jejunostomies in an era of percutaneous endoscopic gastrostomy: A population-based study. *The Mayo Clinic Proceedings, 70*, 829–836.

Blakeley, W., Garety, E., & Smith, D. (1968). Section of the cricopharyngeus muscle for dysphagia. *Archives of Surgery, 96*, 745–762.

Blumberg, D., Prapote, C., & Viscomi, G. (1977). Cervical osteophytes producing dysphagia. *Ear, Nose and Throat Journal, 56*, 15–21.

Buchholz, D. W. (1995). Cricopharyngeal myotomy may be effective treatment for selected patients with neurogenic oropharyngeal dysphagia. *Dysphagia, 10*, 255–258.

Calcaterra, T. (1971). Laryngeal suspension after supraglottic laryngectomy. *Archives of Otolaryngology, 74*, 306.

Calcaterra, T., Kadell, B., & Ward, P. (1975). Dysphagia secondary to cricopharyngeal muscle dysfunction. *Archives of Otolaryngology, 101*, 726–729.

Chodosh, P. (1975). Cricopharyngeal myotomy in the treatment of dysphagia. *Laryngoscope, 85*, 1862–1873.

Cruse, J., Edwards, D., Smith, J., & Wyllie, J. (1979). The pathology of a cricopharyngeal dysphagia. *Histopathology, 3*, 223–232.

Dayal, T., & Freeman, J. (1976). Cricopharyngeal myotomy for dysphagia in oculopharyngeal muscular dystrophy. *Archives of Otolaryngology, 102*, 115–116.

Duranceau, C., Letendre, J., Clermont, R., Levisque, H., & Barbeau, A. (1978). Oropharyngeal dysphagia in patients with oculopharyngeal muscular dystrophy. *The Canadian Journal of Surgery, 21*, 326–329.

Edgerton, M. T., & Duncan, M. M. (1959). Reconstruction with loss of the hyomandibular complex in excision of large cancers. *Archives of Surgery, 78*, 425–436.

Ellis, F., Schlegel, J., Lynch, V., & Payne, W. (1969). Cricopharyngeal myotomy for pharyngoesophageal diverticulum. *Annals of Surgery, 170*, 340–350.

Goode, R. L. (1976). Laryngeal suspension in head and neck surgery. *Laryngoscope, 86*, 349.

Habal, M. B., & Murray, E. (1972). Surgical treatment of life-endangering chronic aspiration pneumonia. *Plastic and Reconstructive Surgery, 49*, 305–311.

Heine, R. G., Reddihough, D. S., & Catto-Smith, A. G. (1995). Gastro-oesophageal reflux and feeding problems after gastrostomy in children with severe neurological impairment. *Developmental Medicine and Child Neurology, 37*, 320–329.

Henderson, R., & Marryatt, G. (1977). Cricopharyngeal myotomy as a method of treating cricopharyngeal dysphagia secondary to gastroesophageal reflux. *Journal of Thoracic and Cardiovascular Surgery, 74*, 721–725.

Jacobs, J., Logemann, J., Pajak, T. F., Pauloski, B. R., Collins, S., Casiano, R. R., & Schuller, D. E. (1997, May). *Failure of cricopharyngeal myotomy to improve dysphagia following head and neck cancer surgery*. Paper presented at American Society of Head and Neck Surgery's Annual Meeting, Scottsdale, AZ.

Kirby, D. F. (1995). Editorial: Surgical gastrostomies versus endoscopic gastrostomies: A tube by any other name . . . *The Mayo Clinic Proceedings, 70*, 914–916.

Kitahara, S., Ikeda, M., Ohmae, Y., Nakanoboh, M., Inouye, T., & Healy, G. (1993). Short communication: Laryngeal closure at the level of the false cord for the treatment of aspiration. *The Journal of Laryngology and Otology, 107*, 826–828.

Kostas, S. P., Karam, F., Langhans, J. J., & Vasquez, A. B. (1995). Treatment of dysphagia resulting from cricopharyngeal dysfunction with BOTOX: Preliminary thoughts and observation. *FLASHA, 15*, 22–26.

Koufman, J. A. (1986). Laryngoplasty for vocal cord medialization: An alternative to Teflon. *Laryngoscope, 96*, 726–731.

Lebo, C., Sang U. K., & Norris, F. (1976). Cricopharyngeal myotomy in amyotrophic lateral sclerosis. *Laryngoscope, 86*, 862–868.

Lewy, R. (1963). Glottic reformation with voice rehabilitation in vocal cord paralysis. *Laryngoscope, 73*, 547–555.

Lindeman, R. A. (1975). Diverting the paralyzed larynx: A reversible procedure for intractable aspiration. *Laryngoscope, 85*, 157–180.

Little, A. G. (1996). Nissen fundoplication for gastroesophageal reflux disease: How does Nissen fundoplication prevent reflux? *Diseases of the Esophagus, 9*, 247–250.

Lund, W. (1968). The cricopharyngeal sphincter: Its relationship to the relief of pharyngeal paralysis and the surgical treatment of the early pharyngeal pouch. *Journal of Laryngology and Otology, 82*, 353–367.

Mendelsohn, M. (1993a). A guided approach to surgery for aspiration: Two case reports. *The Journal of Laryngology and Otology, 107*, 121–126.

Mendelsohn, M. (1993b). New concepts in dysphagia management. *The Journal of Otolaryngology Supplement, 1*, 5–24.

Mills, C. (1964). Dysphagia in progressive bulbar palsy relieved by division of the cricopharyngeus. *Journal of Laryngology and Otology, 78*, 963–964.

Mills, C. (1973). Dysphagia in pharyngeal paralysis treated by cricopharyngeal sphincterotomy. *Lancet, 1*, 455–457.

Mitchell, R., & Armanini, G. (1975). Cricopharyngeal myotomy: Treatment of dysphagia. *Annals of Surgery, 181*, 262–266.

Mladick, R., Horton, C., & Adamson, J. (1961). Immediate cricopharyngeal myotomy: An adjunctive technique for major oral–pharyngeal resections. *Plastic and Reconstructive Surgery, 47*, 6–11.

Mladick, R., Horton, C., & Adamson, J. (1971). Cricopharyngeal myotomy. *Archives of Surgery, 102*(6), 1–5.

Montgomery, W. W. (1975). Surgery to prevent aspiration. *Archives of Otolaryngology, 109*, 809–811.

Palmer, E. (1974). Dysphagia due to cricopharyngeus dysfunction. *American Family Physician, 9*, 127–131.

Park, R. H., Allison, M. C., Lang, J., Spence, E., Morris, A. J., Danesh, B. J., Russell, R. I., & Mills, P. R. (1992). Randomised comparison of percutaneous endoscopic gastrostomy and nasogastric tube feeding in patients with persisting neurological dysphagia. *British Journal of Medicine, 304*, 1406–1409.

Parker, M. D. (1989). Dysphagia due to cervical osteophytes: A controversial entity revisited. *Dysphagia, 3*, 157–160.

Press, H. D., & Leffall, L. D. (1972). Hoarseness and dysphagia secondary to cervical hyperostosis: Report of an unusual case. *Medical Annals of the District of Columbia, 41*, 26–28.

Robbins, J. A., & Levine, R. (1993). Swallowing after lateral medullary syndrome plus. *Clinics in Communication Disorders, 3*(4), 44–45.

Sessions, D., Zill, R., & Schwartz, J. (1979). Deglutition after conservation surgery for cancer of the larynx and hypopharynx. *Otolaryngology, Head and Neck Surgery, 87,* 779–796.

Stevens, K., & Newell, R. (1971). Cricopharyngeal myotomy in dysphagia. *Laryngoscope, 81,* 1616–1620.

Valadka, A. B., Kubal, W. S., & Smith, M. M. (1995). Updated management strategy for patients with cervical osteophytic dysphagia. *Dysphagia, 10,* 167–171.

Ward, P. J., Hanson, D. C., & Abemayor, E. (1985). Transcutaneous Teflon injection of the paralyzed vocal cord: A new technique. *Laryngoscope, 95,* 644–649.

Wilkins, S. (1964). Indications for section of the cricopharyngeus muscle. *American Journal of Surgery, 108,* 533–538.

Yarington, C., & Harned, R. (1971). Polytef (Teflon) injection for postoperative deglutition problems. *Archives of Otolaryngology, 94,* 274–275.

Zinninger, G. (1966). Dysphagia and esophageal dilatation. *Journal of the American Medical Association, 196,* 128–129.

C H A P T E R   1 2

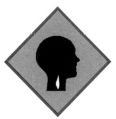

Clinical Decision Making

Throughout the care of each dysphagic patient, the swallowing therapist progresses through a series of clinical decisions. This chapter is designed to identify the major decision-making points and the types of information the clinician should consider in making each decision.

Prerequisites for Good Decision Making

Good clinical decision making depends upon a strong knowledge base regarding the anatomic and physiologic swallow problems exhibited by the patient, the patient's cognitive and behavioral controls, and the nature of the patient's damage or disease process and its potential effects on swallowing. Good clinical decision making also depends upon the clinician's skill in interpreting radiographic studies and other diagnostic procedures, in terms of both the dysphagia symptoms revealed and the physiologic and anatomic swallowing disorders identified. A full range of knowledge about the clinical armamentarium of procedures that can be used in treating dysphagic patients is also necessary.

Clinical Decisions

Is the patient dysphagic or at high risk for dysphagia?

The first decision the swallowing therapist must make upon being consulted to see a patient who may be dysphagic is whether the patient is at risk for oropharyngeal dysphagia. This involves a screening procedure, as described in Chapter 5. The clinician must select the type of screening procedure to be used with the patient. In general, screening should be quick and cost effective, often involving a brief chart review and observations of the patient, and should not be risky for the patient.

Should the patient receive an in-depth diagnostic assessment?

After screening the patient, the clinician must decide whether the patient needs an in-depth diagnostic assessment, such as the videofluorographic study. If the clinician suspects a pharyngeal stage swallowing problem, based on the diagnosis, the patient's history and symptoms, and so forth, a videofluorographic study is generally needed. Other instrumental procedures are available but, as described in Chapter 3, currently each reveals only small segments of the swallow physiology. The diagnostic procedure that provides the most information in a single session is the videofluorographic study known as the modified barium swallow. Sometimes, however, the clinician may have a more specific diagnostic question that needs to be answered regarding a particular patient, and that question may be best answered by the use of another diagnostic procedure. In selecting the instrumental procedures, the clinician should ask, "What is it that I need to know about this patient before I can determine whether swallowing therapy is appropriate and what type of therapy to initiate?" If the question to be answered is, "What is going wrong in the anatomy and physiology of this patient's pharyngeal swallow?" then videofluorography is recommended. However, if the question is, "What does this patient's pharyngeal anatomy look like after head and neck cancer surgery to the pharynx?" a superior view of the pharynx via videoendoscopy may be the technique of choice. If the question is, "Does this patient generate adequate pressure to move the food through the system?" manometry is the procedure of choice. Such a question may arise based on the patient's diagnosis. For example, radiotherapy for cancer of the pharynx usually causes reduced pressure by damaging pharyngeal wall function. Pharyngeal manometry in combination with videofluoroscopy may be selected so that the movements in the pharynx that create the pressure needed for efficient swallowing can be visualized by fluoroscopy while the pressure is being measured by manometry.

Which treatment strategies should be evaluated during the diagnostic procedure?

Once the diagnostic procedure is under way, the clinician should be making determinations about the nature of the patient's swallow anatomy and physiology and about the treatment intervention strategies that may improve the swallow and that can be evaluated during the diagnostic procedure. What postural techniques may improve the patient's swallow? What procedures for heightening sensory input, if any, are appropriate for the patient's disorder? Are there different ways to present the food and feed the patient that will facilitate the patient's swallow? Are there treatment strategies, such as swallow maneuvers, that will improve the swallow? And, finally, are there particular food viscosities that are safest and easiest for the patient to swallow? This clinical decision making is critical during the diagnostic procedure in order to attempt to return the patient to oral intake as quickly as possible, or to maintain oral intake for as long as possible. If a procedure is immediately successful in improving swallowing efficiency or safety, the patient may return to oral intake more quickly.

Is this a patient who will benefit from therapy?

Swallowing therapy is designed to improve the patient's swallowing function and ability to eat orally. There are patients whose swallowing function cannot be rehabilitated with currently available swallowing therapy. For example, advanced motor neuron disease will eventually create severe swallowing impairments that do not respond to swallowing therapy. Similarly, patients with dysphagia resulting from advanced dementia will not be remediable. The clinician must examine the patient's history, medical diagnosis, and reactions to any evaluation procedures and trial therapy techniques, and come to a decision as to whether the patient can benefit from swallowing therapy services. This decision can be difficult for the clinician but must be made in order not to overutilize services or use therapy services inappropriately. The swallowing therapist may still provide counseling to the patient and significant other, and involve members of the multidisciplinary team such as the dietitian.

Should swallowing therapy be scheduled during mealtime or as a part of feeding?

Swallowing therapy, like treatment for speech, is usually designed to retrain muscle function, teach a new sequence of muscle activity, or stimulate increased sensory input. Usually, the treatment session should be separate from mealtimes. If the patient needs a particular treatment strategy in order to eat orally, such as a postural technique, this should be designed by the swallowing therapist and taught to the caregiver to maintain. Some patients, then, will be fed according to a program designed by the swallowing therapist, taught to the caregiver by the swallowing therapist, and implemented by a caregiver. The patient will also receive therapy from the swallowing therapist at another time during the day. Only if the patient is in transition from nonoral feeding to oral feeding using specific therapy strategies should the swallowing therapist be involved in "feeding."

When should the clinician terminate swallowing therapy with a patient who has been making measurable progress?

Generally, when a patient has plateaued in his or her measurable swallow function over a month's time, the clinician should reevaluate whether to continue active therapy with the patient or whether to encourage the patient or caregiver to continue to exercise independently and undergo reevaluation in 6 months to 1 year. Patients who have sustained severe head injury, spinal cord injury, or a large stroke, may plateau in their recovery and exhibit no change in swallow function for a series of months, after which they may suddenly exhibit significant clinical improvement and be able to return to eating. In general, when a patient's function plateaus for 4 weeks, it is suggested that active therapy be terminated, at least temporarily, but practice of exercises continue until a change in status is identified.

When does the swallowing therapist turn a part of the patient's dysphagia care over to an aide?

When a therapy program involves repetitive tasks that need to be presented several times a day, such as thermal–tactile stimulation or range-of-motion exercises, and that can be measured with each trial, these tasks could be performed by an aide. No professional judgment is needed until the patient's performance meets a threshold set by the swallowing therapist, usually a certified speech–language pathologist (SLP) (e.g., "The pharyngeal delay must consistently diminish to only 2 seconds from 10 seconds, or the vertical range of motion of the anterior tongue must reach 1 cm"). When the desired threshold(s) are reached, the certified speech–language pathologist/swallowing therapist would reestablish new goals and exercises for the patient in a therapy session. The certified speech–language pathologist/swallowing therapist would also provide a list of early "stop" signals for each patient (i.e., a list of behaviors that, if observed, would result in the aide's stopping practice with the patient and calling the SLP into the session).

Another situation when aides are involved is the implementation of a maintenance program. If the patient is no longer making progress in active therapy but can eat orally by using therapy strategies, such as postural techniques, the use of these strategies over time is a maintenance program and should be implemented by an aide under supervision of the certified swallowing therapist.

How are the optimal therapy procedures selected for a patient?

The first step in selecting a therapy regimen is to carefully assess the patient's anatomy and physiology in the context of his or her medical status, prognosis, and behavioral and cognitive abilities. Can the patient practice independently? Can he or she follow directions reliably? If so, the patient may be able to participate in such things as range-of-motion exercises and swallowing maneuvers. If the patient cannot follow directions or is uncooperative, then procedures that are under the control of the caregiver, such as postural changes, heightening sensory input via the nature of the food presented, and changing the methods for feeding, may be the most effective procedures. If the patient's anatomic or physiologic swallowing problem does not lend itself to these types of procedures, then the patient's success in swallowing therapy will be significantly compromised. Does the patient fatigue easily? If so, some therapy procedures, such as swallowing maneuvers, may be too tiring. In defining the treatment plan, the clinician must examine the range of treatments for a particular anatomic or physiologic swallowing problem and identify those that are most easily used by each particular patient. For example, patients with Alzheimer's disease and a delay in triggering pharyngeal swallow may achieve success only from presentation of particular bolus types, such as a large sour bolus, and cannot cooperate with thermal–tactile stimulation or apply it to themselves. In contrast, patients with motor neuron disease or who have undergone treatment for head and neck cancer are quite capable not only of accepting thermal–tactile stimulation but of applying it to themselves prior to every third or fourth swallow, depending upon the frequency that is most effective for them.

When and to whom should referrals be made?

In the current health care climate of increasingly restricted referrals to specialists, use of a full team of professionals for every patient with a swallowing disorder is unrealistic. Instead, the swallowing therapist (usually a speech–language pathologist) needs to assess the patient's oropharyngeal anatomy and physiology, overall history, behavior, overall motor control (gait, fine motor coordination), voice production, and so on, to determine whether additional referrals need to be made to assure a complete and accurate medical diagnosis. For those patients referred for a complaint of a swallowing disorder with no known medical diagnosis, referral is critical. Most often, patients with no medical diagnosis and complaints of oropharyngeal swallowing abnormalities have some type of neurologic damage or disease. These patients have exhibited brain tumors (particularly brainstem tumors), motor neuron disease, Parkinson's disease, myasthenia gravis, strokes (particularly brainstem strokes), Guillain–Barré, and oculopharyngeal or myotonic dystrophy. Based on these clinical experiences, a first referral to a neurologist who has knowledge of the neurogenic dysphagia signs and symptoms and cranial nerve assessment should be made. If the patient with complaints of dysphagia is also hoarse, a referral to an otolaryngologist first may be most appropriate. If the first referral is not revealing of an underlying diagnosis responsible for the swallowing problems, then referral to another specialist is needed. Unfortunately, the current health care system will not allow broad referral to a number of specialists. If the patient exhibits complaints of pressure in the chest, a feeling of burning or discomfort in the chest or throat, or waking up in the middle of the night coughing or gagging, a referral to a gastroenterologist is appropriate. These are frequent symptoms of gastroesophageal reflux disease or other esophageal dysfunction requiring a gastroenterologist's expertise.

Ethical Issues for Good Clinical Decision Making

Ethical issues can and should be an important factor in clinical decision making (American Speech-Language-Hearing Association, 1994; Groher, 1990; Logemann, 1996; Sharp & Genesen, 1996). The swallowing therapist seeing a patient with a terminal illness, such as motor neuron disease or Alzheimer's disease, may recommend to the patient or family that oral feeding be discontinued and that the patient move to nonoral nutrition and hydration. The decision, in most instances, belongs to the patient or the family. The patient may indicate a wish to continue to eat orally despite the knowledge that he or she is at high risk for developing a potentially life-threatening pneumonia. Should the clinician provide the patient with information about the safest way to swallow within a range of nonsafe alternatives? For example, the patient aspirates 20% of everything with the chin down and 50% with the head in the normal position. Should the clinician recommend oral feeding with the chin down? I suggest that the clinician provide the information to the patient, family, or caregivers by writing a report in lay terms that clearly specifies all of the situations of eating and their relative safety (i.e., how much the patient aspirates under the various conditions). The clinician does not need to advocate that the patient eat in a particular way. Instead, the patient, family, or caregivers can be given the information needed to make their own informed decision without the clinician's advocating an unsafe oral intake.

Because many swallowing therapists are speech–language pathologists, the speech–language pathologist may become involved in other aspects of ethical decision making, such as assuring that the patient understands fully the choices and risks involved in oral intake and that the patient's wishes are clearly communicated and understood by the medical team. In some cases, patients with swallowing problems may have severe speech and language problems that make their communication with the medical team difficult. The speech–language pathologist may ease this communication difficulty and assist in determining whether the patient understands the information needed in decision making.

References

American Speech-Language-Hearing Association. (1994, March). Code of Ethics/Issues in Ethics. *Asha, 36*(Suppl. 13), 1–27.

Groher, M. E. (1990). Ethical dilemmas in providing nutrition. *Dysphagia, 5,* 102–109.

Logemann, J. A. (1996). Speaking out: Should treatment for pharyngeal swallowing disorders begin before instrumental assessment is completed? *Asha, 38,* 14–15.

Sharp, H. M., & Genesen, L. B. (1996). Ethical decision-making in dysphagia management. *American Journal of Speech-Language Pathology, 5,* 15–22.

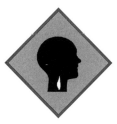

MULTIDISCIPLINARY MANAGEMENT
OF DYSPHAGIA

There are a number of reasons why a variety of health care professionals should be available to the oropharyngeal dysphagic patient, as needed (Logemann, 1983; Logemann, Sisson, & Wheeler, 1980; Newman, Dodaro, & Welch, 1980; Thresher & Kehoe, 1992; Trible, 1967; Tuchman & Walter, 1993). Some dysphagic patients come to a swallowing center for both evaluation of their swallowing problem and a determination of its etiology (i.e., the medical diagnosis causing the swallowing problem). Usually, these patients have a swallowing disorder or complaint that has never been clearly identified. These patients may have neurologic disease (the most common reason for dysphagia of previously unknown etiology), head and neck cancer (more infrequent as an etiology of dysphagia), or other medical disorder (Lazarus & Logemann, 1987; Logemann & Bytell, 1979; Logemann et al., 1993; Pauloski et al., 1993; Robbins, Logemann, & Kirshner, 1986; Veis & Logemann, 1985). In many cases these patients have been seen by a variety of medical and allied health professionals who have been unable to define the reason for the dysphagia, usually because the physiology of the oropharyngeal swallow has not been assessed in detail. Although increased attention has focused on normal and abnormal oropharyngeal swallowing and more medical and allied health professionals are aware of oropharyngeal dysphagia as a symptom of many disease entities, patients are sometimes treated for psychological illnesses when in fact they have a physiologic disorder. Before a dysphagic complaint is labeled as psychogenic, the patient should have a detailed oropharyngeal and esophageal swallowing assessment and a complete evaluation by the entire multidisciplinary team to rule out a physiologic cause.

A second reason for a multidisciplinary approach is the complexity of management of the dysphagic patient. Although the majority of dysphagic patients have a known etiology for their problem, such as stroke, head injury, or head and neck cancer, many have both oropharyngeal and esophageal disorders that require input from both the swallowing therapist for the oropharyngeal dysphagia and the gastroenterologist for gastroesophageal management. Those individuals over age 60 and children with congenital neurologic impairment are at particularly higher than average risk for oropharyngeal and esophageal disorders (Logemann, 1993; Tuchman & Walter, 1993).

Professions Often Included on the Multidisciplinary Team

In the multidisciplinary approach, the initial intake and evaluation of the dysphagic patient is usually done by the swallowing therapist, who is most often a speech–language pathologist (Logemann, 1983; Strandberg, 1982). The intake usually involves a careful history of the patient's symptoms and progression of swallowing complaints, as well as a detailed medical history including medications, and a careful oropharyngeal motor evaluation. Following this history, an oropharyngeal radiographic evaluation is usually completed by the swallowing therapist and radiologist. This examination should involve the introduction of a range of carefully measured bolus volumes of liquid from 1 to 10 ml and cup drinking, as well as the introduction of several food consistencies, including pudding and a cookie, as described in Chapter 5. If a patient has a food-specific dysphagia, that particular food may also be mixed with barium or other radiopaque substance and introduced during the radiographic study.

Following the oropharyngeal radiographic assessment, the patient may then be referred to the gastroenterologist for an esophageal assessment, as well as to other medical or allied health specialists as appropriate. The patient may see a neurologist for careful neurologic evaluation, particularly focusing on those cranial nerves innervating swallow-related musculature and on symptomatology for neurologic diseases that may present with dysphagia symptoms, such as Parkinson's disease, motor neuron disease, and myasthenia gravis. The patient may be referred to the otolaryngologist for a structural evaluation of the head and neck, as well as a sensorimotor assessment of the pharynx and larynx. If the patient has a history of recurrent or recent pneumonia or history of other recurrent pulmonary problems, the patient may need to see a pulmonologist. If the patient is a child, a pediatrician's evaluation is often important. For patients in a rehabilitation center, the assessment by a physiatrist (physical medicine physician) is key to fitting the dysphagia rehabilitation plan into the patient's overall rehabilitation schedule. If the patient is over 80 years old, the participation of a gerontologist is very helpful in assuring that realistic goals are set for the patient, and in determining whether the patient's medications may be contributing to the dysphagia. A maxillofacial prosthodontist should be available to the team for those patients with impaired tongue function needing prosthetic intervention or postoperative surgical defects requiring obturation (Leonard & Gillis, 1982; Wheeler, Logemann, & Rosen, 1980). A general dentist may also be helpful for refitting dentures. Many elderly patients take multiple medications. Interactions of these medications, or effects of single medications, can cause dry mouth or xerostomia, which can contribute to difficulty in initiating the oral and pharyngeal stages of swallow. A pharmacist can provide important information on potential drug interaction effects on swallowing, as well. The occupational therapist can provide assistive devices for eating, as well as direct therapy for arm and hand control for food placement in the mouth. The physical therapist can assist in establishing optimal positioning for the patient during meals. In some settings, the occupational and physical therapists serve as the direct swallowing therapists, providing both evaluation and treatment of swallowing disorders.

The dietitian plays a key role in dietary evaluation of the patient through blood chemistries, weight monitoring, and calorie counts (American Dietetic Association, 1980). Regular communication between the swallowing therapist and the dietitian is essential, as the dysphagic patient progresses from nonoral nutrition to some oral intake on food consistencies best tolerated by the patient, to full oral intake. During these transitions from nonoral to oral intake, the dietitian monitors the patient's daily oral calorie intake and decreases the patient's nonoral intake accordingly. Together, the dietitian, swallowing therapist, and attending physician determine when the patient can safely take adequate intake orally so that nonoral intake can be discontinued completely.

The respiratory therapy service and nursing staff can be critical to early identification of patients with dysphagia in the inpatient setting, as these professionals often identify patients who show symptoms of dysphagia. In-service education should be provided to these professionals regarding signs and symptoms of dysphagia. In some hospitals, nurses also provide direct swallowing therapy.

The staff who serve as feeders for dysphagic patients who cannot feed themselves are critically important to the dysphagia team (Buckley, Addicks, & Maniglia, 1976; Gaffney & Campbell, 1974; Thresher & Kehoe, 1992; Tuchman & Walter, 1993). A patient with dysphagia can begin to aspirate if fed too much food too quickly. The way in which patients are fed can either keep them safe or make them unsafe eaters. The staff members who feed patients with dysphagia should be under the supervision of the swallowing therapist and follow each patient's feeding instructions without deviation. The feeding staff must check the patient's tray to be sure the correct foods are presented and that the food is within the patient's visual field, and must discontinue feeding and notify the swallowing therapist if the patient shows any signs of distress during a meal. The swallowing therapist should provide in-service training to the feeding staff regarding the complexity of normal swallowing physiology, the range of swallowing disorders, and the need for individualized feeding plans for each patient. The important point to emphasize is that each patient's feeding must be individualized, and the swallowing therapist will provide the feeding staff with each patient's specific feeding protocol. The swallowing therapist will then supervise the feeding staff and serve as a consultant to the feeding staff as needed.

Establishing the Radiographic Procedure

To initiate the radiographic procedure, the swallowing therapist should be knowledgeable in the radiographic symptoms of the various anatomic and physiologic disorders of oropharyngeal deglutition (Logemann, 1993). This individual or the chief of his or her department should meet with the chief of radiology in the hospital to discuss establishing the radiographic procedure in which both the swallowing therapist and the radiologist participate, and, preferably, write and sign a single report. The swallowing therapist should be prepared to discuss the necessary radiographic procedure, the rationale for all aspects of the procedure, and the ways it differs from the standard barium swallow or upper gastrointestinal examination (as summarized in Chapter 5).

Once the procedure has been agreed upon, the cost of the procedure should be established. In most institutions three fees are charged: the room fee for use of the equipment, the radiologist's fee, and the swallowing therapist's fee. These fees should be discussed with the administrator of the institution involved, as should the establishment of the new procedure. There are instances in which the swallowing therapist initiating the request for the new procedure should discuss it *first* with referring physicians or the institution's administration before approaching the other professionals involved.

Models of Communication Between the Team Members

There are many methods for communication among team members, including weekly face-to-face meetings, telephone conversations, and electronic mail. The method of communication is less important than the quality of the communication; that is, team members need to respect each other's expertise and communicate easily and quickly with each other. If a particular team member takes a week to respond to another member of the team, the communication will break down. Similarly, if each team member does not respect the expertise of the other team members, poor patient care will result. Each dysphagia team must assess its particular characteristics and determine how to facilitate effective and efficient communication among members.

Efficacy of Multidisciplinary Rehabilitation for Dysphagia

Although multidisciplinary management of dysphagia generally appears necessary from the perspective of the complexity of the patient's swallowing problems, in the context of the specific medical problems and management, only a small amount of data support the efficacy of multidisciplinary intervention from the perspective of establishing reduced rates of pneumonia and improved nutrition and hydration (Bach et al., 1989; Donner & Jones, 1985; Jones & Altschuler, 1987; Lierman, Wolff, Hazelton, Pesquera, & Wilson, 1987; Martens, Cameron, & Simonsen, 1990; Ravich et al., 1985; Thresher & Kehoe, 1992). None of these studies has examined cost of dysphagia care with and without the multidisciplinary approach. This is critical in this era of cost containment.

It is important that each team examine the cost effectiveness of its operations and ask some critical questions regarding team operations. For example, does every dysphagic patient need to be evaluated routinely by every team member, or can some patients be seen by only some members of the team? If the latter model is used, which patients are seen by only selected team members?

In many team settings, only dysphagic patients with no known diagnosis for their swallowing problems are seen by all team members until a diagnosis is made. Then, when the etiology for the swallowing problems is identified, the patient is cared for by selected team members. For example, a patient with a complaint of dysphagia may be diagnosed as having Parkinson's disease. Once that diagnosis is made, the neurologist on the team provides the continuing care for the patient's Parkinson's disease, and the swallowing therapist and gastroenterologist provide rehabilitation as needed for the patient's swallowing problem(s). A patient with swallowing disorders of known etiology, such as secondary to surgical treatment for head and neck cancer, is not seen by all team members, but only by the otolaryngologist–head and neck surgeon (typically serving as the patient's attending physician in this case) and the swallowing therapist. In this era of cost containment, the patient with a pharyngeal dysphagia of no known etiology should usually be referred first to a neurologist on the dysphagia team who is familiar with swallowing problems associated with neurologic problems, because most patients with dysphagia of unknown etiology have neurologic disease or damage.

Staff Education by the Team

When a multidisciplinary team is established, the team should offer a short, systematic educational program for other medical and allied health staff in the facility (Thresher & Kehoe, 1992; Tuchman & Walter, 1993). The purpose of this program should be to increase staff awareness of swallowing problems and their symptoms, and to relate how to refer patients to the team. The kinds of services (diagnostic and rehabilitative) offered by the team should be described and illustrated.

This program is usually best done with a small meeting format, often at departmental staff meetings. The departments of internal medicine, neurology, otolaryngology, and rehabilitation medicine are usually targeted first. In each case, the radiographic diagnostic procedure should be described, highlighting the safety of the procedure for patients who aspirate and the value of the procedure in accurate diagnosis of the anatomic or physiologic swallowing disorder. It is often appropriate to review briefly the various therapy procedures for particular swallowing disorders. Team participants should be available for questions. It is most important that all members of the swallowing rehabilitation team be prepared to handle patients at the time any announcement of the program is made, as patient flow will frequently be heavy from the beginning. A careful audit of the institution's patient population to identify the approximate percentage of patients with swallowing disorders requiring management is helpful in estimating the amount of professional time required to establish and continue the program.

References

American Dietetic Association. (1980). *Study guide—Dysphagia: The dietitian's role in patient care* [Audiocassette series]. Chicago: Author.

Bach, D. B., Pouget, S., Belle, K., Kilfoil, M., Alfieri, M., McEvoy, J., & Jackson, G. (1989). An integrated team approach to the management of patients with oropharyngeal dysphagia. *Journal of Allied Health, 18*, 459–468.

Buckley, J., Addicks, C., & Maniglia, J. (1976). Feeding patients with dysphagia. *Nursing Forum, 15*, 69–85.

Donner, M. W., & Jones, B. (1985). The multidisciplinary approach to dysphagia. *Gastrointestinal Radiology, 10*, 193–261.

Gaffney, T., & Campbell, R. (1974). Feeding techniques for dysphagic patients. *American Journal of Nursing, 74*, 2194–2195.

Jones, P. L., & Altschuler, S. L. (1987). Dysphagia teams: A specific approach to a non-specific problem. *Dysphagia, 1*, 200–205.

Lazarus, C., & Logemann, J. A. (1987). Swallowing disorders in closed head trauma patients. *Archives of Physical Medicine and Rehabilitation, 68*, 79–87.

Leonard, R., & Gillis, R. (1982). Effects of a prosthetic tongue on vowel intelligibility and food management in a patient with total glossectomy. *Journal of Speech and Hearing Disorders, 47,* 25–30.

Lierman, C., Wolff, R., Hazelton, J., Pesquera, K., & Wilson, E. (1987). Multidisciplinary treatment of feeding disorders in the home. *Pediatric Nursing, 13,* 266–270.

Logemann, J. A. (1983). *Evaluation and treatment of swallowing disorders.* Austin, TX: PRO-ED.

Logemann, J. A. (1993). *Manual for the videofluorographic study of swallowing* (2nd ed). Austin, TX: PRO-ED.

Logemann, J. A., & Bytell, D. E. (1979). Swallowing disorders in three types of head and neck surgical patients. *Cancer, 44,* 1095–1105.

Logemann, J. A., Pauloski, B. R., Rademaker, A. W., McConnel, F. M. S., Heiser, M. A., Cardinale, S., Shedd, D., Stein, D., Beery, Q., Johnson, J., Saunders, A., & Baker, T. (1993). Speech and swallow function after tonsil/base of tongue resection with primary closure. *Journal of Speech and Hearing Research, 36,* 918–926.

Logemann, J., Sisson, G., & Wheeler, R. (1980). The team approach to rehabilitation of surgically treated oral cancer patients. *Proceedings of the National Forum on Comprehensive Cancer Rehabilitation and Its Vocational Implications,* (pp. 222–227).

Martens, L., Cameron, T., & Simonsen, M. (1990). Effects of multidisciplinary management program on neurologically impaired patients with dysphagia. *Dysphagia, 5,* 147–151.

Newman, L., Dodaro, R., & Welch, M. (1980, May). *A comprehensive program for dysphagia rehabilitation.* Workshop conducted at Mercy Hospital and Medical Center, Chicago.

Pauloski, B. R., Logemann, J. A., Rademaker, A., McConnel, F., Heiser, M. A., Cardinale, S., Shedd, D., Lewin, J., Baker, S., Graner, D., Cook, B., Milianti, F., Collins, S., & Baker, T. (1993). Speech and swallowing function after anterior tongue and floor of mouth resection with distal flap reconstruction. *Journal of Speech and Hearing Research, 36,* 267–276.

Ravich, W. J., Donner, M. W., Kashima, H., Bucholz, D. W., Marsh, B. R., Hendrix, T. R., Kramer, S. S., Jones, D., Bosma, J. F., Siebens, A. A., & Linden, P. (1985). The swallowing center: Concepts and procedures. *Gastrointestinal Radiology, 10,* 255–261.

Robbins, J., Logemann, J., & Kirshner, H. (1986). Swallowing and speech production in Parkinson's disease. *Annals of Neurology, 19,* 283–287.

Strandberg, T. (1982, January). *Establishment of a swallowing rehabilitation program.* Lecture presented at workshop on swallowing rehabilitation, Sarah Bush Lincoln Health Center, Mattoon, IL.

Thresher, J. C., & Kehoe, E. A. (1992). *Working with swallowing disorders: A multidisciplinary approach.* Tucson, AZ: Communication Skill Builders.

Trible, W. (1967). The rehabilitation of deglutition following head and neck surgery. *Laryngoscope, 77,* 518–523.

Tuchman, D., & Walter, R. (1993). *Disorders of feeding and swallowing in infants and children: Pathophysiology, diagnosis and treatment.* San Diego: Singular.

Veis, S., & Logemann, J. (1985). The nature of swallowing disorders in CVA patients. *Archives of Physical Medicine and Rehabilitation, 66,* 372–375.

Wheeler, R., Logemann, J., & Rosen, M. (1980). Maxillary reshaping prostheses: Effectiveness in improving speech and swallowing of post-surgical oral cancer patients. *Journal of Prosthetic Dentistry, 43,* 313–319.

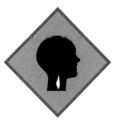

MEASUREMENT OF SWALLOWING
AND INTERVENTION STRATEGIES:
THE FUTURE

Only in the past 10 years have measurements of swallowing physiology been attempted (Jacob, Kahrilas, Logemann, Shah, & Ha, 1989; Kahrilas, Lin, Logemann, Ergun, & Facchini, 1993; Lazarus, Logemann, & Gibbons, 1993; Logemann, Kahrilas, Kobara, & Vakil, 1989; Platt, Logemann, Rademaker, Kahrilas, & Lazarus, 1994). Previously, even research on normal swallowing physiology involved only observations from a variety of imaging studies (Bosma, 1973). Some measurements were made from electromyographic studies, although these studies largely also resulted in descriptions of the onset and termination of muscle activity, and in manometric studies, which were largely done until recently in the esophagus (Doty & Bosma, 1956; Kobara-Mates, Logemann, Larson, & Kahrilas, 1995; Reimers-Neils, Logemann, & Larson, 1994).

Swallowing Measures

In recent years, a number of measures of oropharyngeal swallow physiology have been developed, including measures of bolus movement, of the durations of events in the oral and pharyngeal stages of swallowing, and of the coordination of these events in time. Some of the specific measures that have been used to date are presented in Table 14.1. Some normative data on these measures are now available on adults of various ages (Jacob et al., 1989; Rademaker, Pauloski,

Logemann, & Shanahan, 1994; Robbins, Hamilton, Lof, & Kempster, 1992; Tracy et al., 1989); however, more normative data are needed. Still no normative data are available on the pharyngeal aspects of swallow in normal children of various ages because of the continuing need to use radiographic studies to collect most of these data on the pharyngeal swallow.

Table 14.1
Examples of Measures of Oropharyngeal Deglutition

Bolus Movement

Oral transit time—Interval from onset of the tongue movement propelling the bolus posteriorly until the bolus passes the base of the tongue.

Pharyngeal transit time—Interval from the bolus passing the base of the tongue to the bolus passing through the cricopharyngeal sphincter.

Pharyngeal delay time—Interval from the bolus passing the base of the tongue to the onset of laryngeal elevation indicating the onset of the pharyngeal response (pharyngeal swallow).

Pharyngeal response time—Duration of the pharyngeal motor response (from onset of laryngeal elevation until the bolus passes through the cricopharyngeal sphincter or until the cricopharyngeal sphincter closes).

Esophageal transit time—Interval from the bolus passing the cricopharyngeus (upper esophageal sphincter) to the bolus passing through the lower esophageal sphincter.

Temporal Measures of Movement

Duration of velopharyngeal closure—Length of time the soft palate is in contact with the posterior pharyngeal wall.

Duration of maximum laryngeal elevation—Length of time the larynx is maximally elevated from its rest position.

Duration of laryngeal closure—Length of time the laryngeal entrance is closed (absence of air in the airway entrance).

Duration of cricopharyngeal (CP) opening—Length of time the cricopharyngeal sphincter is open.

Temporal Measures of Swallow Coordination

Onset of velopharyngeal closure in relation to onset of CP opening

Onset of laryngeal elevation in relation to onset of CP opening

Onset of laryngeal closure in relation to onset of CP opening

Also biomechanical measures of various aspects of swallowing have been described using computer analysis (Logemann, Kahrilas, Begelman, & Pauloski, 1989). Computer analysis enables the tracking of movements of structures in the pharynx or oral cavity from the onset to the termination of the swallow or for any portion of the swallow that is of interest. The availability of this technology enables more detailed studies of normal and abnormal swallowing and of treatment effects. Many more studies of treatment effects are needed to further validate current and future intervention strategies used in rehabilitation of patients with oropharyngeal dysphagia.

Criteria for the Measurement of Treatment Effects

All of the measures noted above, and other similar measures, can be used to define the effects of specific treatments on swallowing disorders (Kahrilas, Logemann, & Gibbons, 1992; Kahrilas, Logemann, Krugler, & Flanagan, 1991; Lazarus et al., 1993; Logemann, Kahrilas, Kobara, & Vakil, 1989). When collecting data and designing a study on treatment effects, certain criteria need to be met (Logemann, 1987):

1. *Quantification of the disorder and the outcomes of treatment.* Meaningful measures of the disorder under treatment and the treatment itself must be defined. The clinical investigator or clinician needs to consider the most important aspects of the swallow physiology that need to be measured to reflect the disorder and the effects of its treatment.

2. *Standardization of the testing procedures.* When completing the radiographic study or any other data collection procedure, the test conditions should be calibrated and replicated with each patient and at each data collection point. Such variables as the patient's head position, body posture, food viscosity, bolus size, and order of materials presented should be carefully controlled because differences in any of these variables may change the physiology of the swallow. Randomization of the order of swallows studied should be considered.

3. *Selection of the patient population to be studied.* Patients who are given specific treatments should be homogeneous on a variety of characteristics, including (1) the nature of the physiologic or anatomic swallowing disorder, (2) the nature of the underlying disease entity or dysfunction causing the dysphagia, and (3) the stage of the disease entity or recovery process when the treatment technique is needed. Patient age should also be considered.

4. *Definition of the treatment protocol.* When instituting a treatment protocol to be evaluated, the protocol should be carefully described. This description should include the exact nature and duration of the treatment provided and the direct therapy or contact time given if it is an exercise program, the number of physician visits if it is a drug protocol, the nature and duration of any practice the patient is to complete independently or with family members, the number of sessions provided to the patient, and the frequency and the type of reevaluations provided posttreatment.

In addition to using the temporal measures of food movement and structural movement and the biomechanical measures defined in Table 14.1, measures of the effects of the treatment on overall patient function are critical. Does the treatment improve the patient's ability to eat orally? Does the treatment allow the patient to take liquids orally? How long does it take for the patient to successfully attain full or partial oral intake using the treatment? These are all important questions in order for swallowing therapists to understand the major impact(s) of treatment strategies.

Every Clinician's Role

When treating each dysphagic patient, it is important that the swallowing therapist collect as many of the types of data described in the previous section as are possible and appropriate for the patient's disorder and the treatment under study. Case studies consisting of careful assessments of treatment using some of these measurements are very important additions to the literature. Also, it is essential that each swallowing therapist track the impact of his or her management strategies. It is also critical that each therapist examines each new treatment presented in workshops or in other formats relative to the kinds of data available that validate the procedure. Are there sensible measurements of the effects of the treatment? Does the swallowing therapist understand why the treatment works? Have data been published on the effectiveness of the treatment strategy? If no data are published in peer-reviewed journals regarding the effects of a treatment, therapists may be at risk for not receiving third-party payment when using that treatment. Also, in some cases, patients may be harmed.

The Future

The future of dysphagia assessment and treatment depends, in large part, on the ability of clinicians and researchers to collect even more data to further support current and new treatments developed for patients with oropharyngeal dysphagia. Every clinician's responsibility is to participate in such research and, at the very least, to collect systematic data on the effects of his or her own treatment of each dysphagic patient.

Several areas of research may prove to be particularly productive in the next 10 years. These include further investigations on the sensory assessment and treatment of swallowing disorders. Professionals need to further develop strategies to (1) more systematically examine sensory input and recognition in normal subjects of various ages and in specific groups of dysphagic patients, and (2) heighten sensory input in systematic ways as one form of compensation for sensory deficits contributing to oropharyngeal swallowing problems.

Another important area for future research is the coordination of respiration and swallowing in normal subjects of various ages and in patients with various types of dysphagia, and the relationship of disorders in one function to dysfunctions in the other. Initial reports of patients with pulmonary disorders who also have swallowing problems are beginning to show improvements in swallowing when respiratory problems improve (Loughlin & Lefton-Greif, 1994). Criteria for how and when to intervene in patients of this sort are much needed.

The future for expansion of the field's understanding of normal and abnormal swallowing and the most effective assessment(s) and treatment(s) for various patient groups looks extremely bright if the momentum of research that has begun in the past decade continues. There is every reason to believe that, with the increased clinical interest in dysphagia, there will be a concomitant continued interest in research into these areas.

References

Bosma, J. (1973). Physiology of the mouth, pharynx and esophagus. In M. Paparella & D. Shumrick (Eds.), *Otolaryngology volume 1: Basic sciences and related disciplines* (pp. 356–370). Philadelphia: Saunders.

Doty, R., & Bosma, J. (1956). An electromyographic analysis of reflex deglutition. *Journal of Neurophysiology, 19*, 44–60.

Jacob, P., Kahrilas, P., Logemann, J., Shah, V., & Ha, T. (1989). Upper esophageal sphincter opening and modulation during swallowing. *Gastroenterology, 97*, 1469–1478.

Kahrilas, P. J., Lin, S., Logemann, J. A., Ergun, G. A., & Facchini, F. (1993). Deglutitive tongue action: Volume accommodation and bolus propulsion. *Gastroenterology, 104*, 152–162.

Kahrilas, P. J., Logemann, J. A., & Gibbons, P. (1992). Food intake by maneuver: An extreme compensation for impaired swallowing. *Dysphagia, 7*, 155–159.

Kahrilas, P. J., Logemann, J. A., Krugler, C., & Flanagan, E. (1991). Volitional augmentation of upper esophageal sphincter opening during swallowing. *American Journal of Physiology, 260* (*Gastrointestinal and Liver Physiology, 23*), G450–G456.

Kobara-Mates, M., Logemann, J. A., Larson, C., & Kahrilas, P. J. (1995). Physiology of oropharyngeal swallow in the cat: A videofluoroscopic and electromyographic study. *American Journal of Physiology, 268*, (*Gastrointestinal and Liver Physiology, 31*), G232–G241.

Lazarus, C., Logemann, J. A., & Gibbons, P. (1993). Effects of maneuvers on swallowing function in a dysphagic oral cancer patient. *Head & Neck, 15,* 419–424.

Logemann, J. A. (1987). Criteria for studies of treatment for oral-pharyngeal dysphagia. *Dysphagia, 1,* 193–199.

Logemann, J., Kahrilas, P., Begelman, J., & Pauloski, B. R. (1989). Interactive computer program for biomechanical analysis of videofluorographic studies of swallowing. *American Journal of Roentgenology, 153,* 277–280.

Logemann, J., Kahrilas, P., Kobara, M., & Vakil, N. (1989). The benefit of head rotation on pharyngoesophageal dysphagia. *Archives of Physical Medicine and Rehabilitation, 70,* 767–771.

Loughlin, A. M., & Lefton-Greif, M. A. (1994). Dysfunctional swallowing and respiratory disease in children. *Advances in Pediatrics, 41,* 135–161.

Platt, E. M., Logemann, J. A., Rademaker, A. W., Kahrilas, P. J., & Lazarus, C. L. (1994). Pharyngeal effects of bolus volume, viscosity and temperature in patients with dysphagia resulting from neurologic impairment and in normal subjects. *Journal of Speech and Hearing Research, 37,* 1041–1049.

Rademaker, A. W., Pauloski, B. R., Logemann, J. A., & Shanahan, T. K. (1994). Oropharyngeal swallow efficiency as a representative measure of swallowing function. *Journal of Speech and Hearing Research, 37,* 314–325.

Reimers-Neils, L., Logemann, J. A., & Larson, C. (1994). Viscosity effects on EMG activity in normal swallow. *Dysphagia, 9,* 101–106.

Robbins, J., Hamilton, J. W., Lof, G. L., & Kempster, G. B. (1992). Oropharyngeal swallowing in normal adults of different ages. *Gastroenterology, 103,* 823–829.

Tracy, J., Logemann, J., Kahrilas, P., Jacob, P., Kobara, M., & Krugler, C. (1989). Preliminary observations on the effects of age on oropharyngeal deglutition. *Dysphagia, 4,* 90–94.

Author Index

SUBJECT INDEX